Trauma Intensive Care

DATE DUE

Pittsburgh Critical Care Medicine Series

Trauma Intensive Care

Edited by

Samuel A. Tisherman, MD, FACS, FCCM

Professor
Departments of Critical Care Medicine and Surgery
University of Pittsburgh Medical Center
Pittsburgh, Pennsylvania

Raquel M. Forsythe, MD

Assistant Professor
Departments of Surgery and
Critical Care Medicine
University of Pittsburgh Medical Center
Pittsburgh, Pennsylvania

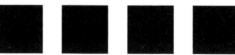

OXFORD
UNIVERSITY PRESS

OXFORD
UNIVERSITY PRESS

Oxford University Press is a department of the University of Oxford.
It furthers the University's objective of excellence in research, scholarship,
and education by publishing worldwide.

Oxford   New York
Auckland   Cape Town   Dar es Salaam   Hong Kong   Karachi
Kuala Lumpur   Madrid   Melbourne   Mexico City   Nairobi
New Delhi   Shanghai   Taipei   Toronto

With offices in
Argentina   Austria   Brazil   Chile   Czech Republic   France   Greece
Guatemala   Hungary   Italy   Japan   Poland   Portugal   Singapore
South Korea   Switzerland   Thailand   Turkey   Ukraine   Vietnam

Oxford is a registered trademark of Oxford University Press in the UK and certain other
countries.

Published in the United States of America by
Oxford University Press
198 Madison Avenue, New York, NY 10016

Library of Congress Cataloging-in-Publication Data
Trauma intensive care / edited by Samuel A. Tisherman, Raquel M. Forsythe.
   p. ; cm.—(Pittsburgh critical care medicine series)
   Includes bibliographical references and index.
   ISBN 978–0–19–977770–9 (alk. paper)—ISBN 978–0–19–977780–8 (alk. paper)
   I. Tisherman, Samuel A.   II. Forsythe, Raquel M.   III. Series: Pittsburgh critical care
   medicine.
   [DNLM: 1. Wounds and Injuries—therapy.   2. Intensive Care—methods.
   3. Intensive Care Units. WO 700]
   LC Classification not assigned
   617.1—dc23
   2012049560

9 8 7 6 5 4 3 2 1
Printed in the United States of America
on acid-free paper

Series Preface

No place in the world is more closely identified with Critical Care Medicine than Pittsburgh. In the late sixties, Peter Safar and Ake Grenvik pioneered the science and practice of critical care not just in Pittsburgh, but around the world. Their multidisciplinary team approach became the standard for how ICU care is delivered in Pittsburgh to this day. The Pittsburgh Critical Care Medicine series honors this tradition. Edited and largely authored by University of Pittsburgh faculty, the content reflects best practice in critical care medicine. The Pittsburgh model has been adopted by many programs around the world and local leaders are recognized as world leaders. It is our hope that through this series of concise handbooks a small part of this tradition can be passed on to the many practitioners of critical care the world over.

John A. Kellum
Series Editor

Preface

The management of critically ill patients who have suffered multiple trauma can be challenging. Optimal management requires rapidly assessing and resuscitating patients, establishing priorities of care, coordinating multiple diagnostic tests and therapeutic interventions, while minimizing complications, all with the goal of achieving the best possible functional outcome for the patient. Most textbooks devoted to trauma care tend to thoroughly cover all of the topics related to management of trauma patients, including out-of-hospital care, initial assessment and resuscitation, and management of specific injuries. The unique issues of management in the intensive care unit tend to be addressed in various ways, but typically not extensively. There are currently no books solely devoted to the critical care management of trauma patients.

This book was developed for all healthcare professionals involved in managing trauma patients in the intensive care unit. The topics are presented in a concise and practical fashion.

By its nature, trauma management must be multi-disciplinary. The physicians involved include emergency physicians, trauma surgeons, and surgical subspecialists (e.g., neurosurgery, orthopedics, plastics), as well as physical medicine and rehabilitation specialists. Fellows, residents, interns, and medical students also are typically involved. Other professionals who are integral to management of critically ill trauma patients include nurses; respiratory, physical, and occupational therapists; social workers; and case managers.

This book was designed to be used by all healthcare professionals interested in the management of critically ill trauma patients. Our hope is that the book will prove valuable at the bedside and will help improve the quality of trauma care and functional patient outcomes.

Samuel A. Tisherman, MD,
Raquel Forsythe, MD

Contents

Contributors

Louis H. Alarcon, MD
Medical Director, Trauma Surgery
Associate Professor of Surgery and
    Critical Care Medicine
University of Pittsburgh
Pittsburgh, Pennsylvania

Aman Banerjee, MD
Trauma Research Fellow
Department of Surgery
Case Western Reserve University
    School of Medicine at
MetroHealth Medical Center
Cleveland, Ohio

Graciela Bauzá, MD
Assistant Professor of Surgery
University of Pittsburgh
Pittsburgh, Pennsylvania

Matthew Benns, MD
Assistant Professor of Surgery
Division of General Surgery
University of Louisville
Louisville, Kentucky

Joshua Brown, MD
Resident, General Surgery
University of Pittsburgh
Pittsburgh, Pennsylvania

Jodie Bryk, MD
Resident, Internal Medicine
University of Pittsburgh
Pittsburgh, Pennsylvania

Jeffrey A. Claridge, MD, MS, FACS
Division Director of Trauma, Critical
    Care, and Burns
Associate Professor, Department of
    Surgery
Case Western Reserve University
    School of Medicine at
MetroHealth Medical Center
Cleveland, Ohio

Alain C. Corcos, MD, FACS
Clinical Assistant Professor of Surgery
University of Pittsburgh
Pittsburgh, Pennsylvania

Kerry Deluca, MD
Assistant Professor, Department
    of Physical Medicine and
    Rehabilitation
University of Pittsburgh
Pittsburgh, Pennsylvania

Lillian L. Emlet, MD, MS, FACEP
Assistant Professor, Department of
    Critical Care Medicine
University of Pittsburgh
Pittsburgh, Pennsylvania

Paula Ferrada, MD
Faculty, Department of Trauma, Critical
    Care, and Emergency Surgery
Virginia Commonwealth University
Richmond, Virginia

Raquel M. Forsythe, MD
Assistant Professor
Departments of Surgery and Critical
  Care Medicine
University of Pittsburgh Medical
  Center
Pittsburgh, Pennsylvania

Barbara A. Gaines
Children's Hospital of Pittsburgh
University of Pittsburgh Medical Center
Pittsburgh, Pennsylvania

Ramesh Grandhi, MD
Resident, Department of
  Neurological Surgery
University of Pittsburgh
Pittsburgh, Pennsylvania

**Lewis J. Kaplan, MD, FACS,
FCCM, FCCP**
Associate Professor of Surgery
Yale University School of Medicine;
  Department of Surgery
Section of Trauma, Surgical Critical
  Care and Surgical Emergencies
New Haven, Connecticut

Kenneth D. Katz, MD
Chief of the Division of Medical
  Toxicology
Medical Director, Pittsburgh Poison
  Center
University of Pittsburgh Medical
  Center
Pittsburgh, Pennsylvania

A. Murat Kaynar, MD, MPH
Associate Professor, Critical Care
  Medicine and Anesthesiology
University of Pittsburgh
Pittsburgh, Pennsylvania

Richard P. Kidwell
Adjunct Faculty
Senior Associate Counsel and
  Director of Risk Management
University of Pittsburgh Medical Center
Pittsburgh, Pennsylvania

Gary T. Marshall, MD
Assistant Professor of Surgery and
  Critical Care Medicine
University of Pittsburgh
Pittsburgh, Pennsylvania

Lauren M. McDaniel, BS
Medical Student
University of Pittsburgh School of
  Medicine
Pittsburgh, Pennsylvania

Deepika Mohan, MD
Assistant Professor of Critical Care
  Medicine and Surgery
University of Pittsburgh
Pittsburgh, Pennsylvania

Matthew D. Neal
Resident, General Surgery
University of Pittsburgh
Pittsburgh, Pennsylvania

Juan B. Ochoa
Professor of Surgery and Critical
  Care Medicine
University of Pittsburgh
Pittsburgh, Pennsylvania
Medical and Scientific Director
Nestle Health Care Nutrition, Nestle
  Health Science
North America

David O. Okonkwo, MD, PhD
Associate Professor of Neurological
  Surgery
University of Pittsburgh
Pittsburgh, Pennsylvania

David M. Panczykowski, MD
Resident, Department of
    Neurological Surgery
University of Pittsburgh Medical Center
Pittsburgh, Pennsylvania

Nimitt Patel, MD
Trauma/Surgical Critical Care/Acute
    Care Surgery Fellow
Department of Critical Care Medicine
University of Pittsburgh
Pittsburgh, Pennsylvania

Andrew B. Peitzman, MD
Mark M. Ravitch Professor
Executive Vice-Chairman,
    Department of Surgery
University of Pittsburgh
Pittsburgh, Pennsylvania

Greta L. Piper, MD
Assistant Professor of Surgery
Yale University School of Medicine,
    Department of Surgery
Section of Trauma, Surgical Critical
    Care and Surgical Emergencies
New Haven, Connecticut

Benjamin R. Reynolds, PA-C
Director of the Office of Advanced
    Practice Providers
Division of Vascular Surgery
University of Pittsburgh
Pittsburgh, Pennsylvania

Matthew Rosengart, MD, MPH
Assistant Professor, Surgery and
    Critical Care Medicine
University of Pittsburgh
Pittsburgh, Pennsylvania

Daniel Rutigliano, DO
Children's Hospital of Pittsburgh
University of Pittsburgh Medical Center
Pittsburgh, Pennsylvania

Babak Sarani, MD, FACS
Chief of Trauma and Acute Surgery
Associate Professor of Surgery
George Washington University
Washington, D.C.

Kai Singbartl, MD, MPH
Associate Professor of Anesthesiology
Penn State Hershey
Hershey, Pennsylvania

Peter A. Siska, MD
Assistant Professor
University of Pittsburgh School of
    Medicine
Department of Orthopedic Surgery
Pittsburgh, Pennsylvania

Jason Sperry, MD, MPH
Assistant Professor of Surgery and
    Critical Care
University of Pittsburgh
Pittsburgh, Pennsylvania

Richard M. Spiro, MD
Assistant Professor of Neurological
    Surgery
University of Pittsburgh
Pittsburgh, Pennsylvania

Ivan S. Tarkin, MD
Chief of Orthopedic Traumatology
University of Pittsburgh School of
    Medicine
Department of Orthopedic Surgery
Pittsburgh, Pennsylvania

**Samuel A. Tisherman, MD,
FACS, FCCM**
Professor
Departments of Critical Care
    Medicine and Surgery
University of Pittsburgh Medical Center
Pittsburgh, Pennsylvania

Amy Wagner, MD
Associate Professor, Physical
    Medicine & Rehabilitation
University of Pittsburgh
Pittsburgh, Pennsylvania

**Gregory A. Watson, MD,
FACS**
Assistant Professor of Surgery and
    Critical Care Medicine
University of Pittsburgh
Pittsburgh, Pennsylvania

Boris A. Zelle, MD
Orthopedic Trauma Fellow
University of Pittsburgh School of
    Medicine
Department of Orthopedic Surgery
Pittsburgh, Pennsylvania

Jennifer Ziembicki, MD
Assistant Professor of Surgery
University of Pittsburgh
Pittsburgh, Pennsylvania

Structure

Chapter 1

Development of the trauma intensive care unit within trauma systems

Deepika Mohan

The modern trauma intensive care unit (ICU) reflects the confluence of two trends: the development of inclusive trauma systems and the rise of subspecialty intensive care units. This chapter will review key historical events that influenced the development of the trauma ICU within trauma systems, as well as some of the literature on the current role of the trauma ICU in the management of trauma patients.

The development of trauma systems

Over 40 years ago, the growing burden imposed by injury and violence prompted a reassessment of how trauma care was delivered in the United States. In 1966, this resulted in the National Academy of Sciences publication *Accidental Death and Disability: the Neglected Disease of Modern Society*. With a stinging indictment of the existing standards of care, the authors offered a call to arms:

> In 1965, 52 million accidental injuries killed 107,000, temporarily disabled over 10 million and permanently impaired 400,000 American citizens at a cost of approximately $18 billion. This neglected epidemic of modern society is the nation's most important environmental health problem. It is the leading cause of death in the first half of life's span.... Public apathy to the mounting toll from accidents must be transformed into an action program under strong leadership.

Initial legislative efforts focused on the need to provide more consistent emergency services in the wake of accidental injuries to reduce the impact of those injuries [see Table 1.1]. The National Highway Safety Act, passed in 1966, authorized the federal government to set and to regulate standards for motor vehicles and highways. Part of the mandate included the creation of guidelines to improve the provision of emergency services. Signing the new bill into law, Lyndon B. Johnson said, "We have tolerated a raging epidemic of highway death...which has killed more of our youth than all other diseases combined.

Table 1.1 Milestones in the development of trauma systems

1966	Publication of *Accidental Death and Disability: the Neglected Disease of Modern Society*—a white paper from the National Academy of Sciences
1966	Passage of the National Highway Safety Act (P.L. 89–564), which provided funds to help states develop and strengthen their highway safety programs
1973	Passage of the Emergency Medical Services Systems Act (P.L 93–154), which provided funding for the development of regional EMS systems
1976	Publication of *Optimal Hospital Resources for Care of Injured Patients*—a set of standards for trauma centers developed by the American College of Surgeons—Committee on Trauma
1986	Passage of the Injury Prevention Act (P.L 99–663), which established the Division of Injury Epidemiology and Control at the Centers for Disease Control to provide leadership for a spectrum of injury-related public health activities
1990	Passage of the Trauma Systems Planning and Development Act (P.L 101–590), which created the Division of Trauma and Emergency Medical Services at the Department of Health and Human Services
1991	Publication of a position paper from the Third National Injury Control Conference at the CDC, which introduced the distinction between exclusive and inclusive trauma systems.
1992	Publication of *Model Trauma Care System Plan* by the Division of Trauma and Emergency Medical Services, to help states develop inclusive trauma systems.
1999	Publication of *Reducing the Burden of Injury* by the Institute of Medicine—a call for a greater national commitment to trauma systems.
2000	Reauthorization of the Trauma System Planning and Development Act provides funds for states to develop regional trauma systems
2006	Publication of a revised version of *Model Trauma System Planning and Evaluation* by the Health Resources Services Administration, to help states develop and evaluate their trauma systems

Through the Highway Safety Act, we are going to find out more about highway disease—and we aim to cure it."

The American College of Surgeons began to view the trauma system primarily as a means of organizing the care provided to the sickest patients. To optimize the use of resources and ensure the best outcomes, patients with moderate to severe injuries should receive care at high-volume, specialty centers, while patients with minor injuries could remain at local hospitals. The first edition of the American College of Surgeons—Committee on Trauma's (ACS-COT) report *Optimal Hospital Resources for the Care of the Injured Patient*, published in 1976, delineated a set of standards for trauma centers and categorized the resources provided by different tiers of centers.

Only in 1991, did the concept of a trauma system as "preplanned, comprehensive, and coordinated statewide and local injury response networks that included all facilities with the capability of care for the injured" emerge. A position paper from the Third National Injury Control Conference at the Centers for Disease Control distinguished between "inclusive" and "exclusive" trauma systems. Exclusive systems, defined as systems dominated by a few specialty trauma centers, did not adequately resolve the public health burden imposed by injury and violence. Instead, effective regionalization required a combination of efforts, beginning with prevention, including the moderation of the impact of injuries, and concluding with optimization of outcomes. Inclusive systems, defined as systems with a network of facilities that coordinated care for the injured, ensured that care extended from prevention to rehabilitation.

The next year, the Division of Trauma and Emergency Medical Services (EMS) within the Health Resources Services Administration published the Model Trauma Care System Plan to aid states in the development of inclusive regional trauma care systems. The plan identified key steps required in the development of a trauma system: (1) public education and support; (2) a needs assessment study; (3) enabling legislation; (4) development of a trauma plan; (5) standards for optimal care; (6) the evaluation, verification, and designation of trauma centers; (7) trauma system evaluation and performance improvement; and (8) external review and assessment of the trauma system.

In the decade that followed, the debate shifted to the influence trauma systems had on outcomes. For example, Utter et al found that moderate to severely injured patients treated in the most inclusive systems had significantly reduced rates of mortality when compared with patients treated in exclusive systems (OR 0.77, CI 0.6–0.99). In the middle of the next decade, however, Shafi et al (2006) compared outcomes between states that did and did not have a trauma system, rather than using a before-after methodology, and found no significant mortality reduction in states with trauma systems. They argued that the mortality benefit described by other investigators reflected secular changes, such as primary seat belt laws and speed limits, rather than the influence of the trauma system itself. To address this controversy, Celso et al (2006) systematically reviewed the literature to determine if the outcome from severe traumatic injury improved following the establishment of a trauma system. The authors found 14 relevant published studies: eight described improved odds of survival associated with trauma systems, three described worsened odds of survival, and three described no difference. In their meta-analysis, published in 2006, the authors concluded that the implementation of a trauma system reduced the risk of mortality by 15%.

Perhaps the most definitive work on this subject came from the National Study on the Costs and Outcomes of Trauma. In a prospective observational cohort, Mackenzie et al (2006) demonstrated that care at trauma centers significantly improved mortality and morbidity. Although the authors did not specifically address the role of systems in improving outcomes, their subsequent analysis focused on the importance of a system that appropriately triaged patients. They argued that the higher incremental cost per life-gained for less severely injured patients treated at trauma centers highlighted the importance of a system that would ensure that patients received the appropriate level of care (i.e., a well-functioning inclusive system).

The development of specialty intensive care units

Walter Dandy organized the first specialty ICU at Johns Hopkins Hospital in 1923 to care for his neurosurgical patients. Whereas *general* ICUs admit patients with a wide range of diagnoses and procedures, *specialty* ICUs manage a few select conditions. In theory, diagnosis-specific care can improve efficiency, reduce diagnostic variability, and concentrate nursing expertise. Specialty ICUs can also exploit the relationship that exists between volume and outcomes. Admission to higher volume hospitals has been associated with a reduction in mortality for numerous surgical conditions and medical procedures. In the critical care literature, patients receiving mechanical ventilation in hospitals with a high case-volume have a 37% reduction in mortality compared to patients receiving mechanical ventilation in hospitals with a low case-volume.

The data on whether or not specialty ICUs improve care, however, remains mixed. Kahn et al have recently shown no difference in risk-adjusted mortality for patients admitted to specialty ICUs compared with patients admitted to general ICUs. Nonetheless, their retrospective analysis concentrated on the outcomes of patients with a few specific illnesses: acute coronary syndrome, ischemic stroke, intracranial hemorrhage, pneumonia, abdominal surgery, and coronary artery bypass graft surgery. In contrast, the trauma literature suggests that specialty ICUs can improve outcomes. For example, patients with traumatic brain injuries managed in neurosurgical ICUs have a 51% reduction in mortality, a 12% shorter length of stay, and a 57% greater odds of being discharged to home or to a rehabilitation facility rather than to a nursing home. When managed in a trauma ICU, patients with moderate-to-severe injuries have a reduced ICU length of stay, as well as fewer ventilator days and total number of consults.

The development of trauma ICUs within trauma systems

Part of the development of trauma systems has included delineating the role of the ICU in the management of trauma patients. Trauma patients receive up to 25% of their care in an ICU, and have clinical issues that can differ from other medical or surgical patients. For example, patients with moderate-to-severe injuries frequently have competing diagnostic and therapeutic priorities. They can require immediate operative intervention, management after damage control procedures, massive transfusion, and monitoring of intracranial pressure. Additionally, they remain at risk of developing acute respiratory distress syndrome and sepsis.

The ACS-COT therefore recommends that trauma patients requiring critical care be transferred to a Level I or II trauma center. As part of the verification of trauma centers, the ACS-COT has established standards for ICUs that manage trauma patients, including a patient-to-nurse ratio of no more than 2:1 and the availability of equipment necessary to monitor and resuscitate patients. Level I trauma centers should have ICUs managed by surgeons, with continuous in-house coverage for all ICU trauma patients. Level II or III centers should have ICUs with a surgeon serving as either a co-director or director, who holds the responsibility for setting policies and administration needs. Physician coverage must be promptly available 24 hours a day. Additionally, the ACS-COT requires that the trauma service assume initial responsibility for all trauma patients, and retain that responsibility throughout the acute-care phase of the hospitalization. In Level II centers, critical care physicians may provide input in the management of these patients, although the final responsibility for coordinating all therapeutic decisions remains that of the trauma team. Again, the ACS-COT recommends that Level III centers transfer the most critically ill patients to higher levels of care.

Using a validated survey to assess practice patterns in ICUs in Level I and II trauma centers, Nathens et al (2006) found that few centers consistently followed the ACS-COT recommendations for the organization of their ICUs. ICUs rarely had a patient to nurse ratio of ≤2:1 at all times and only 16% of units had dedicated attending physicians providing clinical care exclusively in the ICU. Most notably, however, Nathens et al (2006) observed that trauma centers used a variety of staffing models for their trauma centers. The majority of trauma centers relied predominantly on a collaborative model of critical care. The ACS-COT emphasizes the importance of the trauma surgeon retaining responsibility for all trauma patients. However, in only 22% of Level I ICUs did the trauma surgeon act as the primary provider of critical care services; 61% of ICUs described their model as intensivist-led, and 66% allowed the intensivist to take responsibility for all admission and discharge decisions.

The discrepancy between the ACS-COT recommendations and practice patterns may reflect an increasing wealth of evidence that suggests that multi-disciplinary, intensivist-led critical care improves outcomes. A variety of staffing models for ICUs exist [see Table 1.2]. Pronovost et al (2002) performed a systematic review of ICU attending-physician staffing strategies and hospital and ICU mortality. They found that high-intensity staffing (i.e., ICUs that either required an intensivist consult for all patients or transferred patients to the intensivist service) was associated with a 40% reduction in ICU mortality, and a 30% reduction in in-hospital mortality. In the wake of this study, the Leapfrog group, a consortium of healthcare purchasers formed to advocate for improved quality and safety in health care, has recommended that purchasers preferentially refer patients to hospitals that agree to implement intensivist-led physician staffing models.

In the trauma literature, Nathens et al (2006) used prospective data collected for the National Study of the Costs and Outcomes of Trauma to estimate a relative risk reduction in mortality of 0.78 (0.58–1.04) associated with intensivist-led ICUs. The association became significant in subgroup analyses, particular for older patients. Additionally, trauma centers with intensivist-led ICUs had

Table 1.2 Examples of ICU staffing and organizational models

Term	Definition
Low intensity staffing	Intensivists are available for consultation at the discretion of the responsible physician.
High intensity staffing	Closed ICUs or ICUs that mandate an intensivist consult for all patients.
Closed ICU	All patients are cared for by intensivists in collaboration with a primary service. Only intensivists have admitting and ordering privileges in the ICU.
Open ICU	Any physician can admit patients to the ICU and can write orders.

significantly improved outcomes compared with nondesignated trauma centers. These findings may suggest that the ACS-COT recommendations for the configuration of ICUs in trauma systems require amendment.

Key references

Celso B, Tepas J, Langland-Orban B, et al. "A systematic review and meta-analysis comparing outcome of severely injured patients treated in trauma centers following the establishment of trauma systems." *J Trauma*. 2006;60(2):371–378.

Lee JC, Rogers FB, Horst MA. "Application of a trauma intensivist model to a level II community hospital trauma program improves intensive care unit throughput." *J Trauma*. 2010; 69(5): 1147–1153.

Lott JP, Iwashyna TJ, Christie JD, et al. "Critical illness outcomes in specialty versus general intensive care units." *Am J Respir Crit Care Med*. 2009; 179: 676–683.

MacKenzie EJ, Rivara FP, Jurkovich GJ, et al. "A national evaluation of the effect of trauma-center care on mortality." *NEJM*. 2006; 354(4):366–378.

Nathens AB, Rivara FP, MacKenzie EJ, et al. "The impact of an intensivist-model ICU on trauma-related mortality." *Ann Surg*. 2006; 244(4): 545–554.

Nathens AB, Maier RV, Jurkovich GJ, et al. "The delivery of critical care services in US trauma centers: is the standard being met?" *J Trauma*. 2006; 60(4): 773–784.

Pronovost PJ, Angus DC, Dorman T, et al. "Physician staffing patterns and clinical outcomes in critically ill patients." *JAMA*. 2002; 288(17): 2151–2162.

Shafi S, Nathens AB, Elliott AC, et al. "Effect of trauma systems on motor vehicle occupant mortality: a comparison between states with and without a formal system." *J Trauma*. 2006;61(6):1374–1379.

Vaelas PN, Eastwood D, Yun HJ, et al. "Impact of a neurointensivist on outcomes in patients with head trauma treated in a neurosciences intensive care unit." *J Neurosurg*. 2006; 104: 713–719.

Chapter 2

Injury severity scoring systems

Matthew Rosengart

In 1976, in an effort to improve trauma care delivery, the American College of Surgeons developed criteria for the designation of trauma centers and the establishment of regional trauma systems. Since that time, substantial evidence has accumulated that the identification and triage of the most critically injured patients to these regional centers is effective in reducing injury-related mortality. Discerning who these patients are from among the overall population of injured necessitates a method by which to estimate the risk of an outcome, such as death, and thus identify who would benefit from this higher level of care. Injury severity scoring is simply a means by which to do this, to characterize and quantify an injury. It has been extended to estimating the risk of an outcome (e.g., mortality, morbidity, length of stay). Initially developed and utilized by the automotive industry, the scores have been modified so as to be relevant to and incorporated into the practice of emergency medical services (EMS) personnel, clinicians, and injury epidemiologists for field triage, clinical decision-making, epidemiological studies, and quality improvements. The scores themselves draw upon characteristics of the patient (anatomic, physiologic, comorbidity) to construct a summary measure quantifying a patient's condition after injury. These have been incorporated into a fourth type of score that combines these elements to enhance the predictive capacity.

Anatomic scores

Abbreviated Injury Scale (AIS)

Long before the establishment of criteria for the verification/credentialing of trauma centers, efforts to better understand the ramifications of public health initiatives were influencing how we defined trauma. In 1971, in an effort to better understand the shifts in the magnitude and distribution of injuries that occurred with advancements in automotive design (e.g., seatbelts), a coalition of the Society of Automotive Engineers and the American Medical Association (AMA), spearheaded by the Association for the Advancement of Automotive Medicine (AAAM), standardized a score characterizing the type and quantifying the magnitude of organ injury: Abbreviated Injury Scale (AIS). It has

Table 2.1 Abbreviated Injury Score (AIS) severity scale

AIS Components

Grade	Definition	Example (Liver)	AIS
1	Superficial/Minor	Subcapsular hematoma, < 10% surface area	2
		Laceration, < 1 cm parenchymal depth	2
2	Moderate	Subcapsular hematoma, 10–50% surface area	2
		Intraparenchymal hematoma, < 10 cm in diameter	2
		Laceration 1–3 cm parenchymal depth, < 10 cm in length	2
3	Serious	Subcapsular hematoma, > 50% surface area of ruptured subcapsular or parenchymal hematoma	3
		Intraparenchymal hematoma > 10cm or expanding	3
		Laceration, > 3cm parenchymal depth	3
4	Severe	Parenchymal disruption involving 25% to 75% of hepatic lobe or 1 to 3 Couinaud's segments within a single lobe	4
5	Critical	Parenchymal disruption involving > 75% of hepatic lobe or > 3 Couinaud's segments within a single lobe	5
		Juxtahepatic venous injuries	5
6	Universally fatal	Hepatic avulsion	6

since undergone several revisions to make it more relevant to medical audit and research. More recently it was expanded to include Organ Injury Scales (Table 2.1). The AIS classifies each injury in every body region according to its relative importance. Consequently, it has become one of the most widely utilized scoring systems. It has been invaluable in the conduct of epidemiological studies by permitting appropriate risk adjustment, as well as, serving as a validated outcome itself.

The AIS-code itself consists of a 7-digit number. The initial 6-digit predecimal number classifies the injury by body region (e.g., head), type of anatomic structure (e.g., skeletal), specific anatomic structure (e.g., base) and level of injury (e.g., with CSF leak). This is followed by a single digit postdecimal severity designation (range 1 to 6) that describes the severity of the injury: 1 (superficial, universally survivable) to 6 (critical, universally fatal) (Table 2.1). It is this severity designation that has been extensively utilized by the scientific, clinical, and public health community. The scale is ordinal in that the transition between levels is not of equal magnitude. Furthermore, the scores are assigned by expert consensus, implicitly based on four criteria: threat to life, permanent impairment, treatment period, and energy dissipation. Thus, similar scores for different body regions may not have the same risk of death [e.g. AIS 3 (head) ≠ AIS 3 (extremity)]. Nonetheless, AIS correlates well with the magnitude of injury and patient outcome and has been validated in numerous studies. The maximum AIS (maxAIS) is highly associated with mortality, yet ignores concomitant injuries. Additional limitations include the allocation of resources used to screen, abstract, and code injuries, the variability in scoring introduced by the modality used to define the injury (computed tomography [CT] vs. pathology), and the lack of a universally accepted injury aggregation function. The current AIS 2005 Update 2008 represents the collective efforts of hundreds of contributors from the United States, Canada, Australia, New Zealand, and numerous European countries and contains thousands of injury descriptions.

Injury Severity Score (ISS)

The Injury Severity Score (ISS) was first proposed in 1974 to serve as an injury aggregation function that capitalized upon the AIS system. It has subsequently become one of the most widely used anatomical scoring systems. In its current form, six regions (head and neck, face, thorax, abdomen, extremity, external) are scored using the most severely injured organ within that region, as defined by the AIS. When initially developed, an exponential relationship between AIS severity and mortality was observed. Subsequent iterations concluded that a quadratic equation, incorporating the sum of the squares of the largest AIS severity in each of the three most severely injured regions, performed most ideally in prognostication. The addition of a fourth region did not enhance predictive capacity. Any patient sustaining an injury with AIS severity of 6 was automatically given an ISS score of 75.

$$ISS = A^2 + B^2 + C^2$$

where A, B, C are distinct body regions possessing the highest three AIS severity scores.

Though the ISS correlates well with mortality, it, too, does not exhibit a linear relationship; though considered ordinal, it has a more nominal function. There are other limitations of which one must remain aware. The ISS considers only one injury in each of the body regions. In the setting of polysystem trauma, injuries additional to the three of greatest magnitude are ignored. A similar weakness occurs in the circumstance of a severe single-body-region injury (e.g., penetrating abdominal trauma) in which multiple organ injuries are represented by a single AIS score. Thus, the same ISS score would be attributed to an individual sustaining hepatic and splenic injuries with AIS severities of 4 as attributed to an individual with isolated, but similar, hepatic injury. Distinct combinations of AIS squares may yield the same ISS, which ideally should be handled categorically; but such methods are impractical and commonly infeasible. Its foundation, the AIS, rests in subjective estimates of risk of mortality, which perform less well than data-driven scoring systems.

New Injury Severity Score (NISS)

Several additional severity scoring systems have been developed to address the inherent limitations of the ISS. The New Injury Severity Score (NISS) is defined by the sum of the squares of the three highest AIS scores, independent of body region. This modification only addresses the weakness of ISS in assessing the single body region with multiple injuries. Subsequent studies show that it offers only a slight improvement in predictive capacity; and thus, it has not gained widespread favor.

Anatomic Profile Score (APS)

A significant limitation of the scores thus far discussed is the equal weight attributed to different body regions. The Anatomic Profile Score (APS) also incorporates AIS severity in its measure, but attempts to account for the effect of AIS severity by different body regions. APS constructs a single summary measure representing four components: (1) head, brain and spinal cord (mA); (2) the thorax and neck (mB); (3) all other regions (mC); and all others (mD). Components A–C incorporate only significant (AIS > 2) injuries, by contrast to component D (AIS ≤ 2). The score for each component is derived from the square root of the sum of the squares of all AIS scores within the body regions of that component. Weights for each component, developed from multivariate models relating APS components to survival probability using the Major Trauma Outcome Study (MTOS), are incorporated into the final formula:

$$\text{APS} = .3199(\text{mA}) + .4381(\text{mB}) + .1406(\text{mC}) + .7961(\text{max AIS}).$$

Unlike the ISS and NISS, APS incorporates all injuries exceeding a particular magnitude, thereby yielding a more comprehensive measure of the cumulative magnitude of injury. Recently the predictive performance of APS has been demonstrated to exceed that of ISS. However, the APS is more cumbersome to utilize, rendering its use limited to the conduct of outcomes research, rather than time-pressured clinical decision-making.

ICD-9 Injury Severity Score (ICISS)

A tremendous amount of information is collected in the ICD-9 coding of diagnoses; data that would seem ideal for use in injury severity scoring. In 1989, Mackenzie et al first published a validated ICD-9-CM to AIS-85 conversion table that enabled AIS-based injury scoring approaches to be applied to data encoded using ICD-9 codes. They subsequently developed a software program, ICDMAP-90, that translates, or rather "maps" ICD-9 codes to approximate AIS codes for each injury. From this ICD-9 AIS code, an ISS, NISS, APS, or other score can be calculated. The approach has been used extensively for research and administrative data collection.

The initial enthusiasm for ICDMAP-90 has been tempered by significant limitations that stem, in part, from the greater specificity of AIS and the conservative nature in which ICD codes are converted to AIS scores. Due to the specificity of AIS definitions, many ICD-9 diagnoses do not correlate well with an exact AIS injury classification. Recent studies have noted that many ICD-9 codes are ignored in the calculation of important AIS scores, and that ICDMAP-90 underestimates higher ISS scores. Assumptions have been made in the conversion table to best approximate the AIS score; and thus medical-record-based AIS scoring may yield different severity scores. Lastly, the accuracy with which ICDMAP-90 functions depends, in large part, upon the accuracy and extent to which diagnoses are captured, both of which are subject to the number of diagnosis fields and human error.

The International Classification of Diseases Injury Severity Score (ICISS) extends the ICD-9 methodology of severity scoring, but eliminates the AIS conversion and the inherent weaknesses therein. Its foundation is the ICD-9 survival risk ratio (SRR), an ICD-9 code-specific survival probability associated with a particular injury. The SRR is defined simply by dividing the number of times a particular code occurs in surviving patients by the total number of times the code occurs in a population. The product of the SRRs corresponding to the collective injuries of a patient determines the ICISS and ranges from 0 to 1.

$$\text{ICISS} = \text{Prob}_{survival(injury\ 1)} * \text{Prob}_{survival(injury\ n + 1)} * \text{Prob}_{survival(injury\ last)}$$

ICISS deviates from AIS-based systems such as ISS and NISS, and thus, may be used by centers less familiar with AIS scoring. The ICISS-based survival estimates are directly modeled population-based estimates rather than subjective and consensus-derived. Therefore, ICISS exhibits a more smooth, albeit nonlinear, relationship with mortality. The data suggest that it outperforms ISS and NISS. In fact, population-specific estimates can be derived if sample sizes of representative injuries in the index population are sufficient. However, ICISS methodology is complex, rendering bedside use impractical and restricting its application to epidemiological investigation. Though many SRRs are publically available, the generalizability of these database-specific SRRs to other populations has not been validated. Additionally, the SRRs derived contain residual bias due to concomitant injuries. Recent studies highlight that independent SRRs, calculated from patients sustaining an isolated injury, yield better estimates of survival.

Physiologic scores

The physiologic status of a patient, based upon parameters such as systolic blood pressure or base deficit, is one of the most powerful predictors of outcome, as it provides a global assessment of the magnitude of the injury and its interaction with the host response. However, physiology is a dynamic process, sensitive to many aspects, including the response to medical intervention itself. Isolated measurements offer only a static snapshot in time. Thus, many propose that changes over time improve discrimination and prognostication. This is difficult in population-base analyses, as opposed to individual-based treatment algorithms. Care must be exercised when incorporating these parameters as bias/mis-specification may be introduced: similar abnormal (bradycardia due to athleticism vs. hypoxemia) or normal values (normal sinus rhythm due to beta blockade for prior myocardial infarction vs. health), will carry similar risk estimates, yet stem from potentially extreme differences in risk of outcome. Similar to anatomic scores, these parameters are typically treated as linear covariates, yet the relationship with risk is ordinal. Alternatively, they may be categorized, though the threshold value(s) upon which to categorize them is not uniformly accepted. Nonetheless, physiologic parameters are simple to monitor, provide a more sensitive measure of the host response to the injury, and have been shown to prognosticate better than anatomic scoring systems.

Glasgow Coma Scale (GCS)

Developed over 30 years ago as a means to monitor the neurologic outcome of postoperative craniotomy patients, the Glasgow Coma Scale (GCS) has proven its predictive capacity in quantifying neurologic function and outcome in a variety of contexts, including trauma. Three parameters: Eye Opening, Verbal Response, and Motor Response are scored on an ordinal scale and summed (range: 3 [completely unresponsive] to 15 [completely responsive]) to provide a summary measure of overall neurologic derangement that has been shown to be highly associated with survival (Table 2.2). Non-trauma-related causes (e.g., drugs) might depress the score and obfuscate the clinical picture. Recent data from the National Trauma Data Bank (NTDB) demonstrate that the Motor

Table 2.2 Glasgow Coma Scale (GCS)	
Component	
Eyes	
4	Opens eyes spontaneously
3	Opens eyes in response to speech
2	Open eyes in response to painful stimulation
1	Does not open eyes in response to any stimulation
Verbal	
5	Is oriented to person, place, and time
4	Converses; may be confused
3	Replies with inappropriate words
2	Makes incomprehensible sounds
1	Makes no response
Motor	
6	Follows commands
5	Makes localized movement in response to painful stimulation
4	Makes nonpurposeful movement in response to noxious stimulation
3	Flexes upper/extends lower extremities in response to pain (decorticate posturing)
2	Extends all extremities in response to pain (decerebrate posturing)
1	Makes no response to noxious stimuli

Response component exceeds the full GCS score in predicting survival. As such, the Motor score alone has supplanted the full GCS score in many high-impact trauma studies.

Base deficit/lactate

The *sine qua non* of trauma is tissue injury and hemorrhage, which collectively may perturb tissue oxygen delivery and/or extraction and utilization, causing a systemic inflammatory response and shock. It is not surprising, then, that global measures of oxygen delivery and utilization possess considerable utility in severity adjustment. Admission **base deficit** (the amount of base needed to normalize 1 L of blood to pH = 7.4 under standard conditions) correlates linearly and independently with the risk of death and enhances the predictive capacity of the Revised Trauma Score and Trauma and Injury Severity Score (TRISS). Similar conclusions have been drawn for abnormal admission serum **lactate** concentration (> 2 m Mol/L). A recent study demonstrated that prehospital, point-of-care lactate determinations improved prediction of mortality, need for surgery, and organ failure, when added to routine cardiovascular, respiratory, and neurologic parameters. A separate study found that the addition of abnormal base deficit (> 2.0 m Mol/L) or lactate (> 2.2 m Mol/L) concentration to abnormal vital signs (heart rate > 100 beats/min; systolic blood pressure < 90 mm Hg) substantially increased the ability to discern major from minor trauma. The dynamic nature of these parameters and added utility of serial measurements in assessing the response to therapy was highlighted in observational studies that have demonstrated that persistently elevated based deficit or lactate, despite resuscitation to normal vital signs, correlate with an increased rate of organ failure and death. These parameters may also predict the need for transfusions. They seem to be applicable in the elderly and pediatric populations.

Revised Trauma Score (RTS)

Designed as a simplification of the original trauma score described by Champion, which included respiratory rate, respiratory effort, systolic blood pressure, capillary refill and GCS, the revised trauma score (RTS) score was developed over 20 years ago to assist in the triage (T-RTS) of critically injured patients to trauma centers that could provide appropriate definitive care. It has since been expanded to include the prediction of outcome following traumatic injury. The RTS with Major Outcome Trauma Study weights (MTOS-RTS) is currently the standard physiologic severity score in trauma research and quality control. Simplistic in its composition of three ordinal scales representing GCS (range: 0–4), systolic blood pressure (range: 0–4), and respiratory rate (range: 0–4), weighted and summed to a range of 0 to 7.8408, it linearly correlates with the outcome of death.

$$RTS = 0.9368(GCS) + 0.7326(SBP) + 0.2908(RR)$$

A recent comparative study of T-RTS, a population-based RTS (POP-RTS), and MTOS-RTS concluded that the T-RTS provided statistically equivalent discriminatory power for in-hospital mortality, was easier to calculate, and, thus, should be considered a more simplistic means of risk adjustment. More recent data raise concern over its predictive capacity. Specifically the published coefficients may not be broadly applicable to more contemporary populations or those outside the United States. Furthermore, there is little evidence regarding its use for other clinically relevant outcomes (e.g., functional outcome, quality of life). Nonetheless, the RTS is a well-established predictor of mortality in trauma populations, has been successfully utilized in triage and patient-care guidelines, and has been incorporated into several important observational studies for case-mix adjustment.

Comorbidity assessment

There is little doubt, and in fact considerable supportive evidence, that the presence of chronic disease (e.g., prior myocardial infarction, obesity, coagulopathy of liver disease) markedly modifies the host response to injury, and thus affects the risk of nearly every important clinical outcome, including mortality. What varies is the extent to which each disease affects outcome and how to appropriately incorporate chronic disease into a case-mix adjusted analysis of injured patients. No trauma-specific score adjusts for comorbidity, in contrast to Acute Physiology and Chronic Health Evaluation (APACHE) scoring, in which a chronic comorbidity index is incorporated.

Age as a surrogate is directly associated with comorbidity burden, and its simplicity and predictive power necessitate its inclusion into any analysis. It alone serves as an audit filter for American College of Surgeons Committee on Trauma (ACSCOT) triage guidelines. However, age is an indirect measure, and the association between age and outcome exhibits an exponential association at higher ages.

Several risk adjustment scales have been developed that enhance the discriminatory power of age. The modified Charlson-Deyo comorbidity index is widely used in other disciplines and has found widespread applicability in the analysis of administrative databases, particularly those that are ICD-9 based. Incorporating a total of 22 comorbidities, a summary score is generated that is predictive of mortality. It has been successfully utilized in several landmark trauma database analyses. Recent studies highlight the need to modify the weight attributed to certain comorbidities (e.g., Human Immunodeficiency Virus) as advances in medical management have lessened the risk of death. Furthermore, other comorbidities not originally included (e.g., obesity) have been shown to alter the outcome from injury.

By contrast, the Elixhauser score incorporates an individual covariate for each of 30 comorbidities and has been demonstrated to outperform the Charlson-Deyo index. However, the need to incorporate a distinct covariate for each comorbidity renders its use in smaller data sets impractical. In these circumstances, the more parsimonious Charlson-Deyo score is all that is feasible. Both summary measures are subject to the accuracy of chart documentation and coding.

Combined scores

Trauma and Injury Severity Score (TRISS)

In light of the prognostic utility of measures of patient anatomy, physiology, and comorbidity, one could conclude that a combined system incorporating each of these would be ideal. The first such attempt occurred in 1987 and yielded the Trauma and Injury Severity Score (**TRISS**), which has since become the standard tool by which to benchmark trauma fatality outcome. TRISS uses a weighted combination of ISS (anatomic), RTS (physiologic), and an age indicator (comorbidity component) to estimate survival (Table 2.3). Separate models have been constructed for blunt and penetrating trauma. The coefficients used in weighting have most recently been revised using data obtained from NTDB and the NTDB National Sample Project (NSP). From these equations, one can estimate the probability of survival of an individual patient.

However, the TRISS approach has its shortcomings. The calculation of TRISS is cumbersome and requires a large number (8–10) of variables. Estimates can be derived only if all component variables have valid nonmissing values. Unfortunately, about a quarter of trauma cases have missing data. In such circumstances imputation may obviate this problem. TRISS could be improved by replacing ISS with a better anatomic predictor and by accounting for actual comorbidities, rather than the surrogate of age. The existing models ignore variable interactions and make strong linear assumptions between the predictor variables and survival outcomes. A recent study using a large nationally representative database reclassified the predictor variables, relaxed the assumptions of linearity, and incorporated significant interactions to generate a revised TRISS model that demonstrated improved predictive performance.

Table 2.3 Trauma and Injury Severity Score (TRISS)				
Equations for TRISS				
	Major Trauma Outcome Study (MTOS)		**National Trauma Database (NTDB)**	
Mechanism	**Blunt**	**Penetrating**	**Blunt**	**Penetrating**
Intercept	−0.4499	−2.5355	−2.17	−0.36
β ISS	0.8085	0.9934	0.077	0.10
β RTS	−0.0835	−0.0651	−0.49	−0.68
β AGE	−1.743	−1.1360	1.85	1.12

A Severity Characterization of Trauma (ASCOT)

Though TRISS continues to be the principal model used in estimating injury mortality, it carries several weaknesses: use of ISS and dichotomization of age. To address these shortcomings, Champion et al introduced A Severity Characterization of Trauma (ASCOT). ASCOT similarly incorporates anatomic descriptors, physiology, age, and mechanism into the model. However, it substitutes APS for ISS and lessens the restrictive dichotomization of age by creating five ordinal age categories. All the values are statistically weighted in such a manner as to produce a probability of survival. Several trials have demonstrated the improved prognostication of ASCOT over TRISS. However, ASCOT has failed to replace TRISS, in part, because of the complexity of its use.

Key references

Baker SP, O'Neill B, Haddon W, Jr, Long WB. The injury severity score: a method for describing patients with multiple injuries and evaluating emergency care. *J Trauma*. 1974; 14(3):187–196.

Boyd CR, Tolson MA, Copes WS. Evaluating trauma care: the TRISS method. Trauma Score and the Injury Severity Score. *J Trauma*. 1987;27(4):370–378.

Champion HR, Sacco WJ, Camazzo AJ, Copes W, Fouty WJ. Trauma score. *Crit Care Med*. 1981;9(9):672–676.

Charlson ME, Pompei P, Ales KL, MacKenzie CR. A new method of classifying prognostic comorbidity in longitudinal studies: development and validation. *J Chronic Dis*. 1987;40(5):373–383.

Guyette F, Suffoleto B, Castillo JL, Quintero J, Callaway C, Puyana JC. Prehospital serum lactate as a predictor of outcomes in trauma patients: a retrospective observational study. *J Trauma*. 2011;70(4):782–786.

Healey C, Osler TM, Rogers FB, et al. Improving the Glasgow Coma Scale score: motor score alone is a better predictor. *J Trauma*. 2003;54(4):671–678; discussion 678–680.

MacKenzie EJ, Steinwachs DM, Shankar B. Classifying trauma severity based on hospital discharge diagnoses. Validation of an ICD-9CM to AIS-85 conversion table. *Med Care*. 1989;27(4):412–422.

Mohan D, Rosengart MR, Farris C, Cohen E, Angus DC, Barnato AE. Assessing the feasibility of the American College of Surgeons' benchmarks for the triage of trauma patients. *Arch Surg*. 2011;146(7): 786–792.

Moore EE, Moore FA. American Association for the Surgery of Trauma Organ Injury Scaling: 50th anniversary review article of the Journal of Trauma. *J Trauma*. 2010;69(6):1600–1601.

Osler T, Rutledge R, Deis J, Bedrick E. ICISS: an international classification of disease-9 based injury severity score. *J Trauma*. 1996;41(3):380–386; discussion 386–388.

Thompson HJ, Rivara FP, Nathens A, Wang J, Jurkovich GJ, Mackenzie EJ. Development and validation of the mortality risk for trauma comorbidity index. *Ann Surg*. 2010;252(2):370–375.

Patient Management

Chapter 3

The tertiary survey: how to avoid missed injuries

Samuel A. Tisherman

Introduction

The Advanced Trauma Life Support (ATLS) Course of the American College of Surgeons and the development of mature trauma systems have standardized trauma care, both in the out-of-hospital arena and in the emergency department (ED). This standardization has led to improved outcomes in terms of morbidity and mortality. The bulk of the ATLS course focuses on the initial assessment and management of the trauma patient, stressing the importance of the primary and secondary surveys to identify immediately life-threatening injuries. Injuries that are less critical for survival, but perhaps very important for eventual morbidity, may not be identified because of patient instability or urgent need for interventions. Often the primary and secondary surveys are interrupted because of the need to resuscitate the patient or proceed with interventions for management of life-threatening injuries, such as craniotomy, thoracotomy, laparotomy, or angiography. Perhaps as many as two-thirds of patients have injuries not identified by this initial assessment.

In order to optimize the complete care of the patient, standardized patient assessment and management should continue when the patient arrives in the intensive care unit (ICU) or the hospital ward. Major life-threatening issues, including hypoxemia, hypoperfusion, and intracranial hypertension, may still need to be addressed. The goal of management is to promptly restore tissue perfusion and oxygenation, as well as minimize neurologic deficit.

Further evaluation of possible injuries must proceed simultaneously with ongoing resuscitation. The patient should be fully evaluated expeditiously so that all injuries are recognized and managed optimally. This complete evaluation of the trauma patient in the ICU or hospital ward has been called the *tertiary survey*, as first described by Enderson, et al (1990). The survey should be performed in all trauma patients, regardless of whether or not they require intensive care. Either residents or midlevel providers could be charged with completing this survey.

A complete tertiary survey is critical to fully assess the patient and avoid missing important injuries, which can have a significant impact on morbidity as well as mortality. Not surprisingly, the more severely injured patients, particularly those with hemorrhagic shock or head injuries, are at the greatest risk for having occult injuries. The tendency, indeed the training, is to focus only on the immediately life-threatening injuries, while inadvertently ignoring less obvious, but potentially life-threatening or life-altering, injuries.

The tertiary survey is not a one-time evaluation, but a process that includes serial physical examinations and assessments. Ongoing vigilance is critical to preventing missed injuries.

Tertiary survey description

Specific components

The goal of the tertiary survey is synthesize a complete picture of the patient's status. This includes identification of all injuries, as determined by physical examination, radiographic studies, and operative findings, plus understanding the patient's previous medical conditions, medications, allergies, etc. Each institution may develop its own protocol for who completes the survey and how it is documented. In some institutions, the same physicians who have evaluated the patient in the ED will continue to manage the patient in the ICU. In this case, these individuals may only need to "fill in the gaps" during the tertiary survey. In other institutions, other individuals, such as critical care attendings and fellows, will also be involved in patient management or may take on primary responsibility for patient care in the ICU. The most important initial step for the tertiary survey is direct communication among everyone involved. This communication is frequently forgotten when the patient does not go directly from the ED to the ICU. For instance, patients may be transported to the ICU from the operating room by only the anesthesia team or from radiology by a nurse. These individuals typically have focused on a limited number of specific issues in the patient's management. They often miss the "big picture." The importance of direct physician-to-physician contact, as well as accurate and complete written documentation, cannot be overemphasized. Standardized admission forms and orders help improve accuracy of the tertiary survey.

Obtaining an accurate history is often difficult in the critically ill trauma patient. The patient is often unable to provide information and family is usually not immediately available. Mechanism of injury is one of the most important pieces of information, along with observations made at the scene. Unfortunately, this information is passed along between so many different individuals that important details are often lost. The medic "trip sheets," if available, can be very helpful. One should not hesitate to contact the emergency medical providers or a referring hospital if additional information is needed.

In addition to history regarding the injury, one must obtain information regarding the patient's past medical history, medications, allergies, etc. This information is best obtained from the patient or the patient's family. If the family is not clear regarding medications and doses, asking them to bring in the pill bottles may help. It may also be helpful to contact the patient's primary care physician.

The physical examination portion of the tertiary survey should be similar to that of the typical primary and secondary surveys. One should begin with evaluation of the airway, breathing, circulation, and neurologic disability, followed by a complete head-to-toe examination. This must include examination of the patient's back; patients who have not had spinal injuries ruled out can be log-rolled. If possible, sedation should be minimized so that neurologic function can be reassessed. When sedation is required, the use of a very-short-acting agent such as propofol can facilitate serial examinations off sedation. Similarly, pain should be managed with low doses of a short-acting narcotic.

Any abnormal physical findings noted during the initial assessment in the ED should be reassessed at this time. New findings must be documented, communicated to appropriate team members, and followed. If needed, appropriate changes in management should be implemented.

Initial radiographs should be reviewed. At this point, additional radiographic studies may be needed, particularly in cases of blunt trauma. Standard imaging for almost all blunt-trauma victims includes chest and pelvic radiographs, abdominal ultrasound (focused assessment with sonography for trauma), and computed tomography (CT) of the head, spine, chest, abdomen, and pelvis. Additional imaging should be based upon patient symptoms or physical examination findings. Depending upon the time frame from admission to arrival in the ICU, some films may need to be repeated, such as radiographs of the chest and CT of the head. Timing of the studies may depend upon the patient's overall condition, need for ongoing resuscitation, need for transporting the patient off the unit for the study, and the potential adverse effects of delaying the study. In general, studies that require a "road trip" should be delayed until homeostasis has been achieved, unless the study is deemed to be necessary to achieve homeostasis; for example, a pelvic arteriogram to diagnose, and potentially control, bleeding into the pelvis in a patient with pelvic fractures. An experienced physician, for example, senior-level resident or attending, should make these decisions while weighing the risks and benefits of the study.

Once the imaging has been completed, it is imperative that the images are reviewed for adequacy. Ideally, actions should not be taken based on the imaging findings until the final reading has been documented by the attending radiologist.

Concurrent resuscitation issues

Restoring respiratory and cardiovascular stability often takes precedence over completion of the tertiary survey. One should ensure that the patient's natural airway is intact or that the airway has been "secured," usually with an endotracheal tube. If present, endotracheal tube position must be assessed, keeping in mind that tube migration (in or out) may have occurred during patient transport. Adequate ventilation to each lung must be assured by physical examination or repeat chest radiograph.

The circulation should first be evaluated by examining blood pressure, heart rate, and perfusion of the patient's extremities, keeping in mind that a significant number of trauma patients have "occult" hypoperfusion despite relatively normal blood pressure, heart rate, and urine output. Many parameters have been touted as markers of hypoperfusion and endpoints for resuscitation, but measuring arterial base deficit or lactate has become standard. The optimal endpoint is yet to be determined.

Regarding neurologic disability, any intracranial hemorrhage and/or intracranial hypertension must be addressed in conjunction with the neurosurgical service. Spinal immobilization should be continued until the radiographs have been read and the patient has been "cleared" clinically. For patients who have no neurologic impairment, controversy continues regarding the need for a magnetic resonance imaging study of the cervical spine if the CT is normal.

Confounding factors

Examination of the critically injured trauma patient is frequently confounded by a number of factors. First, many trauma patients have a decreased level of consciousness from use of alcohol or illicit drugs, or sedation/analgesia used to treat pain, agitation or combativeness. Intoxication may mask injuries or make the patient's examination unreliable, but could also mimic traumatic brain injury. Intoxication may also alter the response to trauma and hemorrhagic shock.

Second, premorbid conditions, particularly cardiac and pulmonary diseases, may alter the patient's response to trauma. Medications, such as beta-blockers, can prevent tachycardia. Patients with pre-existing cardiac or pulmonary dysfunction respond poorly to hemorrhagic shock or chest trauma. In the elderly, baseline neurologic function is frequently not normal secondary to dementia or previous strokes.

Third, concomitant head or spinal cord injuries can make the physical examination unreliable. Patients with head injuries may not be able to communicate. Similarly, patients with spinal cord injuries may not be able to sense pain distal to the site of injury. In these cases, information regarding the mechanism of injury is critical for focusing on the appropriate potential injuries. Additional radiographic studies may be needed.

Fourth, distracting injuries may make physical examination difficult. Small doses of analgesics may help the patient focus on the physical examination. Patients and healthcare workers frequently focus on the most painful or visually shocking injuries while missing injuries that need more acute attention.

Priorities

The management of critically ill trauma patients is complicated by the need for simultaneous resuscitation, diagnostic evaluation, and therapeutic interventions. Because not all issues can be addressed at once, priorities need to be set. In the early management of the trauma patient, the respiratory, cardiovascular, and neurologic abnormalities (ABCD of the ATLS primary survey) usually take precedence. Identifying and managing immediately life-threatening injuries is critical. One should consider which injury is the most imminent threat to life. Infectious complications and the multiple organ dysfunction syndrome do not manifest until later, but the risk of these complications may be minimized by rapid, appropriate early treatment.

To optimize care, priorities regarding diagnostic workups and therapeutic interventions must be set by the most senior physician involved on the trauma service. These decisions must be communicated to all members of the team, including consultants. All pertinent information must be accurate and available for consideration. Decisions must focus on what is best for the patient, ignoring politics or convenience.

Patient transport

For diagnosis and management of injuries, patients frequently require transport ("road trips") out of the ICU to radiology or the operating room. Unless these trips are a necessary part of resuscitation efforts, for example, a pelvic arteriogram to obtain hemostasis, they should generally be avoided until the patient has been stabilized. Balancing the potential diagnostic or therapeutic value of such studies with the patient's need for ventilatory or hemodynamic support demands expert judgment.

When possible, the patient's time away from the unit should be managed as efficiently as possible, that is, coordinating studies so as to avoid long patient wait times in the radiology department or additional transports away from the ICU . In addition, transporting patients should be done as safely as possible. Optimal timing should be considered. For example, though it may be clear that a fine-cut CT scan of temporal bones is needed for a patient, obtaining this study at 2 AM, when staffing is often decreased, is unlikely to affect patient care. The level of patient monitoring during transport should equal that in the ICU. Accompanying nursing staff should have all necessary drugs, fluids, and oxygen on hand so that care is not interrupted. In some circumstances, for example, when patients have been administered neuromuscular blocking agents, a physician should accompany the patient.

Missed injuries

Contributing factors

Missed or occult injuries may be found in up to two-thirds of trauma patients admitted to the ICU, although a figure of around 10% is more generally accepted. The published incidence depends upon the definition used for missed injuries. Patients with truly missed injuries frequently have higher injury severity scores and lower Glasgow Coma Scales than other patients. Intoxication, shock, spinal cord and head injury, and inability to communicate predispose to missed injuries. Multiple other factors (Table 3.1), both patient and clinician-related, increase

Table 3.1 Contributing factors in missed injuries

Patient factors	Clinician factors
Hemodynamic instability	Inexperience
Altered mental status	Inappropriately low level of suspicion
Ethanol/drug intoxication	Radiologic error
Sedation/analgesia/anesthesia	Failure to obtain study
Head injury	Inadequate films
Neurologic deficit	Misinterpretation of studies
Spinal cord injury	Technical errors
Peripheral nerve injury	Multiple patients
Transfer from an outlying facility	Admission to inappropriate service

the risk. Patients may be distracted by other injuries or may lack symptoms at the time of admission. Physician inexperience and diagnostic oversight may also play a role, particularly when multiple simultaneous patients are being managed. The increasing use of abbreviated initial operative procedures (damage control) increases the likelihood of a delay in diagnosis of all injuries. Radiologic errors are common, bringing up questions regarding the need for 24-hour a day coverage by more senior radiologists, not junior level residents. "Final" radiologic readings should be available as soon as possible. Admission of the patient to an inappropriate service, usually a surgical subspecialty service, may also be an issue. This tends to be rare at dedicated trauma centers in which there is a policy that all trauma patients are admitted to the trauma service (or are at least seen by the trauma service) initially.

Many missed injuries are orthopedic. Ward et al analyzed 24 missed orthopedic injuries found in 111 patients. Seventy percent of the injuries were diagnosed by physical examination and plain radiographs. Only 27% required sophisticated imaging techniques. They identified the following risk factors for missed injuries: another more apparent orthopedic injury within the same extremity, patient too unstable for orthopedic evaluation, altered sensorium, hastily applied emergency splint obscuring a less apparent injury, poor-quality or inadequate initial radiographs, and inadequate significance assigned to minor symptoms or signs in a major trauma victim. Laasonen et al noted similar reasons for missed bony injuries, but added unnoticed radiologists' reports, fracture visible at the outermost corner of a radiograph, fracture hidden by other fractures, and obesity.

Nonorthopedic radiographic studies also contribute to missed injuries. Hirshburg et al at Ben Taub in Houston found that difficulties in the diagnostic workup led to 46 of 123 missed injuries. This included failure to obtain the correct investigation and inherent limitations of the modality. The great majority of injuries missed on radiographic studies involved specialized studies such as angiography and CT. Incomplete surgical exploration resulted in 43 missed injuries.

Missed injury patterns

Missed injuries in blunt-trauma patients most commonly include orthopedic injuries, particularly extremity injuries. With routine CT imaging of the head, spine, chest, and abdomen, missed injuries in these body regions have decreased. In contrast, missed vascular and hollow visceral injuries are more common after penetrating trauma.

Preventing missed injuries

The search for occult injuries should first focus on those that may present a threat to life or limb. High-priority occult injuries include brain and spinal cord injury, cerebrovascular injury, thoracic aortic injury, pneumothorax, aerodigestive tract injury, abdominal compartment syndrome, peripheral vascular injury or compartment syndrome, major joint dislocation, and eye injury. Early complications of injuries, such as abdominal or extremity compartment syndromes, should also be sought.

The Ben Taub group proposed a useful classification system for patterns of missed injuries. In type I, which occurred in 20% of cases with missed injuries, the missed injuries were outside the body area that was the focus of clinical attention or surgical activity, suggesting that the standard initial workup protocol may not have been adequately followed. To avoid this type of error, one needs to be compulsive and assume that, based on the mechanism of injury, an injury is present until proven otherwise. A systematic and cautious approach is needed.

In type II, an injury within the body area of interest was missed. This was identified in 69% of cases with missed injuries. These errors occur as a result of improper selection or sequencing of diagnostic tests or from inherent limitations of the studies. Of perhaps greater concern, inadequate surgical exploration accounted for some of the missed injuries. Although the patient's instability and/or number of injuries may contribute to this type of error, the surgeon must try to avoid this error by obtaining adequate exposure of all possible body compartments that may be involved.

The remaining missed injuries, type III, resulted from the surgeon's decision to curtail the diagnostic workup or surgical exploration because of the patient's instability. In contrast to the other types of errors, this is usually due to the surgeon's correct decision to terminate diagnostic studies, or a particular procedure, in the patient's best interest and thus may not be an "error" at all. The importance of discussing the potential for these "missed" injuries is to alert the surgical team to thoroughly explore the patient during the planned reoperation and to maintain a low threshold for early reoperation if the patient is not doing well. Also, the remainder of the tertiary survey must be completed within a reasonable time frame, depending upon the patient's condition.

Preventing missed injuries requires compulsiveness during the assessment of the patient in the ICU and in the operating room. Continued vigilance throughout care of the patient is needed. During operations, a thorough and complete exploration is mandatory. One should avoid focusing only on the known injuries.

Knowledge of the mechanism of injury and maintaining a high index of suspicion are essential.

Because injuries can be missed at any point during the management of multiple trauma patients, including primary, secondary, and tertiary surveys, and in the operating room, clinicians need to be attentive to subtle signs of injury.

Avoiding specific missed injuries

Table 3.2 lists commonly missed injuries and the studies that could be done to decrease the risk of missing these injuries.

Table 3.2 Missed injuries and best tests for diagnosis	
Diagnosis	**Key test**
Facial fractures	Sagittal and coronal CT
Spinal fractures/spinal cord injuries	CT MRI
Blunt cerebrovascular injury	CT angiography or 4-vessel arteriography
Diaphragm injury	CT Thoracoscopy or laparoscopy
Esophageal injury	Esophagram and/or esophagoscopy
Aortic injury	Chest CT Angiography
Cardiac wounds	Echocardiography Pericardial window
Abdominal hollow viscus injuries	Abdominal CT Serial exams Laparoscopy Laparotomy
Pancreatic injuries	Abdominal CT Laparotomy
Biliary ductal injuries	Abdominal CT HIDA ERCP
Rectal injuries	Proctoscopy
Renal artery occlusion	Abdominal CT Angiography
Extremity fractures	Specialized plain radiographs, including proximal and distal joints
Ligamentous injuries	Complete physical examination CT MRI
Arterial injuries	Low threshold for angiography
Pelvic fractures	Pelvis CT

CT = computed tomography, MRI = magnetic resonance imaging, HIDA = hepatic imidoacetic acid, ERCP = endoscopic retrograde cholangiopancreatography

The use of CT scans of the head has significantly decreased the risk of missing an intracranial injury that requires neurosurgical intervention. Any suspicion at all of a head injury based on mechanism of injury, history, or physical examination should be sufficient indication for obtaining the scan. When these scans are delayed because of patient instability, they should be obtained as soon as the patient can be safely transported. Rarely, patients have evidence of a traumatic brain injury and severe extracranial injuries necessitating intracranial pressure monitoring without the benefit of a CT. Some institutions have portable CT scanners to facilitate head CTs in patients otherwise too sick for transport.

Because of the tremendous consequences of a missed spinal injury that leads to a neurologic deficit, spine fractures need to be identified early. Thus radiographs of the spine should be obtained early in the workup of trauma patients. The patients should be immobilized until spinal injuries can be ruled out. At times, however, these concerns may be overemphasized. Obtaining radiographs, for example, should not take precedence over airway management or resuscitation from hemorrhagic shock. Maintaining cervical spine immobilization is similarly important during any airway manipulation, but if the airway is not secured and the patient asphyxiates, the theoretical effects of manipulating an unstable cervical spine injury and causing a neurologic deficit become mute.

Reasons for missed spinal injuries include: (1) not obtaining the appropriate film; (2) misinterpretation of appropriate films; (3) injuries at multiple levels; (4) altered level of consciousness; and (4) patient refusal. Until all necessary films have been obtained and ligamentous injury ruled out by exam or imaging (e.g., magnetic resonance imaging), patients should remain immobilized. As an aside, there is an increasing amount of data suggesting that a normal CT of the cervical spine rules out a significant ligamentous injury. Completion of the cervical spine evaluation should not, however, prevent the patient from undergoing any other important diagnostic tests or procedures.

For thoracic trauma, CT of the chest has become the most important modality to rule out subtle injuries not revealed by physical examination and plain chest radiographs. Computed tomography can readily identify occult pneumothoraces and aortic injuries. The appropriate management of the small pneumothorax found only on CT scan is unclear. Even if the patient is on positive pressure ventilation, a chest tube does not seem to be necessary.

Missed injuries in the abdomen are of particular concern, particularly for the victim of blunt trauma. Initial management of patients who have penetrating trauma or are unstable is usually straightforward as these patients typically undergo prompt laparotomy. The difficulty is with the stable blunt-trauma victim. One must have a high level of suspicion based on the mechanism of injury. Injuries to the bowel and retroperitoneum are notoriously difficult to diagnose. Physical examination is difficult because of decreased mental status or distracting injuries. Ultrasound and CT may not reveal the injury.

One should also keep in mind that physical examination and various diagnostic tests are all complementary. Serial physical examinations, and sometimes radiologic studies, are critical to avoiding missed injuries during the tertiary survey. In general, the risk of a missed intra-abdominal injury is much greater than that of a negative laparotomy.

Musculoskeletal injuries are the most commonly missed injuries. During the initial resuscitation, the typical physical findings may be subtle or may be missed because of the patient's instability, decreased level of consciousness, neurologic deficit, or distracting injuries. The most common reason for missing such an injury is not obtaining the appropriate radiographs, including the joints proximal and distal to a recognized injury. Any complaints by the patient or ecchymosis or swelling on examination should be taken seriously. If complaints continue despite initially negative films, repeat films should be obtained.

Considering the mechanism of injury, specific injuries should be sought. For example, patients with a fall from a height should have a calcaneal fracture ruled out. Patients with one spinal injury should have the remainder of the spine examined closely.

There has been increased interest in early diagnosis of blunt carotid or vertebral injuries. These injuries are thought to be secondary to hyperextension of the neck, resulting in a dissection with an intimal flap, or direct injury related to direct trauma to the neck or a spinal fracture. There may be no physical findings until the patient suddenly develops a significant neurologic deficit. Arteriography remains the gold standard, but the indications remain controversial in the asymptomatic patient given the risks and costs involved. CT angiography has become the screening imaging modality of choice. Indications for CT angiography to rule out cerebrovascular injuries include LeFort II or III facial fractures, complex mandibular fractures, basilar skull fracture, diffuse axonal injury, cervical spine fractures in proximity to the vertebral arteries or involving substantial subluxation or rotation, and near-hanging with anoxic brain injury. Evidence of direct blunt trauma to the neck should also be considered.

System issues

Because many missed injuries are related to mistakes made in interpretation of radiologic studies, the question arises regarding the need for higher level radiologist coverage for trauma patients. Ideally, radiologic studies should be immediately read by attending radiologists or at least senior housestaff. This is frequently not the case in the middle of the night, leaving the ED and trauma staffs to interpret films independently. Review of the films the next morning by the radiologist with the trauma team can help prevent missed injuries and improve education of housestaff.

The benefit of in-house attending trauma surgeon coverage remains controversial. It has been difficult to prove that in-house coverage is better than if the trauma surgeon can respond within 15 minutes of the patient's arrival.

To avoid missed injuries, it is critical for members of the trauma team to discuss missed injuries and complications openly and honestly. System issues that might decrease the incidence of missed injuries, including additional training of personnel, should be addressed.

Despite appropriate primary and secondary surveys, missed injuries still occur. Introduction of a protocolized tertiary survey may decrease the number of missed injuries, particularly when this survey is completed in a timely fashion.

Family issues

Because of its sudden and unexpected nature, trauma is understandably stressful for both the patient and the family. For victims of penetrating trauma, issues related to the violent crime add to the stress. Mistrust of authorities and medical professionals is common. This should be kept in mind when discussing the patient's status with the family. Establishing a good rapport with them can greatly facilitate obtaining the necessary personal health information regarding the patient. Social workers and nursing staff often obtain bits and pieces of information. Communication and documentation, as part of the tertiary survey, is critical to putting together the complete picture of the patient's past medical history and the circumstances of the injury. This issue has both medical and medicolegal implications.

Legal issues

Legal action frequently occurs following traumatic incidents, particularly when violence is involved. The police (and the medical examiner's office in homicide cases) need evidence to prosecute the crime. The staff in the ICU must keep in mind that the medical record may be used during legal proceedings. Any specific observations regarding the injuries need to be as precise and nonjudgmental as possible. For example, descriptions of bullet wounds should only describe the findings and location; one should not attempt to define a wound as an "entrance" vs. "exit" wound. It is also critical to assist the authorities in maintaining the chain of evidence. Anything related to a possible crime that is found on, or removed from, a patient needs to be handled appropriately so that it can be directly linked back to the victim. Hospital security should be involved.

Given our current atmosphere of culpability, there is concern that any errors (real or perceived) on the part of healthcare providers could lead to malpractice lawsuits. This fear has lead many physicians to avoid care of the injured. For radiologists, the most common cause of lawsuits is missed diagnoses, about half of which occur in trauma patients. Claims against Level I trauma centers may be more defensible because of the use of established protocols, a high index of suspicion for injuries, and careful follow-up.

Even with appropriate care, errors can occur and injuries can be missed. A standardized, comprehensive approach can help minimize the risk that life-threatening and disabling injuries will be missed.

Key references

Biffl WL, Harrington DT, Cioffi WG. Implementation of a tertiary trauma survey decreases missed injuries. *J Trauma*. 2003;54:38–44.

Bromberg WJ, Collier BC, Diebel LN, et al. Blunt cerebrovascular injury practice management guidelines: the Eastern Association for the Surgery of Trauma. *J Trauma*. 2010;68:471–477.

Enderson BL, Reath DB, Meadors J, et al. The tertiary trauma survey: a prospective study of missed injury. *J Trauma*. 1990;30:666–669.

Fulda GJ, Tinkoff GH, Giberson F, Rhodes M. In-house trauma surgeons do not decrease mortality in a Level I trauma center. *J Trauma*. 2002;53:494–500.

Hoff WS, Sicoutris CP, Lee SY, et al. Formalized radiology rounds: the final component of the tertiary survey. *J Trauma*. 2004;56(2):291–295.

Huynh TT, Blackburn AH, McMiddleton-Nyatui D, et al. An initiative by midlevel providers to conduct tertiary surveys at a Level I trauma center. *J Trauma*. 2010;68(5):1052–1058.

Lawson CM, Daley BJ, Ormsby CB, Enderson B. Missed injuries in the era of the trauma scan. *J Trauma*. 2011;70:452–458.

Velmahos GC, Fili C, Vassiliu P, et al. Around-the-clock attending radiology coverage is essential to avoid mistakes in the care of trauma patients. *Amer Surg*. 2001;67:1175–1177.

Chapter 4

Monitors and drains in trauma patients

Greta L. Piper and Lewis J. Kaplan

Monitors

Introduction

Monitors are essential for assessment of the critically ill patient. It is necessary to understand the basics, as well as the intricacies, of when and why to use certain monitors, as well as how to interpret the results within the context of other clinical signs and symptoms. Intensive-care patient monitors are constantly evolving to better, faster, and more automated technology, but the human physiology behind the newer tools remains the same.

The purpose of monitoring a patient is to detect abnormalities in physiologic markers that indicate the presence of pathology that requires further evaluation or intervention, and to monitor the progress of interventions. Monitors may be invasive or noninvasive, continuous or intermittent, and may provide absolute values as well as trends. The most basic vital signs of temperature, heart rate, blood pressure, respiratory rate, and oxygen saturation (SaO_2) are only a small part of the spectrum of available physiologic markers.

Temperature

Body temperature is considered one of the basic vital signs and is an indicator of physiologic integrity. Normothermia in perioperative patients is associated with improved outcomes. Increased temperature, typically greater than 38.5°C, indicates a fever, which serves as a warning sign of infection or stress. Hypothermia (core temperature < 35°C) in trauma patients is part of the deadly triad that also includes acidosis and coagulopathy.

Core body temperature is narrowly maintained and differs from the temperature of peripheral tissues by 3–4°C in the hemodynamically normal patient. Because it is not possible to measure the temperature of blood as it enters the hypothalamus, pulmonary artery temperature obtained via a pulmonary artery catheter (PAC) is considered the "gold standard" for core body temperature. As few patients need PACs, urinary bladder, esophageal, or rectal temperature probes clearly suffice. Other less precise sites for temperature measurement include oral, axillary, inguinal, tympanic membrane, and temporal artery locations.

Peripheral temperature reflects tissue perfusion that is affected by varying degrees of vasoconstriction or vasodilatation. Cool extremities may relate to vasoconstriction, decreased cardiac output, peripheral arterial disease, use of an alpha-agonist, or even sympathetic response to pain or anxiety. Alternatively, warm extremities may correlate with the vasodilated, hypoperfused state of sepsis, anaphylaxis, or neurogenic shock, as well as use of a direct vasodilating agent.

For most of the last century, rectal temperatures have been a preferred method because of speed, ease of use, and lack of expense. Although rectal temperatures correlate well with core temperature in patients with relatively constant temperature, they lag behind measured changes at other core sites. Other disadvantages include the risk of rectal injury, the challenge of use in obese or difficult to move patients (including those with axial skeletal injury), difficulty in the presence of rectal-stool collecting systems, and patient discomfort.

Sublingual oral temperatures are also practical, accessible, and used in a region of rich blood supply. In nonintubated patients measurements can be affected by ingestion of warm or cold beverages, or mouth breathing. Some controversy exists as to whether intubation changes the accuracy of oral temperatures. Axillary and inguinal temperatures are easily obtained but tend to underestimate core temperature and do not allow for continuous monitoring.

Tympanic membrane thermometry is widespread because it is convenient, rapid, and noninvasive. The ear canal is well-vascularized by internal carotid artery branches and so is an indirect measure of cerebral vascular temperature. One disadvantage is that it is user dependent, particularly because variable ear tugging to obtain better access to the actual tympanic membrane leads to different measurements. Variability between a patient's left and right ears has been noted. In addition, cerumen occlusion of the tympanic membrane has been identified as a factor that lowers the temperature measurement. This suggests that if a patient's tympanic membrane cannot be visualized, tympanic membrane thermometry should not be used.

Continuous temperature monitoring can be performed via more invasive esophageal, rectal, or urinary bladder temperature probes. Bladder and esophageal temperature measurements may correlate best with PAC temperatures.

A newer addition to measuring core temperatures is the temporal artery thermometer, placed on the skin of the forehead over the temporal artery. The accuracy of this device is still to be determined.

Cardiac/Perfusion

Electrocardiography

Continuous monitoring of electrocardiography (ECG) is standard in the ICU using standard 3-lead and 5-lead configurations. The more detailed 12-lead ECG is generally printed as a snapshot of the cardiac activity at a given time. The three basic features elucidated by ECG monitoring are rate abnormalities, rhythm disturbances, and ischemic patterns. ECG monitoring of patients with acute coronary syndrome or blunt cardiac injury is essential because cardiac dysrhythmias can be lethal. Interpretation that was individual competency specific has been complemented by automated computer-generated readings of continuous ECG tracings, as well as 12-lead ECGs. Nonetheless, continuous rhythm strips or intermittent 12-lead ECG analysis may miss myocardial ischemia. Accordingly, technologic advancements have made possible both continuous 12-lead ECG monitoring as well as ST-segment analysis.

Up to 90% of episodes of myocardial ischemia events are transient and therefore clinically silent and may often be missed with isolated 12-lead ECG or limited 3-lead or 5-lead monitoring. Transient and clinically silent myocardial ischemia developed in 20% of the patients during weaning. The frequency of silent myocardial ischemia during ventilator weaning suggests that unanticipated myocardial ischemia may be related to weaning failure.

The physiologic stress of critical illness increases myocardial oxygen demands. At-risk groups include postoperative surgical patients and patients with sepsis, electrolyte imbalances, or intermittent hypoxia.

Arterial blood pressure

Noninvasive blood pressure measurement

The sphygmomanometer remains the standard for noninvasive measurement of arterial blood pressure. It is essential to use an appropriate cuff size as a too-small cuff will cause falsely elevated readings while a too-large cuff will cause falsely low readings. The cuff is inflated to compress the inflow artery of interest and stop flow. As the cuff is slowly deflated the pressure at which flow returns through the vessel is the systolic blood pressure. This can be determined via auscultation of Korotkoff sounds, most often over the brachial artery, or via detection of plethysmographic oscillations (see below). Palpation, a Doppler stethoscope, or a pulse oximeter may also be used to determine when flow has been re-established.

Automated blood pressure devices have largely replaced manual devices in the critical care setting because they are capable of performing timed serial measurements via a menu setting or on-demand with the press of a button or touch screen. Often these automated measurements are projected directly onto a computer screen and inserted into electronically captured nursing documentation. Rather than using the auscultatory method, these machines rely on oscillometry, recognizing low-frequency signals in the 16–80 Hz range that correlate with Korotkoff sounds or by detecting ultrasonic waves emitted with movement of the arterial wall. Automated oscillometric blood pressure measurements may not be as accurate as manual auscultatory blood pressure measurements, especially in hypotensive, hypovolemic patients. In general, manual blood pressure assessments should be performed for prehospital and triage situations and in all patients with blood pressures < 110 mm Hg.

Photoplethysmography

Photoplethysmography is another noninvasive method for arterial blood pressure measurements in which infrared light is transmitted through a finger placed in an inflatable cuff to estimate the volume of hemoglobin that flows with each heart-beat. The cuff adjusts its compression pressure to keep the volume of blood flow constant. This pressure reflects the digital artery pressure, which may or may not correlate with more central blood pressure, depending on a variety of factors. This technique is not regularly utilized in the inpatient setting due to poor accuracy.

Invasive arterial blood pressure monitoring involves inserting a catheter directly into the lumen of an artery, most commonly the radial or femoral artery. The catheter is then connected to a pressure transducer via fluid-filled tubing. The transducer signal is converted to an electrical signal that is processed and amplified and displayed on a monitor. The most frequent indication for invasive blood pressure monitoring is hemodynamic instability. Beat-to-beat measurements make this method more ideal for patients whose condition is expected to change rapidly or for patients who require blood pressure control with vasoactive agents. Although the intra-arterial catheter also offers the benefit of repeated blood sampling, it is invasive and has been associated with a host of complications;it is therefore only employed in a closely monitored setting, where acute fluctuations in blood pressure are anticipated. Continuous pH monitoring via arterial catheter blood sampling has undergone limited study but is not currently the standard of care.

The radial artery is the most common site due to its accessibility and consistent anatomy as well as its lack of atherosclerotic changes. The femoral artery may be chosen for its lower rate of mechanical complications. Mean arterial pressure tends to correlate between these two sites better than systolic or diastolic pressures. When the radial or femoral arteries are not available, the axillary or dorsalis pedis artery may be used. The brachial artery can also be used. The belief that it is a functional end artery and its thrombosis may lead to limb-threatening ischemia of the forearm and hand is controversial.

Complications of arterial catheters include bleeding, hematoma, pseudoaneurysm, infection, nerve damage, and distal-limb ischemia. Risk factors for vascular occlusion include catheter size (the smallest possible should be used), hypotension, high-dose vasopressors, and presence of hematoma leading to occlusion. Possible risk factors include the number of puncture attempts, duration of catheter placement, and patient gender. The value of the Allen test to determine adequacy of ulnar blood flow and, thereby, the risk of hand ischemia with a radial catheter, seems limited.

Waveform analysis requires an adequate waveform. Damping is a phenomenon whereby anything that reduces the energy in an oscillating system will reduce the amplitude of the oscillations. Bubbles or clots, arterial vasospasm, and catheter kinks cause damping that under-reads systolic pressure and over-reads the diastolic pressure. Catheter whip (or fling) is the oscillating movement of the catheter that creates changes in hydrostatic pressure at the catheter tip. This usually occurs in large diameter arteries such as the femoral or pulmonary arteries, causing the systolic blood pressure to vary by as much as 20 mm Hg.

Analysis of an arterial waveform allows for important insight into a patient's physiology. The systolic upstroke or anacrotic limb reflects the pressure pulse produced by left ventricular contraction. The systolic pressure is measured at the peak of the waveform. The dicrotic (or downward) limb is demarcated by the dicrotic notch, representing closure of the aortic valve and subsequent retrograde flow. The location of the dicrotic notch varies according to the timing of aortic closure in the cardiac cycle. For example, aortic closure is delayed in patients with hypovolemia. Consequently, the dicrotic notch occurs farther down on the dicrotic limb in hypovolemic patients. The dicrotic notch also appears lower on the dicrotic limb when arterial pressure is measured at more distal sites in the arterial tree.

Normal respiration leads to changes in intrathoracic pressure, which affect cardiac output and systemic pressure. With spontaneous inspiration, intrathoracic pressure decreases. The decreased pressure is recognizable on the blood pressure tracing as a downward displacement of the waveform baseline. Concurrently, during inspiration, venous return to the right side of the heart is increased, augmenting right ventricular stroke volume. The increase in right ventricular stroke volume is offset by increased pulmonary vascular compliance and blood pooling during inspiratory thoracic expansion. Consequently, left ventricular stroke volume is decreased. When the pressure in the vena cava is lower than normal due to hypovolemia, the surrounding pressure collapses the veins earlier, further decreasing cardiac preload and creating greater beat-to-beat variation in systolic blood pressure. Thus, relative increases in systolic pressure variation can be an indicator of fluid responsiveness.

Invasive hemodynamic monitoring
Use of the PAC for invasive hemodynamic monitoring has been decreasing because of a lack of conclusive benefit, except for cardiac and some vascular surgery procedures and orthotopic hepatic transplantation. No controlled trials have proved the benefit of PAC in injured patients.

The PAC is most commonly inserted through a central venous sheath introducer in the subclavian, internal jugular, or femoral vein. With the distal balloon inflated, the catheter undergoes flow-directed distal advancement identifying typical waveforms indicative of central venous, right ventricle, pulmonary artery, and then pulmonary artery occlusion pressure tracings (Figure 4.1). The balloon is deflated, the catheter is secured, and its position is confirmed using standard portable chest X-ray (CXR).

The standard PA catheter measures central venous pressure (CVP), pulmonary artery pressure (PAP), and pulmonary artery occlusion pressure (PAOP). Blood samples can be drawn from the PA port to intermittently measure mixed venous oxygen saturation (SvO2). A thermistor located on the outer surface 4 cm from the catheter tip measures temperature. By assessing the rate of change of temperature of a fluid bolus (cold or room temperature) injected into the proximal port of the catheter as a function of time, flow (i.e., cardiac output) may be derived; this technique is termed thermodilution. The PAC may also have additional features including an extra infusion channel, a fiberoptic system that allows continuous monitoring of SvO_2, a rapid response thermistor

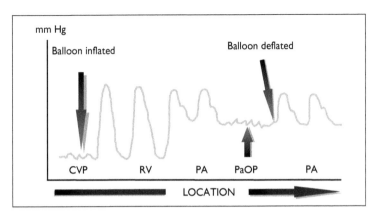

Figure 4.1 Pulmonary Artery Catheter Waveforms

to measure right ventricular ejection fraction (RVEF), or a thermal filament that allows continuous cardiac output monitoring (CCO).

Two main categories of complications are associated with PA catheters: technical complications and misinterpretation of data. Establishing central venous access can cause hematoma, bleeding (venous or arterial), pneumo/hemothorax, puncture or laceration of surrounding structures, thoracic duct injury, or air embolism. Intracardiac passage of the PA catheter frequently induces minor arrhythmias including premature atrial or ventricular contractions. Other dysrhythmias include ventricular tachycardia, ventricular fibrillation, or right bundle branch block. "Knotting" of the PA catheter is another rare but described complication associated with catheter insertion. Once the catheter is in place, complications include venous thrombosis, pulmonary embolism, cardiac mural thrombus, valve injury, catheter-related infection and sepsis, and pulmonary artery rupture.

Misinterpretation of the data provided by the PAC is perhaps more dangerous and pervasive than most technical complications. Interpretation errors frequently derive from obtaining and not recognizing faulty data. Such data is related to improper placement, location, connection, or calibration. Because catheters require hand injection for CO determination, vagaries of the rapidity of infusion lead to substantial variability in the data. Additionally, the determination of PAOP requires the bedside clinical provider to obtain an appropriate tracing and then adjust the threshold line to the end of expiration. High levels of positive end-expiratory pressure (PEEP), nonstandard ventilator modes, and nonstandard positioning will introduce significant errors in PAOP determination—a value that is repetitively used in clinical decision-making as well as a host of derived indices.

Less invasive cardiac performance monitor alternatives
There are now several methods to ascertain CO that do not require PAC placement. These devices use either ultrasound, proprietary analyses of an arterial waveform, or flow assessment using detection of a tracer.

Ultrasound devices range from a standard transthoracic 2-D ECHO to transesophageal echocardiography both of which provide an assessment of left ventricular ejection fraction, PAP, a relative assessment of chamber size, valvular competence, and the presence or absence of a pericardial effusion. Cardiac output can also be assessed. An Esophageal Doppler Monitor (EDM), an ultrasound-based probe that is much smaller, can assess cardiac output via real-time measurements of changes in volume of the aorta as a function of time. These measurements correlate well with PAC data. It is, however, difficult to maintain in the correct position, is readily dislodged, and requires oral insertion and therefore an intubated patient. Although nasal insertion has been utilized, it has not been validated. Also, those who have aortic prosthetic grafts may not be suitable for this tool. Use in the morbidly obese has not been validated.

One less invasive alternative, the FloTrac/Vigileo (Edwards Lifesciences, Irvine, CA) uses arterial pressure signal monitoring to assess variations in stroke volume on a beat-to-beat basis. Although it still requires arterial catheterization, continuous blood pressure monitoring is usually warranted in high-risk patients so no increased invasiveness or risk is incurred. No external calibration is needed, although demographics of height, weight, age, and gender are entered and the device is connected directly to the arterial catheter. Lithium dilution cardiac output (LiDCO) measurement requires a central venous catheter and an arterial catheter. The device assesses the rate of transit of a lithium tracer injected from the central vein and its appearance in the artery. A related system, the peripherally inserted cardiac output device (PICCO) uses a femoral arterial catheter, a CVP and a proprietary algorithm to similarly derive cardiac performance measures. In this way, it uses features of both the LiDCO system and the FloTrac/Vigileo devices. To date, no system has demonstrated superiority compared to one another or the PAC.

The first completely noninvasive cardiac output assessment method involved transthoracic bioimpedence. This was inconsistent in its accuracy. A new signal processing method using chest bioreactance is known as Noninvasive Cardiac Output Monitoring (NICOM). Four double electrode stickers are placed on the patient's thorax. Upper thoracic electrodes deliver small alternating currents with specific propagation characteristics to their corresponding lower thoracic electrodes, providing a measure of bioreactance. When compared to CO measured via PAC, NICOM has acceptable accuracy, precision, and responsiveness.

In a combined study of postoperative cardiac surgery patients, both the FloTrac/Vigileo and the NICOM devices were similar in their accuracy and precision compared to the PAC. Responsiveness of both methods was faster than that of the continuous thermodilution technique.

Respiratory

In all critically ill patients, important goals are hemodynamic optimization and support of oxygen delivery and utilization. Many ICU patients require mechanical ventilation to achieve these goals. Assessment parameters that allow one to follow the progress of ventilator therapy, assess readiness for weaning and liberation from mechanical ventilation, and rapidly recognize clinical deterioration or adverse events are important tools. At a minimum, these parameters include physical examination, respiratory rate, and pulse oximetry. Additional data may be readily gleaned from real-time analysis of CO_2 (capnography and capnometry) as well. Although it is recognized that the ventilator will provide a host of airway pressure measurements, their interpretation and utilization are both beyond the scope of this chapter and have been extensively reviewed elsewhere in detail. Tidal volume (VT) and exhaled minute ventilation (VE) can also be measured.

Respiratory rate

The simplest means of determining respiratory rate is counting the number of breaths a patient at rest takes in 1 minute. The absolute number is as important as the trend. The value lies in understanding how the rate relates to the minute ventilation of the patient. Certainly, a declining respiratory rate that is below the lower limit of normal may be predicted to result in ineffective and inadequate CO_2 clearance and should prompt both investigation as to the root cause and therapy to correct the likely rising pCO_2. One should be cognizant of the following definitions:

Tachypnea: increased RR, decreased VT, normal VE
Hyperpnea: increased RR, increased VT, increased VE

The importance is that only hyperpnea is associated with increased CO_2 production reflecting increased metabolic demand; hyperpnea is highly correlated with sepsis.

Pulse oximetry

Prior to the introduction of pulse oximetry, arterial oxygen saturation could be determined only by obtaining an arterial blood gas. Pulse oximetry is a continuous noninvasive measurement of arterial hemoglobin oxygen saturation using a probe on the finger or ear; the forehead and nasal septum may be sampled as well using specialized probes. The Beer-Lambert Law states that optical absorbency is proportional to the thickness of the medium and the concentration of the substance being measured. Light with red and infrared wavelengths is sequentially passed from one side of a patient's finger or ear lobe to a photodetector on the other side. Oxygenated hemoglobin absorbs more infrared light while deoxygenated hemoglobin absorbs more red light. Changing absorbance of each of the two wavelengths is measured and, based upon the changing ratio, a measure of arterial hemoglobin oxygenation can be made.

Pulse oximeters maintain reasonable accuracy down to a patient hemoglobin of 5 mg/dL, but falsely low readings occur with hypoperfusion of the extremity being evaluated, incorrect sensor application, severely calloused skin, shivering, and methemoglobinemia. Falsely high readings occur with carbon monoxide poisoning. Additionally, the pulse oximeter will record heart rate. The ECG-monitored heart rate should match that of the pulse oximeter; cardiac arrhythmias do not usually affect accuracy.

Near-infrared spectroscopy

Cohn et al (2007) showed that Near-Infrared Spectroscopy (NIRS) is a noninvasive technique, similar to pulse oximetry, of measuring peripheral muscle tissue oxygen saturation (StO$_2$). The device is applied to the patient's thenar eminence and StO$_2$ readings are generated every 4 seconds. Subsequent studies established a correlation between decreased thenar muscle StO$_2$ and hypoperfusion, and found that in trauma patients, the device can predict patients who are likely to develop multi-organ-dysfunction syndrome or die. Although further studies are needed, NIRS-derived StO$_2$ also has potential as an endpoint of resuscitation.

Capnometry/Capnography

Capnometry is a direct measure of exhaled carbon dioxide (CO$_2$). End-tidal CO$_2$ (ETCO$_2$) is commonly used to detect correct placement of an endotracheal tube using colorimetric intermittent sample devices that indicate presence or absence of CO$_2$ but do not provide quantitation. It can also be used as an in-line sidestream analyzer that provides a continuous readout of the concentration of arterial CO$_2$; confirmation of agreement between the indirect monitor and an arterial blood gas should occur. Capnometry has been well-studied in cardiac arrest patients. The absence of detectable CO$_2$ correlates closely with death and restoration of CO$_2$ generally signals the return of spontaneous circulation.

Although the absolute concentration and trend of ETCO$_2$ is useful, perhaps more useful is the analysis of the waveform by capnography, indicating changes in concentration over time. The CO$_2$ waveform can be divided into segments that represent different phases of the respiratory cycle. At the start of normal expiration, gas expelled from the anatomic dead space contains very low CO$_2$ concentrations. As more perfused alveoli empty, the increasing proportion of alveolar to dead-space gas results in greater concentrations of exhaled CO$_2$. As remaining areas with different ventilation-perfusion ratios and CO$_2$ concentrations empty, a nearly constant CO$_2$ concentration, called the alveolar plateau, is noted. When this alveolar plateau is achieved, the ETCO$_2$ closely approximates the mean alveolar concentration and the PaCO$_2$. With inspiration, the CO$_2$ concentration returns to the baseline level as there is no CO$_2$ in the inspired gas. Deviation from the normal tracing (Figure 4.2) is indicative of specific clinical conditions (Figure 4.3).

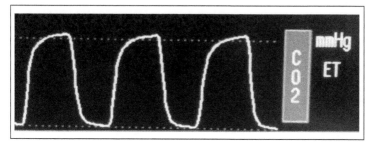

Figure 4.2 Capnography Monitor

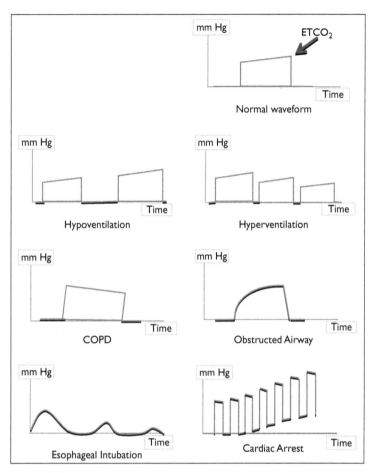

Figure 4.3 Capnography Waveforms

Although capnography was initially used for patients undergoing general anesthesia procedures, its use has broadened to include nonintubated patients undergoing sedation to identify respiratory depression and airway obstruction. Capnography is more sensitive than pulse oximetry in detecting respiratory abnormalities.

Another use of capnography is in the prehospital setting for determining appropriate endotracheal tube placement and adequacy of ventilation.

Renal

Bladder pressure

Increased intra-abdominal pressure (IAP) affects organ function in critically ill patients and may progress to abdominal compartment syndrome (ACS), defined by IAP > 20 mm Hg in the setting of an attributable organ failure. When elevated IAP reduces venous return, cardiac output is compromised, and renal hypoperfusion occurs. Renal perfusion is further decreased by increased renal vein pressure. IAP is measured by assessing intravesical (bladder) pressure. There are multiple devices to assess bladder pressure but an indwelling Foley catheter attached to a transducer apparatus is most commonly utilized. It is important to instill only 25 mL of sterile saline into the decompressed bladder prior to IAP measurement as larger volumes falsely elevate the reflected pressure.

Glucose monitoring

Patients in the ICU commonly develop hyperglycemia as a result of their baseline diabetes, stress-induced hyperglycemia, or iatrogenic hyperglycemia. Glucose variability in critically ill patients requires prompt recognition and frequent, accurate, and timely glucose measurements for appropriate insulin dosing. Concern has been raised over the optimal target glucose concentration, the accuracy of measurements, the resources required to attain tight glycemic control, and the impact of strict control across a heterogeneous ICU population. Increased variability in glucose concentrations alone, regardless of the severity of hyperglycemia, may be deleterious, perhaps because of iatrogenic hypoglycemia.

Blood glucose results vary with the measurement technique (central laboratory, arterial blood gas machine, or point of care [POC]). A major advantage of POC glucose-monitoring devices is rapid measurement using minimal blood volumes. In hemodynamically appropriate and non-critically ill patients, POC measurements correlate with laboratory reference values. In critically ill patients with poor peripheral tissue perfusion, POC measurements may vary significantly with laboratory references.

Neurologic

Electroencephalogram

Assessment of the neurologic state of a patient is ideally performed by a thorough clinical exam. Patients requiring critical care are often unable to be evaluated in this way due to sedative medications or their underlying neurologic illnesses. Electroencephalography (EEG), monitoring neuronal electrical activity at standardized points on the scalp, is one means of assessing global and focal cerebral function, particularly subclinical seizures. Continuous EEG monitoring is sometimes used to detect seizures during therapeutic hypothermia after resuscitation from cardiac arrest and for monitoring burst-suppression during barbiturate-induced coma.

Bispectral index score (BIS) monitoring, utilizing simple bifrontal electrodes, utilizes proprietary manipulation of the EEG signal to determine level of sedation and arousal. Originally designed for monitoring in the operating room to prevent recall, it can be used in the ICU, particularly when neuromuscular blockade is utilized.

Intracranial pressure monitoring

One of the most potentially catastrophic aspects of brain injury and other central neuraxial conditions is elevated intracranial pressure (ICP). The Monro-Kellie hypothesis states that the cranial compartment is incompressible, and the volume inside the cranium is therefore a fixed combination of blood, cerebral spinal fluid (CSF), and cerebral parenchyma. Any condition that increases the volume of one must be met with a decrease in at least one of the other or an increased pressure will result from the increased volume. A normal ICP is < 15 mm Hg, while multiple retrospective studies have identified ICP > 20–25 mm Hg as a predictor of poor outcomes. In fact, even transient episodes of high ICP correlate with poor outcome. Monitoring ICP allows one to adjust the cerebral perfusion pressure (CPP) by either addressing the ICP directly or by increasing mean arterial pressure (MAP). CPP is defined as MAP-ICP; normal is > 50 mm Hg. Maintenance of CPP > 60 mm Hg is similarly associated with improved outcome after traumatic brain injury (TBI).

There are multiple techniques for monitoring ICP. The gold standard is placement of an external ventricular drainage (EVD) catheter, which provides fluid coupled pressure monitoring as well as the ability to externally drain CSF to reduce ICP. A fiberoptic-tipped intraparenchymal pressure monitor is placed directly into brain tissue. This monitor only measures pressure and does not offer any therapeutic intervention to directly decrease ICP. However, this catheter does not require intraventricular placement and is therefore easier to insert and reliably use when there are small ventricles. These catheters may also be modified to provide additional data such as tissue oxygen saturation. The subdural/subarachnoid "bolt" is a device that is placed via a burr hole and screwed into the bone with a tip that resides in the subdural/subarachnoid space. This device is similar to the fiberoptic catheter in that the ventricular system does not need to be accessed.

Transcranial Doppler

Transcranial Doppler assessments (TCD) employ ultrasound to interrogate blood flow velocity in vessels supplying the cerebral parenchyma. This technique relies on the presence of an appropriate insonation window, requiring that the cranium in the region of interest is sufficiently thin to allow vascular interrogation. Alternatively, the cornea provides a clear window to the ophthalmic artery and has also been used as an alternate window. Vessels with increased velocity measurements correlate with vasospasm and decreased flow through that vascular region. TCDs may have the greatest utility following aneurismal subarachnoid hemorrhage (SAH) where vasospasm is prevalent and is a leading cause of death in patients who survive the initial insult. TCDs may provide readily repeatable assessment and trend analysis of blood flow that initiates a change in therapy. Cerebral angiography remains the gold standard for the diagnosis of cerebral vasospasm.

Jugular venous oxygen saturation

In a fashion similar to monitoring SvO_2, placement of a catheter retrograde in the internal jugular vein allows one to obtain jugular venous oxygen saturation ($SjvO_2$), which can provide information about the relationship between global cerebral oxygen supply and demand. A low $SjvO_2$ (< 55%) may indicate hypoperfusion but may also indicate cerebral hypermetabolism (increased cerebral metabolic rate for oxygen [$CMRO_2$]). Conversely, high $SjvO_2$ (>75 %) can indicate hyperemia or failure of O_2 utilization and inappropriately low $CMRO_2$. The arterial-venous O2 difference (arterial O_2 content—jugular vein O_2 content) is another parameter that can give similar information.

Near infrared spectroscopy

Near infrared spectroscopy is an evolving technology for noninvasive monitoring of cerebral blood flow. The technique of NIRS is based on the principle of light attenuation by the oxyhemoglobin, deoxyhemoglobin, and cytochrome-oxidase. Changes in the detected light levels can therefore represent changes in concentrations of these chromophores. Early experience with NIRS has shown that in patients with head injury, changes in oxyhemoglobin correlate well with changes in jugular bulb oximetry and transcranial Doppler.

Fetal monitoring

Although injuries are relatively common during pregnancy (especially the third trimester), it is rare for a gravid female to require intensive care for injury, for complications of pregnancy, or for exacerbations of comorbid conditions. Although pregnancy does not change the overall goal of hemodynamic stabilization and oxygenation, patients do have an altered physiologic state. The clinician should bear in mind that the optimal method to assure fetal health and viability is to address maternal physiologic derangements with alacrity.

Consultation with an obstetrics specialist, particularly subspecialists in maternal-fetal medicine is invaluable. The bare minimum for fetal viability is usually at 20 weeks gestation. Fetal monitoring, except for evaluation for presence of a fetal heart rate is usually not employed prior to this time point. Transabdominal fetal ultrasound provides important information about viability and potential complications of pregnancy. Once viability is confirmed, continuous external fetal monitoring includes using Doppler ultrasound to continuously interrogate the fetal heart rate (FHR) in conjunction with toco-dynamometry to assess for uterine contractions. FHR decelerations as well as the frequency and amplitude of contractions are the main aberrations for which one monitors.

Drains

Introduction

The use of drains after operative procedures is often shrouded in religion, habit, or anecdote. Clearly identified and scientifically supported indications for drain placement includes (1) removing fluid, exudates, and or gas; (2) promoting tissue apposition to facilitate wound healing and cavity collapse; (3) monitoring leakage from an internal organ; (4) diverting fluids away from a surgical site; and (5) allowing subsequent access to a cavity.

Physiology

Drain construction requires an understanding of Poiseuille's law that states that the flow (F) of fluid through a drain lumen is proportional to the suction (ΔP) applied to the drain and to the fourth power of the drain radius (r). Furthermore the flow of the fluid (F) is inversely proportional to the viscosity (n) and the length of the drain (L). For example, doubling drain diameter may increase flow by a factor of 16. Poiseuille's law is depicted below:

$$F = \Delta Pr^4/8nL$$

Gravity may be utilized as an important driving force for fluid flow. Accordingly, inserting the tip of a drainage catheter in the most dependent portion of a cavity and locating the collection container below the level of the patient improves wound drainage. Negative pressure, created either manually or from mechanically generated suction, will also facilitate flow through a drain.

Because they are foreign bodies, all drains induce some amount of tissue reaction, including inflammation, thrombosis, or fibrosis. Although this physiologic reaction is often undesired, in some circumstances it may serve a purpose, including promoting the formation of a durable tract. In general, the softer the drain, the less likely it is to create tissue erosion. Also, drain material frequently incorporates a radio-opaque strip along its length to allow localization on radiographic imaging.

Drain type

Drains may be categorized as open or closed depending on whether the system is open to the environment or not. Open drains, such as a Penrose drain, direct their effluent into a gauze pad or other wound management system using only gravity or capillary action. The wound effluent may be irritating to the skin especially if the effluent is rich in bacteria or activated proteolytic enzymes. Fluid drains through and around the Penrose, and a fibrotic tract usually forms within 7 to 10 days. However, open drains allow fluid and bacteria to travel in both directions. They do not control the odor associated with actively infected beds.

Closed drains (such as a Jackson-Pratt drain) are preferable to open drains because they are associated with lower infection rates, more accurate measurement of drainage output, and protection of surrounding skin from irritating drainage fluid. Closed drains can then be classified as either active suction or passive drainage systems, based on whether or not a negative pressure system is employed. Active suction drains allow for more effective evacuation of effluent, and promote tissue cavity collapse, at times minimizing bleeding or seroma formation. The negative pressure may also retard drain occlusion by debris. The disadvantages of active suction systems include the collapse of tissue surrounding the drain or of the drain itself that may lead to drain obstruction. High-pressure suction (i.e., wall suction) applied across the drainage system can cause tissue erosion and may increase the likelihood of persistent anastomotic leaks and continued drainage from fistulae.

Table 4.1 Commonly used drains in the intensive care unit

	Drain	Type of action	Methods of placement	Purpose
Cardiothoracic				
	Thoracostomy tube	Closed active suction	In OR—under direct visualization	Prevention or treatment of pneumothorax, pleural effusion, hemothorax, or empyema
		Water seal	Outside OR—using anatomic landmarks	
	Pleural pigtail	Closed active suction	Ultrasound guidance	Treatment of pneumothorax or serous pleural effusion
		Water seal	Using anatomic landmarks	
	Mediastinal drain	Closed active suction	In OR—under direct visualization	Prevention of mediastinal hematoma
Gastrointestinal				
	Nasogastric tube	Sump suction	Blind—confirmed by auscultation or x-ray	Aspiration of gastric contents
		Closed passive drainage		Gastric feeding
	Surgical gastrostomy	Closed intermittent active suction	In OR	Drainage of gastric contents
		Closed passive drainage		Gastric feeding
	Percutaneous gastrostomy	Closed intermittent active suction	Endoscopically (PEG)	Drainage of gastric contents
		Closed passive drainage	Fluoroscopic guidance	Gastric feeding
	Nasojejunal tube		Blind—confirmed by x-ray	Jejunal feeding
		Closed passive drainage	Magnetic direction	Decompression of obstructed small bowel
	Jejunostomy tube		In OR	Jejunal feeding

(continued)

Table 4.1 (Continued)

Drain	Type of action	Methods of placement	Purpose
	Closed passive drainage		Decompression of obstructed small bowel
T tube	Closed passive drainage	In OR	Biliary tree drainage to protect distal biliary anastomosis
Cholecystostomy tube	Closed passive drainage	Ultrasound guidance	Decompression of cholecystitis gallbladder in nonoperative patients
Neurosurgical			
External ventricular drain (EVD)	Closed passive drainage	Using anatomic landmarks based on CT	Intracranial pressure (ICP) monitor
			Drainage of CSF to reduce ICP or for sampling
Lumbar drain	Closed passive drainage	Blind using anatomic landmarks	Drainage of CSF
		Fluoroscopic guidance	
Mutipurpose			
Vacuum-Assisted Closure System (VAC)	Closed active suction	Direct visualization	Facilitation of wound granulation
			Removal of wound secretions
			Reduction of wound bacterial load
Urological			
Foley catheter	Closed passive drainage	Blind	Decompression of bladder
			Urine drainage and output monitor
Suprapubic catheter	Closed passive drainage	In OR—under direct visualization	Decompression of bladder
		Blind or ultrasound guided Seldinger technique	Urine drainage and output monitor
Nephrostomy tube	Closed passive drainage	Ultrasound guided	Decompression of obstructed ureter
		Fluoroscopic guidance	Urine drainage and output monitor

Active suction drains can then be further subdivided into closed suction or sump suction systems. Closed suction involves negative pressure applied to one end of a single lumen drain that pulls fluid into the drainage catheter and a collection canister. As the canister gradually fills with drained fluid, the negative pressure decreases until the reservoir is fully inflated to its original shape.

Sump suction drains have both a main drainage lumen as well as a small vent lumen. When suction is applied via wall suction, fluid is removed via the drainage lumen while external air enters the cavity through the vent lumen; the vent lumen typically incorporates a filter to ensure that particulate debris is not actively drawn into the cavity. Sumped external air enters the drainage lumen, eliminating negative pressure trauma to the tissue or organ surrounding the drain tip, and decreasing the risk of occlusion of the drainage lumen. To ensure proper function, the vent lumen must remain patent and open to air.

Most drains have multiple holes or channels to prevent blockage caused by tissues collapsing on the drain holes.

The pigtail catheter is a multi-purpose drain with a spiraled tip that straightens during insertion with the use of a guidewire. Once the catheter is in position, the guidewire is withdrawn and the tip is curled into position by an internal tether that is under tension. The pigtail catheter has multiple side holes for drainage generally spaced 1 cm apart from the catheter tip. Pigtail catheters may be limited by the viscosity of the fluid to be drained.

The table demonstrates the most commonly used drains in the ICU. (Table 4.1)

Key references

Abalos A, Leibowitz AB, Distefano D, Halpern N, Iberti TJ. Myocardial ischemia during the weaning process. *Am J Crit Care.* 1992;1(3):32–36.

Cohn SM, Nathens AB, Moore FA, et al. Tissue oxygen saturation predicts the development of organ dysfunction during traumatic shock resuscitation. *J Trauma.* 2007;62:44–55.

Davis JW, Davis IC, Bennink LD, Bilello JF, Kaups KL, Parks SN. Are automated blood pressure measurements accurate in trauma patients? *J Trauma.* 2003;55(5):860–863.

Frank SM, Fleisher LA, Breslow MJ, et al. Perioperative maintenance of normothermia reduces the incidence of morbid cardiac events: a randomized clinical trial. *JAMA.* 1997;277:1127–1134.

Lawson L, Bridges EJ, Ballou I, et al. Accuracy and precision of noninvasive temperature measurement in adult intensive care patients. *Am J Crit Care.* 2007;16:485–496.

Marque S, Cariou A, Chiche JD, Squara P. Comparison between Flotrac-Vigileo and Bioreactance, a totally noninvasive method for cardiac output monitoring. *Crit Care.* 2009;13(3):R73.

Shinohara T, Yamshita Y, Naito M, et al. Prospective randomized trial of a closed-suction drain versus a penrose after a colectomy. *Hepatogastroenterology.* 2010;57(102–103):1119–1122.

Squara P, Denjean D. Estagnasie P, et al. Noninvasive cardiac output monitoring (NICOM): a clinical validation. *Intensive Care Med* 2007;33(7):1191–1194.

Chapter 5

Airway management in the intensive care unit

Lillian L. Emlet

Introduction

Airway management in the Intensive Care Unit (ICU) requires a systematic, comprehensive approach to manage the anticipated and unanticipated difficulties that arise from critical illness and respiratory failure. It is similar in many ways to other emergent airway management situations in the emergency department (ED) and in-hospital cardiopulmonary arrest due to its unanticipated, emergent nature. In contrast, the situation may be different, however, due to progressively decreased cardiopulmonary physiologic reserve, anatomic difficulties, and variable injury complex of each trauma patient.

Airway management requires careful thought, taking global patient decision-making into account. These decisions include considering (1) the reason for airway management; (2) the urgency and speed of securing the airway; (3) the method used to secure the airway; (4) possible sequential alternative methods to secure the airway in the event of failure; and (5) the potential expected unintended downstream problems that may occur after securing the airway. Clear team communication is critical. Rapid, careful, well-prepared planning in airway management allows for a comprehensive plan for airway management (Figure 5.1).

Assessment of the airway and physiology

Assessment of the airway anatomy should be performed to assess for difficulty of ventilation via bag-valve-mask (BVM), difficulty of intubation via traditional laryngoscopy, difficulty of supraglottic rescue devices for intubation or ventilation, and difficulty of subglottic rescue (Table 5.1). Assessments include inspection of the mouth and oropharynx, as well as external examination of face and neck. Mallampati assessments and thyromental distance inspection allow some limited prediction of difficulty of intubation, with only moderate degrees of sensitivity and specificity. Full evaluation of the airway anatomy should be performed prior to any attempt at securing the airway. Despite the published limitations in airway assessments, quick examination of the face and airway with identification

Does the patient need to be intubated? How quickly?
Can the patient move to a safer location with backup equipment?
Is bag-valve-mask-ventilation and oxygenation adequate?

Does the patient have predictors of difficulty?
Assess for difficulty in ventilation, intubation, supraglottic rescue, and subglottic rescue
Assess for difficulty in rescue ventilation and oxygenation

What should the patient receive for analgesia, sedation, and muscle relaxation?
Predicted difficult airways, consider "awake" topical analgesia
Conscious sedation vs. full anesthesia ± muscle paralysis
Prepare for anticipated physiologic side effects

What sequence of methods will be used when failed airway attempt occurs?
Rescue bag-valve-mask-ventilation vs. rescue laryngeal mask airway
Double set-up for surgical cricothyroidotomy
Location and preparation of airway adjuncts
Pre-identify sequence of methods for failed airway

Figure 5.1 Decisions in airway management

of anatomy that predicts difficulty is necessary. Explicit, specific instructions to airway assistants (usually other members of the Trauma or ICU team, respiratory therapists, and nurses) on assessment of difficulty, plans, and backup plans early in the management allows the team to have a collective understanding of how the airway will be managed.

Assessment of physiology should be performed to assess for difficulty of oxygenation and hemodynamic tolerance for induction. Inability to preoxygenate predicts a difficult airway due to the rapidity of falling off the oxygen saturation curve. Patients who are already severely hypoxic despite significant non-invasive support will have worsening hypoxia during induction, possibly with hemodynamic compromise. Alternatively, patients with severe hemodynamic

Table 5.1 Airway assessments

Difficult Ventilation	Difficult Intubation	Difficult Supraglottic	Difficult Subglottic
Facial hair/beards	Mallampati score	Restricted mouth opening	Short thick neck
Disrupted facial anatomy-trauma	Disrupted facial anatomy-trauma	Disrupted facial anatomy-trauma	Prior radiation and surgical dissection
Angioedema	Angioedema	Disrupted larynx	Coagulopathy
Ludwig's angina	Ludwig's angina	Pulmonary fibrosis	Disrupted larynx
Pharyngeal abscesses	Congenital abnormalities	ARDS	Laryngeal tumors
Age	Retrognathic mandible	Oropharyngeal bleeding	Neck abscesses
Edentulous			Expanding hematoma
Pulmonary fibrosis			Disrupted anatomy
ARDS			Subcutaneous emphysema
Abdominal compartment syndrome			Obesity

ARDS = acute respiratory distress syndrome

compromise (e.g., hypovolemia on one hand or right ventricular heart failure or pulmonary hypertension on the other) do poorly with induction, with significant risk for cardiac arrest. Both situations require careful attention to first-pass intubation success with simultaneous preparation and administration of medications to prevent cardiovascular compromise.

In trauma patients, the mechanism of injury is an important component of airway assessment, because each injury can contribute to difficulties or special considerations for management. Most injuries worsen with tissue edema and swelling over the ensuing 48 hours. This may be one more factor to consider regarding timing to secure the airway to facilitate trauma workup, plan operative management, and orchestrate care of the multiply injured patients.

Airway management in the emergency department or trauma resuscitation room

Rapid sequence induction (RSI) remains the cornerstone of airway management in the ED, given that all patients are assumed to have a full stomach at the time of injury. Even with the multiply injured patient, rapid securing of the airway on the first pass with little to no desaturation is the ideal management strategy. Assessment for first-pass success usually entails RSI. There are, however, situations where awake tracheostomy or cricothyrotomy is indicated. Most patients are presumed to have potential for cervical spine injury and are immobilized, making jaw thrust extremely important in rescue mask ventilation and direct laryngoscopy more difficult due to inability to move the neck from the neutral position. In addition, cervical collar immobilization can limit mouth opening. Although all airway manipulations have been shown to cause some movement (1–3 mm movement and 2°–5° angulation) of the cervical spine in cadaver spine injury models, it is unclear what clinical significance this may have. Generally, rigid indirect and video laryngoscopes have less cervical spine motion but take greater time to achieve endotracheal intubation. Secretions or blood in the airway further limit the utility of these devices.

Airway management in the trauma intensive care unit

Although most airways are secured early in the evaluation of the trauma patient, some patients decompensate later in the natural course of injury and require intubation in the ICU. Swelling from tissue injury and patient-specific physiologic status will determine the likelihood of requiring airway and respiratory support for each injury. The natural course of each injury may require adequate access to the airway to assess for injury and provide pulmonary support. Secondary complications, such as sepsis or pulmonary embolism, may also necessitate intubation in the ICU. Generally, at this point, the patient's cardiopulmonary physiology has less reserve, as further physiologic deterioration has occurred, including malnutrition, atelectasis, and nosocomial infection. Early prediction and continuous assessment of the clinical course in the ICU is necessary to time airway management, prevent secondary injury, and time operative management.

Facial trauma

Facial trauma can distort anatomy such that BVM and orotracheal intubation become impossible, elevating the surgical airway into the primary mode for securing the airway. Early airway management is of paramount importance in facial trauma, with consideration of potential concomitant cervical spine or brain injury. Hutchison et al (1990) described six injury patterns that may be highly associated with airway compromise:

1. Inferoposterior displacement of the maxilla in parallel to the skull base, obstructing the nasopharynx
2. Bilateral anterior mandible fracture obstructing the oropharynx
3. Fractured teeth, bones, blood, or debris obstructing the upper aerodigestive tract
4. Soft-tissue swelling and edema
5. Hemorrhage from face, nose, wounds obstructing the airway
6. Swelling and displacement of larynx and trachea (with associated structures of arytenoid cartilage and vocal cords) from direct trauma

Blunt trauma to the face, such as unstable midface LeFort IV fractures, can present with patent airways with variable amount of blood in the oropharynx. These airways can usually still be secured early with RSI and direct laryngoscopy for potential airway compromise to facilitate trauma workup and eventual surgical fixation. Severe blunt trauma and penetrating trauma to the bony and soft tissue of the face, particularly to the mouth and oropharynx can make RSI and orotracheal access impossible. Surgical cricothyroidotomy is typically the backup procedure when laryngoscopy fails. In some circumstances, however, awake tracheostomy or surgical cricothyroidotomy is a better first choice than direct laryngoscopy, particularly when the injury complex precludes BVM. Videolaryngoscopes and fiberoptic bronchoscopes have limited utility in airways with significant bleeding and direct oropharyngeal trauma.

Significant facial injury can be associated with brain and cervical spine injury, requiring early airway stabilization to facilitate safe injury diagnosis, transport, resuscitation, and repair. Associated brain, cervical spine, or pulmonary injuries may also affect the modality and sedation used during airway management.

Neck trauma

Subcutaneous emphysema of the neck is an important finding, suggestive of laryngeal or tracheal trauma, or significant pulmonary and thoracic trauma.

Signs of laryngeal trauma also include pain, ecchymosis across the anterior neck, hoarseness or stridor, although subcutaneous emphysema is the primary clinical sign. Examination of the neck can be limited by temporary cervical spine immobilization, but early palpation of the thorax, face, and neck is necessary. Depending upon the urgency of the patient's other injuries, awake (or semiawake) orotracheal intubation via videolaryngoscopy versus awake fiberoptic intubation are the primary modalities to secure the airway. Topicalization of the airway with viscous lidocaine or cetacaine spray, followed by minimal conscious sedation with small doses of propofol or midazolam is preferred. With the advent of video laryngoscopes, improved visualization of distorted anatomy makes it the clear method of choice for practitioners who do not perform frequent awake fiberoptic intubations. In the hands of a skilled provider with adequate topical anesthesia, fiberoptic intubations may allow greater flexibility to traverse significant injury, although both methods are limited by the quantity of secretions or brisk bleeding in the hypopharynx.

Cervical spine trauma

Patients with cervical spine injuries often have other injuries. Although 2%–10% of patients with traumatic brain injury have cervical spine injuries, 25%–50% of patients with cervical spine injuries have associated brain injury. Both hypoxia and hypotension are unwanted events in management of these patients. Approximately 0.9%–3% of blunt-trauma patients have cervical spine injury. The most common level of injury is C2, followed by C6 and C7, most commonly injuring the vertebral body.

Securing the airway of trauma patients with unstable cervical spine injuries may be best managed by topical anesthesia and awake fiberoptic intubation. Although most trauma patients immobilized with cervical collars are assumed to have possible cervical spine injury, usually these airways are secured with direct laryngoscopy with RSI and cervical spine immobilization. There is variability in the amount of movement in the cervical spine even with immobilization and manual in-line stabilization. The advent of videolaryngoscopy allows the advantages of direct laryngoscopy with minimal distraction of the cervical spine, as the angulation and field of view is widened by 60°–80°. In patients with spinal cord injury, attention to hemodynamics is important to prevent secondary injury in preparation for urgent fixation and stabilization.

Thoracic trauma

Blunt thoracic trauma results in a wide range of injuries, including rib fractures, pneumothorax, hemothorax, pulmonary contusions, mediastinal injuries (pneumomediastinum, esophageal injury, and hematomas), thoracic spine fractures with and without cord injury, cardiac contusions, cardiac tamponade, and blunt aortic injury. The majority of these injuries result in respiratory insufficiency of variable severity. Some patients may respond to temporary noninvasive ventilatory support until treatment can be initiated (thoracostomy tube, epidural or paravertebral blocks, early operative fixation to allow mobilization). However, multiple rib fractures with flail segments and pulmonary contusions generally will require endotracheal intubation and mechanical ventilation. Early consideration of injury trajectory allows for placement of properly sized tubes, assessment of pneumonia, and appropriate ventilator support.

Pulmonary contusions, flail chest, rib fractures, hemopneumothoraces, and sternal fractures all cause structural chest-wall dysfunction and impaired pulmonary function. Cardiac contusions and tamponade can exhibit hemodynamic compromise. The goal of airway management in the ICU is to provide adequate time for recovery and prevent secondary injury, notably pneumonia. Devitalized tissue and chest wall mechanics contribute to a high rate of pneumonia and a need for early tracheostomy in this population of trauma patients.

Thermal trauma

The need for early management of the airway in burn patients has long been recognized, given the wide range of presentations of inhalational injury and continued evolution of airway and pulmonary injury for up to 72 hours. Inhalational injury is caused by direct thermal injury, systemic effects from reduced oxygenation, inhalation of toxins (e.g., carbon monoxide and hydrogen cyanide), tracheobronchial damage from inhaled smoke particulates, deeper lung parenchyma injury, and systemic inflammatory response. All of these can affect airway management. Early placement of appropriately sized endotracheal tubes is usually performed in the ED. Peak edema occurs at 24 hours and resolves over the next few days.

Equipment preparation

Equipment should be prepared and checked prior to induction. Basic equipment includes oxygen source, suction source, pulse oximetry, cardiac monitoring, endotracheal tube with stylet, and laryngoscope handle and blade (Table 5.2). If using video laryngoscope or flexible bronchoscopy, power, fiberoptics, and image quality should be checked. Backup equipment and devices should be readily accessible in or immediately outside the patient's room. Everyone involved should be aware of their locations around the patient. Dosages of drugs for induction should be drawn up ahead of time (Table 5.3). Closed-loop communication prior to administration is critical to prevent premature induction. Vasopressors such as phenylephrine are useful to have prepared prior to induction, because ablation of the sympathetic drive of work of breathing often causes transient hypotension immediately postintubation that resolves as induction agents wear

Table 5.2 Airway equipment	
Routine Airway Equipment	**Difficult Airway Equipment**
Endotracheal tubes (6.0, 7.0, 7.5, 8.0)	Videolaryngoscope
10 cc slip-tip syringe (2)	Intubating laryngeal mask airway
End tidal CO_2 detector	Flexible fiberoptic bronchoscope
Endotracheal tube holder device	Transtracheal jet ventilation equipment
Endotracheal tube stylet	Berman airway
Intubating stylet (gum elastic bougie)	Cetacaine (benzocaine) spray
Lubricant	Lidocaine preparations (2%, 4%)
Laryngoscope handle	Phenylephrine nasal spray
Batteries for handle (if not rechargeable)	Tongue depressors
Mac & Miller # 3 & #4 laryngoscope blades	Magill forceps
Laryngeal mask airway	Scalpel
Oral airway	
Nasal airway	
Magill forceps	
Scalpel	
Suction device	

off. Predefined mechanisms to activate backup assistance (i.e., equipment and personnel) are important to prevent disastrous complications.

Airway methods and techniques

Several other comprehensive textbooks describe the methods used to secure the airway, and limitations of space preclude a comprehensive description here (Table 5.4). Familiarity with each device as well as understanding of the limitations and advantages each device are important. Routine practice with all devices during intubations that are expected to be easy is important to develop technical skill and expertise. All airways should be approached as though the initial attempt with RSI will fail, therefore warranting preparation for use of a secondary airway device. Care should always be taken, time and clinical situation permitting, for the most optimized first attempt at orotracheal intubation, with specific attention to positioning and preparation of additional equipment, medications, and assistants.

Management of the difficult and failed airway

Discussion of difficult airways can be divided into the predicted and the unanticipated difficult airway. This can be further divided into difficult ventilation, difficult intubation, difficult supraglottic rescue, and difficult subglottic rescue. Predictors of difficult bag-valve-mask ventilation include problems with mask

Table 5.3 Airway medications

Agent	Dose	Onset	Duration	Considerations
Premedication				
Fentanyl	1–3 mcg/kg IV	2–3 min	30–60 min	To blunt sympathetic response & ICP
Midazolam	1–2 mg	60–90 sec	30 min	Adjunct sedative amnestic for conscious sedation
Lidocaine	1.5 mg/kg IV	45–90 sec	2 h	To blunt ICP increase & bronchospasm in asthma,
				Note: all can cause worsened shock state
Induction				
Etomidate	0.3 mg/kg IV	14–45 sec	3–12 min	Myoclonus side effect, temporary cortisol suppression, hemodynamic stability
Ketamine	1.5 mg/kg IV	45–60 sec	10–20 min	Hemodynamic stability, preserved respiratory drive
Propofol	1.5 mg/kg IV	15–45 sec	5–10 min	Hypotension
Thiopental	3 mg/kg IV	< 30 sec	5–10 min	Ultrashort-acting, vasodilator, reduced dose
Dexmedetomidine	1 mcg/kg IV, followed by 0.4–0.7 mcg/kg/hr gtt	10 min	10–15 min	α2 receptors locus ceruleus, hypotension, bradycardia, preserved respiratory drive, slow-loading dose
Neuromuscular Blocking Agents				
Succinylcholine	1.5 mg/kg IV	45 sec	6–10 min	Depolarizing, caution hyperkalemia, rhabdomyolysis, neuromuscular disorders beyond 5 days, malignant hyperthermia
Rocuronium	1–1.2 mg/kg IV	60 sec	60 min	Approximates RSI conditions when correctly dosed, non-depolarizing
Vecuronium	0.15 mg/kg IV	90 sec	60 min	Non-depolarizing
Cisatracurium	0.1 mg/kg IV	7 min	60 min	Non-depolarizing, Hoffman degradation independent of liver or renal dysfunction
Vasopressor				
Phenylephrine	80 mcg/mL IV	2–5 min	15 min	Postsynaptic α1 agonist

ICP = intracranial pressure, RSI = rapid sequence induction

Table 5.4 Airway techniques

Device/Method	Pearls	Considerations
Laryngeal Mask Airway (LMA, I-LMA, iGel, AirQ)	Convert to a situation of "can ventilate, can't intubate." Requires practice but quick to insert. Advance LMA against hard palate until resistance. Convert to fiberoptic intubation through intubating LMA.	Will not work for postextubation stridor and severe upper airway obstruction. Will not work if unable to open mouth or in pharyngeal disruption. Will not work in ARDS or peak pressures > 20 cm H2O. Watch for folding over of LMA with inadequate seal; deflate and reinflate.
Videolaryngoscopes (Glidescope, C-MAC, Pentax)	Improves visualization for anterior airways. Allows videorecording for quality and teaching. Useful for predicted difficult airways or cervical spine injury.	Copious bleeding in oropharynx and airway will not allow visualization. Will not work if unable to open mouth. Watch technique and force used to prevent pharyngeal and laryngeal trauma.
Fiberoptic Bronchoscopes	Able to maneuver around sharp difficult angles of patient anatomy. Requires practice and skill. Awake or minimal sedation, otherwise may need assistant. Not a quick procedure, usually upwards of 20 minutes.	Requires time for anesthesia and cooperative patient. Copious bleeding in oropharynx and airway will not allow visualization. Not indicated for emergent intubations. Use assistant for gentle jaw thrust to improve difficult visualization. Spray-as-you-go technique to provide adequate anesthesia.

(continued)

Table 5.4 (Continued)

Device/Method	Pearls	Considerations
Rigid Fiberoptic Scopes (Levitan, Shikani, Bonfils, Bullard)	Improves visualization for anterior airways. Requires practice for visualization through eyepiece rather than video screen.	Useful for extremely small mouth openings. Copious bleeding in oropharynx and airway will not allow visualization.
Intubating stylets (Gum Elastic Bougie, Eschmann, Frova)	Keep laryngoscope blade in mouth during placement, which is by feel on angulated tip. Tracheal rings may not be felt occasionally even during correct placement. Useful for anterior airways and to assist cricothyrotomy.	Can cause tracheal tears if placement too vigorous. Not completely reliable.

Excludes Blind orotracheal or nasotracheal intubation, Optical stylets, Retrograde intubation, Mirror/Prism blade/scopes, and surgical cricothyrotomy

ARDS = acute respiratory distress syndrome

seal, obesity, upper airway obstruction, age, edentulous mouth, and restrictive lung pathology. Predictors of difficult intubation have traditionally been assessed through the 3-3-2 rule for assessment of thyromental and mentohyoid distances, Mallampati, obstruction, and neck mobility. Predictors of supraglottic rescue include restricted mouth opening, upper airway obstruction, disrupted anatomy, and neck mobility. Predictors of difficult subglottic rescue include prior neck surgery, coagulopathy, obesity, tumors, and anatomic deformities.

When an initial intubation attempt has failed, the primary rescue is bag-valve-mask ventilation. The primary assessment in managing the difficult and failed airway is determining whether ventilation is successful. The ability to ventilate is of paramount importance in airway management. The rescue device to achieve adequate ventilation in the prehospital world remains the King LTD airway, while in the inpatient and ICU setting, a variety of intubating laryngeal mask airways remain the preferred devices to stabilize ventilation. In rescue of the difficult intubation, achieving adequate ventilation allows time to secure a surgical airway under controlled fashion or rescue with an alternative supraglottic method.

Extubation difficulties

Extubating the trauma patient requires some consideration of postextubation stridor and difficulty of potential need for reintubation, depending on the difficulty of initial intubation and reason for intubation. Significant thoracic trauma, neurologic compromise, and repeated abdominal or orthopedic surgical procedures can often be better managed through early tracheostomy. In those patients for whom extubation is indicated, there are limitations in determining postextubation stridor with the cuff-leak test. Sensitivity and specificity of the cuff-leak test range from 75% to 100%. Additional considerations for predicting extubation difficulties also include secretion volume, neurological arousal, and ventilatory support. Proper technique for performing a cuff-leak test includes placing the patient on a controlled mode of ventilation (AC volume cycle, AC pressure control), deflating the endotracheal tube cuff, and measuring the loss in exhaled tidal volume. A loss in tidal volume of only 10% or 110 cc absolute value suggests a higher possibility of postextubation stridor.

Careful extubation requires having multiple contingency plans for resecuring the airway and clear communication to the entire ICU team (nurses, respiratory therapists, intensivists, and surgeons, if needed). Extubation can be performed over endotracheal tube exchanger for a brief trial if there is concern for vocal cord or supraglottic edema in the immediate extubation phase. Treatments for immediate postextubation stridor include racemic epinephrine and, occasionally, closely monitored noninvasive positive-pressure ventilation. Most commonly, postextubation stridor requires a low threshold for reintubation with consideration for requiring a smaller size endotracheal tube. Awake fiberoptic intubation may be a safe approach in this circumstance.

Summary

Airway management in the multiply injured patient requires assessment of airway anatomy with consideration of difficulty in mask ventilation, intubation, supraglottic rescue, and surgical airway. Critical decision points remain the urgency in securing the airway, physiologic reserve, personnel and equipment availability, and contingency plans for airway complications. Airway management should be tailored to each individual trauma patient with unique combinations of injuries.

Key references

Crosby ET. Airway management in adults after cervical spine trauma. *Anesthesiology.* 2006;104(6):1293–1318.

Hagberg CA. *Benumof's Airway Management.* 2nd ed. Mosby; Philadelphia, PA, 2007.

Hutchison I, Lawlor M, Skinner D. (1990). ABC of major trauma. Major maxillofacial injuries. *BMJ.*1990;301(6752): 595–599.

Jaber S, Chanques G, Matecki S, et al. Post-extubation stridor in intensive care unit patients. *Intensive Care Med.* 2003;29:69–74.

Niforopoulou P, Pantazopoulos I, Demestiha T, Koudouna E, Xanthos T. Video-laryngoscopes in the adult airway management: a topical review of the literature. *Acta Anaesthesiologica Scandinavica.*2010;54(9):1050–1061.

Orebaugh SL, Bigeleisen PE. *Atlas of Airway Management Techniques and Tools.* 2nd ed. Lippincott Williams & Wilkins; Philadephia, PA, 2012.

Sandhu RS, Pasquale M D, Miller K, Wasser TE. (2000). Measurement of endotracheal tube cuff leak to predict post-extubation stridor and need for reintubation. *ACS.* 2000;190(6):682–687.

Turner CR, Block J, Shanks A, Morris M, Lodhia KR, Gujar SK. (2009). Motion of a cadaver model of cervical injury during endotracheal intubation with a Bullard laryngoscope or a Macintosh blade with and without In-line stabilization. *J Trauma.* 2009;67(1):61–66.

Verschuren D, Bell R, Bagheri S, Dierks E, Potter B. Management of laryngo-tracheal injuries associated with craniomaxillofacial trauma. *J Oral Maxillofac Surg.* 2006;64(2):203–214.

Walls R, Murphy M. *Manual of Emergency Airway Management.* 4th ed. Lippincott Williams & Wilkins; Philadelphia, PA, 2012.

Chapter 6

Resuscitation from hemorrhagic shock

Benjamin R. Reynolds and Gregory A. Watson

Introduction

Shock from massive hemorrhage can be one of the most difficult, yet reward-ing, problems to manage in the intensive care unit (ICU). Severe hemorrhagic shock and the resulting "lethal triad" of coagulopathy, hypothermia, and acidosis are associated with a very high morbidity and mortality. Achieving a good out-come requires prompt recognition of hemorrhage and institution of measures to stop bleeding, as well as timely resuscitation and reversal of coagulopathy, hypothermia, and acidosis. This mandates a team approach with involvement of surgeons, intensivists, nursing staff, the blood bank, and laboratory person-nel. In this chapter, we will differentiate hemorrhagic from other types of shock and describe its pathophysiology. Treatment will be emphasized, utilizing the extreme example of "damage control" to guide the discussion.

Definition and classification of shock

Simply stated, shock is defined as tissue oxygenation that is inadequate to maintain normal cellular structure and function. Shock may result from a vari-ety of causes, commonly classified on the basis of its etiology as hypovolemic, cardiogenic, obstructive, distributive, or traumatic (see Table 6.1).

Hypovolemic shock results from a diminished circulating volume of red blood cells, plasma, and/or extracellular fluid. This is the most common cause of shock in trauma patients and is responsible for 50% of deaths in the first 24 hours fol-lowing injury. Almost invariably this results from acute blood loss. Cardiogenic shock may result from direct cardiac injury (contusion) or intrinsic cardiac dis-ease (myocardial infarction). Obstructive shock occurs when cardiac function is compromised from either direct compression (cardiac tamponade) or impair-ment of venous return (tension pneumothorax). Distributive shock leads to decreased vascular resistance and may be the result of a high spinal cord injury (neurogenic) or infection (septic). Traumatic shock includes elements of some or all of the above-mentioned causes, which may not in isolation lead to impaired

Table 6.1 Types of shock

	Hypovolemic	Cardiogenic	Obstructive	Distributive	Traumatic
Neck veins	Flat	Distended	Distended	Flat	Flat
Skin	Clammy	Clammy	Clammy	Warm or cold	Clammy
Pulse	Fast	Fast	Fast	Fast or Normal/low	Variable
Response to volume	Rapid	Little to none	Little	Little	Moderate

tissue perfusion, but when combined can result in shock. For example, a patient suffering blunt trauma with a minor splenic laceration, tension pneumothorax, and an open femur fracture may have elements of hypovolemic (splenic laceration), obstructive (tension pneumothorax), and vasogenic (femur fracture resulting in inflammatory cytokine release) shock.

Pathophysiology

The body's response to hemorrhagic shock and injury is to preserve organ blood flow and maintain homeostasis as much as possible and, if the hypovolemia is severe, preferentially preserve flow to the vital organs (heart and brain). This response involves a complex interplay of numerous neurohumoral mediators involving nearly every organ system in the body. A thorough discussion is beyond the scope of this chapter, but the major effects are highlighted below.

Hemorrhage results in intravascular hypovolemia, activating baroreceptors in the aorta and carotid bodies as well as stretch receptors in the atria triggering the sympathoadrenal axis and the hypothalamic-pituitary-adrenal (HPA) axis. Catecholamine release resulting from sympathetic nervous system and adrenal activation results in an immediate increase in blood pressure (peripheral vasoconstriction), heart rate, myocardial contractility, and minute ventilation. As the shock state progresses, metabolic acidosis and hypothermia develop, which stimulate chemoreceptors in the carotid bodies and aorta further augmenting the responses of the sympathoadrenal and HPA axes. Catecholamines, in addition to their cardiovascular effects, also alter metabolic pathways leading to increased glucose availability.

Other important mediators include vasopressin (antidiuretic hormone), the renin-angiotensin-aldosterone system, and numerous other hormones. Vasopressin is released from the posterior pituitary in response to increased plasma osmolality and decreased circulating plasma volume. It increases peripheral vasoconstriction and enhances renal water resorption. It also has metabolic effects geared toward increasing glucose availability.

Decreased renal arterial blood flow (from hemorrhage) and increased β-adrenergic stimulation activate the juxtaglomerular cells of the renal afferent arteriole, which release renin. Renin, in turn, converts angiotensinogen to angiotensin I (in the liver) and ultimately angiotensin II (in the lung). Angiotensin II leads to aldosterone release from the adrenal, which has the net effects of enhancing renal distal tubular sodium and chloride (and hence water) resorption. In addition, angiotensin II itself is a potent peripheral and splanchnic vasoconstrictor. Other important hormones involved in the stress/shock response include corticotrophin, thyroxine, growth hormone, insulin, and glucagon. Each has varying effects on metabolic pathways that enhance substrate availability.

In addition to the neurohormonal responses outlined above, a number of immunologic and inflammatory mediators are released after injury and shock, which have both local and systemic effects. These include complement, cytokines (tumor necrosis factor, interleukins, and interferons), oxygen radicals, eicosanoids (prostaglandins, thromboxanes, and leukotrienes), nitric oxide, and others. In general, these compounds induce a proinflammatory state that may vary widely in its degree and severity. When excessive, terminal shock, acute respiratory distress syndrome, and multiple organ dysfunction syndrome may result. Though discussed separately, it is important to note that the neural, hormonal, and immune responses are intimately related via redundancy and cross-talk.

At the cellular level, shock and hypoperfusion lead to decreased oxygen delivery resulting in oxygen debt. The magnitude of the oxygen debt correlates with the severity and the duration of the shock state; the magnitude of the oxygen debt, its rate of accumulation, and the time taken to correct it correlate with survival. With oxygen deprivation, cells switch to anaerobic respiration. As a result, energy (ATP) production drops, lactate levels rise, and intracellular acidosis ensues. As pH decreases, the oxygen-hemoglobin dissociation curve is shifted farther to the right reflecting decreased affinity for oxygen. This results in an increased extraction of oxygen by the tissues. The combination of decreased energy availability and worsening intracellular acidosis causes alterations in cellular metabolism, enzymatic function, ion transport, and gene expression, and may ultimately lead to cellular death. Unchecked, cellular acidosis eventually becomes systemic acidosis.

Oxygen debt is difficult to determine clinically. Similarly, the commonly obtained parameters of heart rate, blood pressure, cardiac output, urine output, and central venous pressure (CVP) are poor surrogates for the adequacy of tissue perfusion. Clinically, the serum lactate and base deficit have been the most useful indicators of the degree of oxygen debt (and hence shock) and have been useful for monitoring the response to resuscitation. Elevation of both serum lactate levels and base deficit have been shown in animal models and human studies to correlate with increased mortality; failure to clear lactate within 24 hours has been associated with mortality as high as 85%.

Decompensated shock develops when these compensatory mechanisms fail, resulting in hypotension and concomitant end-organ dysfunction. If decompensated shock is not rapidly reversed, oxygen delivery to the heart becomes critically low, eventually resulting in cardiac arrest. Short of that, ongoing inadequate resuscitation may result in renal failure, liver failure, and respiratory failure. Severe hemorrhage and resuscitation, in addition to resulting in loss of blood and development of coagulopathy and metabolic acidosis, leads to hypothermia. The risk of hypothermia may be further increased by efforts to control the hemorrhage, namely the opening of body cavities in the operating room (OR). These three factors; coagulopathy, acidosis, and hypothermia are classically referred to as the "lethal triad" and are the main components of the "bloody vicious cycle." This cycle must be recognized early and efforts to reverse it must be swift. A "damage control" approach may be warranted (discussed further below).

Diagnosis and severity assessment

Signs of shock vary depending on the severity. Tachycardia, diminished urine output, decreased pulse pressure, altered mental status, and cool clammy extremities may variably be present. Hypotension is a relatively late manifestation of shock; its absence does not mean that shock is not present. However, a hypotensive patient should always be considered to be in shock. Differentiation of hemorrhagic from other types of shock is important because treatment will vary depending upon the type of shock. Hemorrhage must always be part of the differential diagnosis in any trauma patient who presents with acute shock physiology. The severity of shock depends not only upon the degree of blood loss but also the duration of the shock state. Prolonged duration of a mild degree of shock can be just as harmful as major blood loss. Prompt recognition and treatment are paramount to achieve a good outcome, as the more severe the shock state the greater the difficulty with treating it. The degree of shock may be quantified by the amount of blood lost, as depicted in Table 6.2.

Table 6.2 Classes of hemorrhagic shock

	Class I	Class II	Class III	Class IV
Blood lost (mL)	750	750–1500	1500–2000	> 2000
% of circulating blood volume	15%	15%–30%	30%–40%	> 40%
Pulse	< 100	100–120	120–140	> 140
Blood pressure	Normal	Normal	Decreased	Decreased
Pulse pressure	Normal or increased	Decreased	Decreased	Decreased
Respiratory rate	14–20	20–30	30–40	> 35
Urine output	Normal	Slightly decreased	Oliguria	Anuria
Skin appearance	Warm	Cool	Cool, pale	Cold, mottled, cyanotic
Thirst	None	None	Moderate	Severe
Mental status	Slight anxiety	Mild anxiety	Anxious, confused	Lethargic, obtunded

Low blood pressure and tachycardia are strongly associated with the degree of shock but may be confounded by underlying preexisting illness, age, pain, or medications. Antecedent beta blocker and calcium channel blocker use, for example, can blunt reflex tachycardia. Even with severe blood loss, children and young adults may display near-normal vital signs (sometimes referred to as "compensated" shock) then become unstable with little to no warning. Ongoing anticoagulant use (warfarin, aspirin, or clopidogrel) even in the presence of a normally mild injury inactivates the normal clotting cascade, potentiating hemorrhage. Furthermore, patients with preexisting cardiovascular disease can have diminished compensatory mechanisms and may be difficult to resuscitate and manage.

As a rule, laboratory testing is a helpful adjunct to diagnosing hemorrhagic shock, but is not a replacement for the physical examination. Obtaining results of these tests should not delay treatment. As mentioned earlier, biochemical markers of hemorrhagic shock include lactate and base deficit. Hemoglobin and hematocrit are unreliable indicators of early hemorrhage because of volume contraction and lack of time for the resultant shifts in body fluid compartments, but their trend is helpful as resuscitation goes forward. Also important is the measurement of baseline coagulation factors including prothrombin time, international normalized ratio (INR), partial thromboplastin time, fibrinogen levels, and platelet count,. These tests not only help identify medication-induced coagulopathy, but they may also identify acute traumatic coagulopathy. More recently, thromboelastography (TEG) has been used to identify coagulopathy and guide its correction. This rapid, point-of-care test has the advantage of measuring the entire coagulation cascade, including fibrinolysis. Four values are analyzed; the reaction time or "R" value is the amount of time from initiation of the test until the first clot forms. The "K" value is time from beginning of clot formation until the amplitude of thromboelastogram reaches 20 mm. The alpha angle is representative of the kinetics or acceleration of fibrin buildup and crosslinking. The maximum amplitutide or "MA" value represents the strength of the clot. The "MA 60" reflects the strength of the clot after 60 minutes. Increasingly, TEG is being utilized to guide goal-directed hemostatic resuscitation.

Treatment

Treatment begins at the time of recognition, often before a diagnosis has been established. As with all acutely ill patients, evaluation and management should begin with the ABCs. In the case of hemorrhagic shock, once the airway and breathing have been addressed, the clinician's goals are quite simple: (1) arrest ongoing hemorrhage; (2) restore intravascular volume; and (3) correct hypothermia, acidosis, and coagulopathy.

In the case of trauma (either blunt or penetrating), the search for the source is very standardized (per Advanced Trauma Life Support protocol) and involves an assessment of five main areas: (1) chest; (2) abdomen; (3) retroperitoneum/pelvis; (4) long bones (femur) or significant soft tissue trauma; and (5) external. Methods to control hemorrhage vary depending upon the specific site of bleeding, but almost always include operative or angiographic/endovascular intervention, or a combination of these.

From the intensivist's perspective, the focus should be on resuscitation of the patient and monitoring for ongoing bleeding and complications following initial hemorrhage control. The most challenging cases are those that involve a damage control approach, though these represent a small fraction, perhaps 3%–5%, of the injured population.

Damage-control surgery and resuscitation describes the process by which a critically ill patient undergoes initial surgery and/or angiographic/endoscopic intervention(s) aimed at controlling hemorrhage and contamination (phase I), followed by resuscitation in the ICU (phase II), and ultimately by definitive repair of injuries once the patient's physiology has been corrected (phase III). Key tenets of this approach include permissive hypotension until hemostasis has been achieved, preferential use of blood and blood products over isotonic fluids, and prevention/correction of the "lethal triad" (coagulopathy, hypothermia, and acidosis). Ideally, this process is initiated in the emergency room and continued through the OR and into the ICU.

The goal of permissive hypotension is to achieve a blood pressure adequate enough to maintain organ perfusion while not disrupting hemostasis prior to surgical control. There is no "magic number" though most authors suggest a systolic pressure in the 80s is acceptable. Definitive studies of permissive hypotension are lacking, however. Permissive hypotension should not be utilized once hemorrhage control has been attained and the patient has arrived in the ICU.

In theory, the best resuscitative fluid for the bleeding patient is blood, specifically fresh whole blood. It contains a hematocrit of 38%–50%, 150 k–400 k platelets, 1500 mg fibrinogen, and 100% coagulation activity. It has been used extensively in specialized situations (namely the military). For logistical reasons of blood banking, fresh whole blood is not readily available in the civilian setting. Packed red blood cells (pRBCs) remain the mainstay of transfusion therapy. Each unit has a shelf life of around 40 days. Unlike fresh whole blood, it lacks platelets and coagulation factors. In addition, it is stored cold. Ideally, type-specific blood will be available, but it takes time to perform a crossmatch. For a patient in extremis, uncrossmatched blood should be used.

Any coagulopathy should be treated as needed with fresh frozen plasma (FFP), platelets (PLTs), or cryoprecipitate. Fresh frozen plasma, once thawed, is available for immediate use. However, the process of thawing takes about 30 minutes; consequently, an increasing number of busy centers are keeping limited quantities of thawed plasma available for emergent use. Each bag contains 200 mL and maintains 100% clotting activity for about 24 hours (although many centers will use it for up to 5 days after thawing). Platelets are available as either pooled, random-donor platelets (4–6 units) or single-donor apheresis platelets.

Each unit is expected to result in an increase in the platelet count of about 20,000 and has a shelf life of about 5 days.

For patients who require a massive transfusion (> 10 units pRBCs/24 hrs), administration of blood, FFP, and PLTs in a 1:1:1 ratio seems to be beneficial in terms of improved survival, reduction in organ failure, decreased crystalloid and component use, and lower costs. The optimal ratio of product administration continues to be debated, yet increasing numbers of centers have developed their own massive transfusion protocols. Identification of patients at risk for massive transfusion remains challenging.

Although crystalloids have traditionally been administered liberally to patients with severe hemorrhagic shock, large amounts of crystalloids seem to mainly contribute to tissue edema. There is no indication for the use of hypertonic fluids or colloids during hemorrhagic shock resuscitation. Thus the mainstay of fluid resuscitation for these patients should be blood products.

In addition to volume resuscitation, other adjuncts are available that may be helpful in the exsanguinating patient. Recombinant activated factor VII is a procoagulant that is believed to function through activation of factor X, stimulating the common coagulation pathway and culminating in fibrin plug generation. The drug appears to be safe for use in trauma patients and has been shown to reduce transfusion requirements, particularly in victims of blunt trauma. However, it has been difficult to demonstrate a clear survival benefit and initial enthusiasm for its use has been tempered somewhat, in part because of excessive costs. Tranexamic acid (TXA) is an antifibrinolytic agent that has recently been shown to reduce overall mortality and the risk of death from hemorrhage in trauma patients. It is administered as a 1 gram dose and is most beneficial when given within the first 3 hours following injury. A second 1 gram dose should be infused over the next 8 hours. Cryoprecipitate is rich in fibrinogen, von-Willebrand factor, factors VIII and XIII, and fibronectin. Currently there is no consensus on whether or not it is beneficial to include cryoprecipitate in a massive transfusion protocol, but most clinicians support its administration if fibrinogen levels are below 100 mg/dL and the patient is bleeding.

Once the patient arrives in the ICU, it is important for the intensivist to gather detailed information from the surgical and anesthesia teams. It is imperative to understand the patient's total injury burden, what exactly was done in the OR (e.g., the type of temporary closure employed and the location of drains), and what the plan for the next several hours should be. Knowledge of the intraoperative course, complications experienced, amount of blood products transfused, and the general trend of laboratory values is essential. The goal of resuscitation is to rewarm the patient, correct the acidosis and coagulopathy, and monitor for ongoing bleeding and complications. This is labor-intensive and requires frequent communication between the surgical team, intensivist, blood bank, and laboratory.

The patient should have adequate vascular access (at least two large-bore peripheral IVs). One should have a low threshold for placing central access, such as an introducer. In addition, it is often prudent to replace central lines that were inserted hastily during the initial resuscitation;these are often done in suboptimal circumstances and the risk of subsequent infection is high. New invasive catheters should be inserted as early as possible given that tissue edema is expected, making the procedures much more challenging later on.

Invasive hemodynamic monitoring is not helpful during the immediate phase (phase I) of resuscitation and should not delay efforts to arrest ongoing hemorrhage. Once hemostasis has been achieved, arterial catheters are critical to allow continuous arterial blood pressure monitoring, as well as serial arterial blood gas analysis for trending of lactic acidosis and base deficit correction. The placement of advanced central monitoring devices, such as pulmonary artery catheters, adds little to the resuscitation of most patients but may be indicated in patients with intrinsic cardiac dysfunction and failure, those with a mixed-shock picture (cardiogenic with hemorrhagic shock), or patients who fail to respond to resuscitation as expected. Many patients who have suffered prolonged hemorrhagic shock have some degree of vasoplegia, necessitating the use of vasopressors despite adequate volume resuscitation.

Vigilance and frequent monitoring of the adequacy of resuscitation must be performed. This involves an assessment of vital signs, urinary output, and serial monitoring of the arterial blood gas, lactic acid level, hemoglobin, coagulation system, and platelets. Particular attention should be paid to surgical drains, external wounds, and open abdominal dressings because these can represent a significant source of volume loss. It is not uncommon for these patients to require in excess of 20 L in the first day to maintain adequate intravascular volume. In addition, frequent monitoring of electrolytes, in particular calcium, should be performed as large volumes of blood transfusion may deplete calcium levels, further impairing coagulation. Vasopressors may be required but should be started cautiously and only after adequate volume loading has occurred. In general, the INR should be returned to < 1.5 and the platelet count should remain above 100 until the patient has stopped bleeding. As mentioned earlier, the use of TEG can be a valuable adjunct to guide resuscitation and coagulopathy reversal. Standard triggers for pRBC transfusion (Hgb < 7.5) may not apply early as the hemoglobin level correlates poorly with transfusion requirements in the setting of acute blood loss. If the patient is actively bleeding, blood should be administered regardless of hemoglobin level. In instances where a "massive transfusion protocol" has been initiated, it is imperative that the surgeon, intensivist, and blood bank communicate regularly regarding the patient's resuscitation so that appropriate and timely implementation and, later, cessation of the protocol may be undertaken.

Determining the adequacy of fluid resuscitation is complicated by the fact that many patients with significant hemorrhage have "compensated" shock at some point during their resuscitation. These patients have compensated for ongoing hypovolemia via vasoconstriction, allowing normalization of blood pressure, heart rate, and urine output. Detecting this state is critical because ongoing, inadequate resuscitation can worsen outcomes. Looking for evidence of anaerobic metabolism by measuring base deficit or lactate levels has become standard.

Higher base deficit or lactate levels, or failure to normalize these values by 24 hours postinjury, correlates with increased mortality. Mixed venous oxygen saturation has also been used frequently. Traditional invasive hemodynamic monitoring using the pulmonary artery catheter, with or without measurements of continuous cardiac output or right ventricular end-diastolic volume, does not seem to be superior to less invasive monitoring techniques. The optimal endpoint for resuscitation remains unclear. Researchers have been exploring a number of potential endpoints, including tissue oxygenation (measured by near-infrared spectroscopy), stroke volume variability (measured by pulse contour cardiac output determination), heart rate variability, and inferior vena cava collapsibility by ultrasound measurements.

In addition to restoration of intravascular volume and correction of coagulopathy, the intensivist must make every effort to maintain or return the patient to normothermia and correct the underlying acidosis. Rewarming efforts begin in the OR by "closing" body cavities as quickly as possible and terminating the operation. It has been shown that the average heat loss during laparotomy is 4.6°C per hour and mortality is clearly associated with worsening hypothermia. The ambient temperature in the room should be increased, fluids and ventilator gases warmed as much as possible, and the patient covered with blankets or warming blankets. Extracorporeal circulation and body cavity lavage may be used in more severe cases. Ideally, the patient should be warmed to 37°C within 4 hours of arrival to the ICU. Once the red cell mass has been restored and hemostasis achieved, acidosis should essentially correct itself. However, in the case of severe hemorrhagic shock or following cardiac arrest, acidosis may be severe. A pH < 7.2 from a metabolic acidosis is associated with decreased cardiac output and contractility, vasodilation, hypotension, dysrhythmias, and diminished hepatic and renal perfusion in addition to its deleterious effects on coagulation. In general, treatment of metabolic acidosis with bicarbonate or other bases (tromethamine [THAM]) is not undertaken unless the pH is severely acidemic (< 7.2). Even then, the effect on patient outcomes remains unclear.

Completion of damage control phase II, re-establishing "normal" physiology, typically can take 24–48 hours. Vital signs should be improving, coagulopathy reversing, and lactic acidosis should be resolving. It is at this point that further, definitive surgical procedures (phase III) may be more safely undertaken. Failure to clear or worsening of the lactic acidosis should clue the intensivist in to potential problems. Ongoing bleeding is a very real possibility as one should never assume that a patient in hemorrhagic shock who has returned from the OR or angiography suite has stopped bleeding. Open lines of communication among all team members is critical during this phase. Other possible reasons for ongoing lactic acidosis include missed visceral injury or development of abdominal compartment syndrome (ACS). The onset of ACS is often insidious and may be difficult to detect. Hypoxemia refractory to increasing oxygen concentration or positive end-expiratory pressure, hypercarbia, and increased peek inspiratory pressures may already be present as a result of underlying chest injury or the large volume resuscitation. Abdominal distention can be difficult to detect, particularly in the obese. A high index of suspicion must be maintained and, if one is contemplating ACS, intra-abdominal (bladder) pressure should be monitored. In general, a bladder pressure > 25 mmHg should prompt laparotomy.

In summary, hemorrhagic shock is the most common type of shock present in injured patients. The diagnosis is primarily clinical with laboratory tests being useful mostly for defining the severity and monitoring the adequacy of resuscitation. Successful resuscitation begins with prompt recognition and initiation of measures to arrest the hemorrhage, restore effective circulating volume, and correct the underlying coagulopathy, acidosis, and hypothermia. Maintaining open lines of communication between and among all team members is critical to achieving good outcomes.

Key references

Alarcon LH, Puyana JC, Peitzman AB. Management of shock. In: Mattox KL, Moore EE, Feliciano D, eds. *Trauma*. 7th ed. New York: McGraw-Hill; 2013.

Duchesne JC, McSwain NE, Cotton BA, et al. Damage control resuscitation: The new face of damage control. *J Trauma*. 2010;69(4):976–990.

Hauser CJ, Boffard K, Dutton R, et al. Results of the CONTROL trial: efficacy and safety of recombinant Factor VII in the management of refractory traumatic hemorrhage. *J Trauma*. 2010; 69(3):489–500.

Nunez TC, Cotton BA. Transfusion therapy in hemorrhagic shock. *Curr Opin Crit Care*. 2009;15(6):536–541.

Sagraves SG, Toschlog EA, Rotondo MF. Damage control surgery—the intensivist's role. *J Intensive Care Med*. 2006;21(1):5–16.

Shakur H, Roberts I, Bautista R, et al. Effects of tranexamic acid on death, vascular occlusive events, and blood transfusion in trauma patients with significant haemorrhage (CRASH-2): a randomized, placebo-controlled trial. *Lancet*. 2010; 364(9442):1321–1328.

Spinella PC, Holcomb JB. Resuscitation and transfusion principles for traumatic hemorrhagic shock. *Blood Reviews*. 2009; 23(6):231–240.

Chapter 7

Massive transfusions and coagulopathy

Matthew D. Neal, Lauren M. McDaniel,
and Raquel M. Forsythe

Blood transfusion is a ubiquitous component of the care of medical and surgical intensive care unit (ICU) patients. In the United States alone, nearly 40,000 units of blood are required in hospitals on a daily basis. According to the American Association of Blood Banks, over 30 million units of blood and blood products are transfused annually. Frequently, large volumes of blood are required for the treatment of uncontrolled hemorrhage. Numerous definitions of massive transfusion (MT) exist, but it is most commonly defined as the administration of ≥10 units of packed red blood cells (pRBCs) to a patient in a single 24-hour period. The need for MT in the ICU arises most commonly in the setting of traumatic injury because 3%–5% of all civilian trauma patients go on to require MT. Postoperative hemorrhage, postpartum complications, complex elective vascular and transplantation surgery, and acute gastrointestinal bleeding are also frequent triggers for massive transfusion. Despite the dramatic differences among these patient populations, the current approaches to initial resuscitation from hemorrhagic shock are quite similar and are mostly taken from the trauma literature where the abundance of research exists. This chapter will discuss the approach to MT for the patient presenting with hemorrhagic shock, with a focus on the evidence-based approach to hemostatic resuscitation as well as the important consequences and complications that must be closely monitored by the ICU clinician.

Identification

The concept of identifying patients who would go on to require MT was popularized due to the recognition of dilutional complications that arise from patients requiring large volumes of pRBCs. The definition of MT is by nature a retrospective one—patients only qualify as having received "massive transfusion" after they have received essentially an entire blood volume in the initial 24 hours. However, this presents an inherent limitation in designing protocols to prospectively optimize the resuscitation of patients in hemorrhagic shock. In order to design the best approach to MT, it is critically important to identify early the patients who are most at risk for severe ongoing hemorrhage. This is especially critical in rural areas or in those facilities without immediate access to a blood bank or to large volumes of stored blood products.

Multiple attempts have been made to predict the need for MT, including a combat-casualty-based model by McLaughlin et al, which identified tachycardia (HR > 105), hypotension (SBP < 110), acidosis (pH < 7.25), and anemia (hematocrit < 32%) as the combination of variables that allowed the accurate prediction of MT in 66% of patients after retrospective review. Similar results are obtained by using the more involved Trauma Associated Severe Hemorrhage (TASH) score, which incorporates hemoglobin, base excess, degree of hypotension and tachycardia, gender, focused assessment with sonography for trauma (FAST) findings, and injury pattern. The most straightforward method to date for predicting the need for MT in civilian trauma was developed at Vanderbilt University Medical Center by Nunez et al (2009) and benefits from a reliance on clinical findings rather than laboratory values. The Assessment of Blood Consumption (ABC) score, which was recently validated in a multi-center study, is calculated by assigning a value (0 or 1) to each of the four parameters: penetrating mechanism, positive FAST for fluid, arrival blood pressure < 90 mm Hg, and arrival pulse > 120 bpm. The cut-off for a "positive" score for predicting massive transfusion was a value of 2, which resulted in a 75% sensitivity and an 86% specificity. The above-listed predictive methods were all developed in either civilian or military trauma practices; little information is available about predicting the need for MT in nontrauma settings.

Hemostatic resuscitation and outcomes of massive transfusion

Many patients with hemorrhagic shock are coagulopathic upon presentation due to a unique but poorly understood entity called the acute coagulopathy of trauma and/or prehospital factors such as hypothermia, acidosis, or prescription anticoagulant use. Previous resuscitation strategies that included large volume crystalloid and plasma-poor pRBC administration resulted in a worsening of these underlying coagulopathies through a dilutional effect. With this in mind, modern MT protocols have been designed to intervene in the so-called "bloody vicious cycle" of acidosis, hypothermia, and coagulopathy that develops following massive hemorrhage (Figure 7.1) by using various procoagulant factors. Although warm whole blood transfusion has been shown to reduce mortality in military settings, resource availability and the need for large-volume and long-term storage makes it impractical in a civilian setting. Thus, the focus of a large body of recent research has centered on the optimum ratio of blood and blood product administration in MT. Unfortunately, a common denominator in this field is the lack of randomized controlled trials, due in large part to patient heterogeneity and difficulty in designing such a study. The major blood products studied as part of MT protocols are fresh frozen plasma (FFP), platelets,

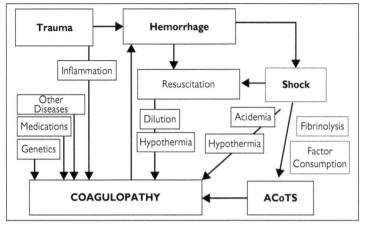

Figure 7.1 "Bloody Vicious Cycle" Involving Acidosis, Hypothermia, and Coagulopathy. ACoTs = acute coagulopathy of trauma-shock. Adapted from Sihler and Napolitano (2010).

cryoprecipitate (fibrinogen), and factor VII. A review of the evidence for each of these is presented here below.

Fresh frozen plasma

Fresh frozen plasma (FFP) provides the largest number of clotting factors to replace the deficiencies encountered from using pRBCs. Its use has increased ten-fold from 2000–2010 with nearly 3 million units used annually. Factors II, V, VII, IX, X, and XI are effectively replaced when using FFP. A recent review of the literature by Phan et al identified 11 trauma studies evaluating the effect of plasma to pRBC transfusion rates on mortality. The largest multi-center study to date to assess the role of FFP in massive transfusion was a retrospective analysis of the trauma registry created by the German Society of Trauma, nearly 18,000 patients. The authors identified 713 patients who underwent MT and discovered that early (< 6 hrs), 24-hour, and late (30-day) mortality rates were reduced in patients who received more FFP in a dose-dependent fashion. An additional large multi-center study by Holcomb et al, published in 2008 supported the observation that higher ratios of FFP were associated with a survival benefit. The authors measured 30-day mortality at varying ratios of FFP to pRBC (FFP:pRBC) at all centers and found that any FFP:pRBC ratio > 1:2 demonstrated an improved survival. Following the application of modeling based on their study results, the authors recommended a transfusion ratio of 1:1 for FFP:pRBC. Similar results were obtained in studies performed in trauma centers by multiple different groups. Gonzalez and coauthors documented a survival benefit in transfusion at a 1:1 ratio of FFP:pRBC; however the most significant benefit was observed with pre-ICU intervention and earlier administration of FFP.

In their analysis, the severity of coagulopathy at ICU admission was associated with survival outcome. The finding of a benefit to early use of high-ratio FFP transfusion was supported by Sperry et al (2008) who documented an increased mortality risk in severely injured blunt trauma patients presenting with signs and symptoms of hemorrhagic shock who received < 1:1.5 of FFP:pRBC in a large retrospective study. A common limitation in most of the studies was the inability to exclude unintended biases. Additionally, all of the analyses that use mortality as an outcome are at risk of what has been termed "survivor bias," meaning that patients who survived longer had more opportunity to receive plasma transfusion, thus increasing the FFP:pRBC ratio. Recognizing these important limitations, the abundance of studies with similar findings of improved survival with 1:1 FFP:pRBC make this a compelling resuscitation strategy.

Despite these strong observational results, not all authors have identified a benefit to high-ratio FFP transfusion in MT. The studies by Scalea and Snyder showed no survival advantage for the plasma ratio. Although Teixiera et al did show a survival advantage associated with plasma transfusion, there was no benefit after the ratio reached 1:3. Due in part to these conflicting analyses, and due largely to the absence of randomized prospective data on the subject, the evidence-based practice guidelines for plasma transfusion released by the American Association of Blood Banks in 2010 could not recommend *for* or *against* transfusion of FFP to pRBC at ratios exceeding 1:3.

Platelets

Nine studies specifically addressing the role of platelets in MT have been published, with the earliest being in 2008, demonstrating the novelty of this resuscitation strategy. Eight of the nine studies assessed the ratio of platelets to pRBCs (platelets:PRBC) and the effects on mortality. The largest of these studies was by Inaba et al in 2010. A retrospective analysis of over 32,000 trauma patients identified 657 who required MT and assessed the mortality according to platelets:pRBC ratio, with the highest ratio assessed being ≥1:6. The authors found that high ratios (1:12–6) were independently associated with improved survival at 24 hours. Given approximately six individual donor units per apheresis unit of platelets, this suggests a transfusion ratio of 1:1 for platelets:pRBC. In 2011, in another large retrospective multi-center study, Holcomb et al (2011) analyzed 643 massively transfused trauma patients and found that high ratios of platelets:pRBC not only improved 24-hour and 30-day survival, but also decreased the incidence of truncal hemorrhage. They did note, however, that high ratios were associated with increased incidence of multiple organ failure. Others have had similar findings of improved survival, with the absolute risk reduction for death in a study by Zink et al reaching 16% in the 1:1 group. Three of the studies that addressed FFP:pRBC ratios also looked at platelets:pRBC transfusion. Holcomb et al (2011) found that platelet transfusion in a ratio ≥ 1:2 platelets to pRBCs was associated with an increased 30-day survival, while Gunter et al demonstrated that a ratio > 1:5 (individual donor units) resulted in an improved 30-day survival. Rowell et al found that although high platelets:pRBC ratios were associated with improved survival in patients who had sustained blunt traumatic injuries, there was no difference in mortality in patients with penetrating traumatic injuries. In the study by Perkins et al (2011), fresh whole blood was compared to apheresis platelets in a combat setting; no significant difference in mortality was observed.

The studies assessing platelet transfusion ratios suffer from the same limitations as mentioned for FFP, including the retrospective design. However, an appropriate level of enthusiasm exists in the trauma and transfusion literature for the use of high-ratio apheresis platelet to pRBC strategies, approaching 1:1, in massive transfusion.

The "Pragmatic, Randomized Optimal Platelets and Plasma Ratios" study (NCT01545232), sponsored by the U.S. Department of Defense, the National Heart, Lung, and Blood Institute and Defence Research and Development Canada, is designed to prospectively study the effects of different ratios of pRBC, FFP, and platelet administration.

Cryoprecipitate

Cryoprecipitate is frequently used to replace clotting factors not contained in FFP (factor VIII, factor XIII, von Willebrand factor, fibronectin, and fibrinogen) and is frequently used as an adjunct to hemorrhage control when fibrinogen levels are depleted (< 100mg/dl). Ten units of cryoprecipitate contain 2.5 grams of fibrinogen. Multiple authors have suggested the benefit of early transfusion of cryoprecipitate/fibrinogen as part of an algorithm for MT.

Fenger-Eriksen et al studied the use of fibrinogen in massive transfusion in a civilian setting. They found that a mean of 2 grams of fibrinogen was transfused as part of an implemented MT protocol. Using historical controls, they documented lower overall blood loss as well as decreased total volume of pRBCs, FFP, and platelets used. In a retrospective military study by Stinger et al (2008), the fibrinogen:RBC ratio appeared to influence patient survival. A high (≥ 0.2 g fibrinogen/RBC unit) versus low (< 0.2 g fibrinogen/RBC unit) fibrinogen:RBC ratio was associated with a statistically significant improvement in overall survival (76% vs. 48%).

Shaz et al demonstrated that 1 unit of cryoprecipitate for two or less RBC products was associated with significantly improved 30-day survival, when compared to less aggressive cryoprecipitate use (66% vs. 41%). The overall incidence of death in those receiving cryoprecipitate as part of massive transfusion was reduced by 41% in this study.

Thus, although the optimum ratio of cryoprecipitate to pRBC remains unclear and complicated by studies using fibrinogen concentrate (available in Europe) rather than full cryoprecipitate, it appears that a trend towards 1:2 or 1:1 cryoprecipitate:pRBC may help to reduce overall blood product administration and potentially reduce the risk of mortality.

Factor VII

Recombinant factor VIIa (rFVIIa) has emerged as an additional tool in the control of massive hemorrhage following not only trauma but a number of both surgical and nonsurgical causes of bleeding. Although only currently approved for the control or prevention of hemorrhage in patients with hemophilia with inhibitors to Factor VIII products or with congenital FVII deficiency, rFVIIa has been used "off-label" for other causes of massive hemorrhage. The physiological effect of rFVIIa is to increase tissue factor binding, binding of activated platelets, and activation factor X, all of which aids in the formation of a platelet aggregate and hemostasis.

Although the use of rFVIIa has been controversial due to high cost as well as the concern for potential thromboembolic events, a number of studies have addressed its use in controlling bleeding after various insults. Most of these have been observational, uncontrolled studies. However, there have been two randomized, placebo-controlled, double-blind trials by Boffard et al (2005) to assess the safety and efficacy of the use of rFVIIa in trauma, one for penetrating trauma and one for blunt trauma. Patients were randomized to receive one of three doses of rFVIIa or placebo in addition to their standard resuscitation after the 8th unit of pRBCs. In penetrating trauma patients, there were no differences in total pRBCs transfused, mortality, need for MT (defined in this study as > 20 units of pRBCs), and incidence of complications, including thromboembolic events. However, in blunt trauma victims, there was a significant reduction in the number of pRBC units transfused (reduced by 2.6 units) as well as the need for MT (reduced by 19%) compared to patients who received placebo. Importantly, there were no significant increases in rate of complications. Most recently, results from the CONTROL trial, a multi-center randomized placebo-controlled phase III study analyzing 560 trauma patients, demonstrated no difference in overall mortality, organ failure, or adverse events between patients administered rFVIIa and patients who received placebo. The authors additionally demonstrated reductions in transfusion of other component products following rFVIIa administration. Although rFVIIa has been deemed to be safe for use with a potential to reduce overall need for blood transfusion, the role of rFVIIa in massive transfusion remains unclear, as rFVIIa does not appear to reduce overall mortality in trauma patients.

The ideal timing of rFVIIa administration is unknown, although a study by Perkins et al (2011) found that the overall reduction in pRBC use was most significant when rFVIIa was given early, that is, before 8 units of pRBCs were transfused.

Although there are additional studies and recommendations for the use of rFVIIa in other types of hemorrhage (obstetrics, etc), none are as robust as those denoted above. The extraordinary expense of rFVIIa and limited prospective data showing any benefit significantly temper the enthusiasm for its use in massive transfusion.

Tranexamic acid

Tranexamic acid is an antifibrinolytic that may be beneficial for bleeding trauma patients. The Clinical Randomization of an Antifibrinolytic in Significant Hemorrhage (CRASH-2) trial found that a short course of tranexamic acid safely reduced the risk of death in bleeding trauma patients. Although a majority of these patients (nor the placebo group) did not receive massive transfusion, the success of tranexamic acid in this trial as well as others in elective surgery and postpartum hemorrhage suggests that it may play a role as an adjunct to MT protocols. Ongoing studies (including the proposed CRASH-3 trial) are assessing the role of tranexamic acid in patients with traumatic brain injury. Importantly, administration of tranexamic acid should occur within 3 hours of injury, as delayed administration may actually increase the risk of death due to bleeding.

In addition to FFP, platelets, cryoprecipitate, and rFVIIa, standard resuscitation tools such as crystalloid and colloid are commonly used to increase volume status in massive transfusion. In a recent secondary analysis of a multi-center prospective cohort study evaluating outcomes in blunt-injured adults with hemorrhagic shock, crystalloid resuscitation in a ratio in excess of 1.5:1 increased the risk of multiple organ failure by 70% and was associated with a two-fold higher risk of acute respiratory distress syndrome and abdominal compartment syndrome. These results support the consensus opinion that the lowest volume of crystalloid possible should be used in patients requiring these additional factors due to the adverse effects associated with high-volume crystalloid use. In fact, a recent trend towards "hypotensive" resuscitation has emerged, which focuses on prehospital minimization of crystalloid use and a lower target SBP until hemostasis has been achieved. Studies to determine the optimum guidelines for prehospital and trauma resuscitation are ongoing.

Protocol design and outcomes

The design and implementation of MT protocols with a predetermined ratio of blood product transfusion have recently become common, especially in Level I trauma centers. In a recent survey, these MT protocols vary significantly in the protocol activation parameters and specific components to be administered. As many as 50% of centers still did not recommend immediate use of FFP with the first batch of pRBC units (ranging from 5–8 units). However, when FFP was recommended, the predominant recommended ratio was 1:1. Similar findings held true for platelet transfusion. Thirty-seven percent of surveyed institutions included rFVIIa as part of their MT protocol, however, the situations leading to request for and administration of the product were variable. The use of cryoprecipitate was not specifically queried, although calcium was included in the protocol by 20% of surveyed institutions. The capacity to activate the MT protocol rested most commonly with trauma surgeons (80%), followed by anesthesiologists (66%), other surgeons (32%), blood bank physicians (17%), and automatic activation (24%).

Implementation of specific MT protocols may result in improved outcomes for patients presenting with massive hemorrhage. Riskin et al reviewed their single-center experience with massive transfusion pre- and post-implementation of a MT protocol calling for 1:1.5 FFP:pRBC transfusion. Expecting a potential reduction in morbidity and mortality due to the increased use of hemostatic resuscitation strategy, the authors were surprised to find that there was, in fact, a significant reduction in mortality, but the overall ratio of FFP:pRBC and the overall mean number of transfusions were the same pre- and post-protocol. They hypothesized that improved product availability and improved communication may have been factors that influenced the survival benefit following the implementation of a MT protocol. Other studies have had similar results.

The ideal MT protocol appears yet to be defined; however, multiple authors and institutions recommend early transfusion of FFP, platelets, and pRBCs in a 1:1:1 ratio, with use of cryoprecipitate as needed (approaching 1:1 or 1:2 relative to pRBCs) and rFVIIa in the setting of blunt trauma when the definition of

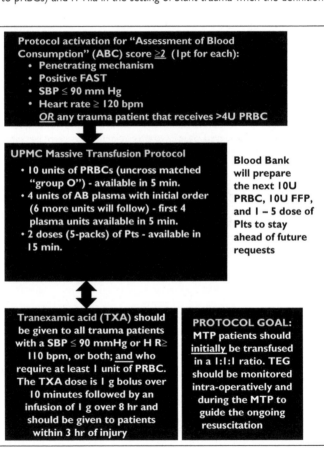

Figure 7.2 University of Pittsburgh Medical Center Massive Transfusion Protocol

MT has been met, and ongoing bleeding and/or transfusion is possible or anticipated. One thing that is clear in the design of such protocols is the need for a multi-disciplinary approach, involving emergency department personnel, trauma and/or acute care surgeons, medical or surgical intensivists, anesthesiologists, and blood bank physicians. An example of a MT protocol along with the multi-disciplinary team of responders taken from the University of Pittsburgh Medical Center appears in Figure 7.2.

Complications

Although potentially lifesaving in its application, and despite documented reductions in morbidity and mortality associated with protocol driven implementation, MT carries with it a number of serious and even life-threatening complications that must be anticipated and avoided if possible by the astute clinician.

The specific risks associated with blood transfusion (independent of massive transfusion) are beyond the scope of this chapter. Although transfusion of blood and blood products has been shown to be of benefit in resuscitation following hemorrhagic shock, it is important for the clinician to recognize that transfusion of pRBCs, especially in trauma patients, has been shown to be an independent risk factor for multiple organ failure, systemic inflammatory response syndrome, postoperative and nosocomial infections, and increased overall mortality. These risks are in addition to one of the most common transfusion associated morbidities: transfusion-related acute lung injury (TRALI) which occurs within 6 hours of transfusion. TRALI occurs after approximately 1/5,000 units of pRBCs, 1/2,000 units of FFP, and 1/400 units of platelets transfused, making it the most common complication associated with blood transfusion and a frequent component of ICU care in these patients. Given all of these underlying risks, the decision to transfuse blood or blood products, whether as part of massive transfusion or for any other indication, must be made judiciously and with an educated analysis of the risks and benefits.

Three major groups of complications exist that appear specific to the large amount of blood utilized in massive transfusion. A brief description and recommendation for prevention are listed below.

Hypothermia

Independent of massive transfusion, hypothermia is common in patients with hemorrhagic shock. This occurs secondary to exposure, cold operating rooms and intensive care units, and impaired thermoregulatory control (effects of anesthesia, sedation, alcohol or drug intoxication, and traumatic brain injury). Transfusion of pRBCs can exacerbate this problem, as pRBCs are stored at approximately 4°C. Hypothermia has profound implications for coagulation because there is a 10% drop in coagulation factor activity for every 1°C drop in core temperature. However, because laboratory clotting assays are typically performed at 37°C, the effects of hypothermia may not be obviously manifest in laboratory abnormalities. In addition, hypothermia causes overall decrease in hepatic metabolism, which can negatively affect drug clearance and acute phase responses.

Keys to avoiding hypothermia after MT include increasing room temperatures, surface warming with warming blankets, using heated and humidified gases for ventilation, and, importantly, using blood and fluid warmers, when time permits, for resuscitation.

Dilutional coagulopathy and thrombocytopenia

More than 25% of severely injured patients, and likely a similar percent of medical patients with hemorrhagic shock present with coagulopathy, either preexisting or acutely acquired from endogenous factors. It is important to recognize that even 1:1:1 transfusion of pRBCs to FFP to platelets still results in hemodilution. When 1 unit of pRBCs, 1 unit of FFP, and 1 unit of platelets are combined, the mean hematocrit is ~30%, while the mean platelet count of 1 apheresis unit is 85,000/ul. A single unit of FFP contains only ~60% of the mean coagulation factor activity of a comparable normal volume of plasma due to dilution in acellular fluid. As a result, clinicians must closely monitor blood counts and coagulation profiles with ongoing bleeding or post-massive-transfusion. Factor VII remains an available tool in most centers, as well as the use of fibrinogen/cryoprecipitate, for persistent coagulopathy after definitive control of hemorrhage.

Following definite control of bleeding and correction of coagulopathy, expert guidelines and the results of randomized studies suggest the implementation of restrictive transfusion strategies, with a hemoglobin of <7 g/dL having been identified as a target for transfusion. These recommendations stem largely from the Transfusion Requirements in Critical Care (TRICC) and the Anemia and Blood Transfusion in the Critically Ill (ABC) trials.

Electrolyte abnormalities

The storage process for pRBCs can lead to important post-transfusion perturbations in various electrolytes and acid-base status. pRBCs are stored in citrate, and the stored blood initially has a pH of 7.0. The latter can decrease with prolonged blood storage. The storage of blood for longer periods of time can also result in increased concentrations of CO_2 as well as an increase in potassium concentration secondary to RBC membrane ion pump activation. Given these findings, the most common electrolyte and acid-base abnormalities seen following massive transfusion are: hypocalcemia, hyperkalemia, hypomagnesemia, metabolic acidosis, and metabolic alkalosis. These conditions and the physiologic explanations for them are detailed in Table 7.1.

Frequent monitoring of serum electrolytes is warranted following massive transfusion, and abnormalities should be corrected as needed. Severe metabolic acidosis is a marker of poor tissue perfusion and may be caused by elevated lactate levels. Obviously, definitive control of hemorrhage is warranted, but

Table 7.1 Electrolyte and metabolic abnormalities after massive transfusions

Abnormality in MT	Mechanism of Abnormality
Hypocalcemia	Stored blood contains citrate, which binds Ca^{2+} and facilitates anticoagulation. Each unit of pRBC contains approximately 3 grams of citrate. If infusion of blood exceeds the liver's ability to metabolize citrate (3 grams/5 min in a healthy adult liver), hypocalcemia may develop related to citrate toxicity. The liver's ability to metabolize citrate may be compromised by liver disease or hypothermia.
Hypomagnesemia	Hypomagnesemia results from the infusion of large volumes of fluid containing low concentrations of magnesium, as well as from the ability of citrate in stored blood to bind magnesium.
Hyperkalemia	Potassium concentrations in stored pRBCs increase as a function of storage duration and can range from 7 to 77 mEq/L. The inactivation of the Na^+/K^+ pump in the red blood cell membrane contributes to this increase. Hyperkalemia has also been associated with rapid transfusion, renal insufficiency, renal failure, and severe tissue injury, particularly muscle damage.
Metabolic acidosis	Lactic acidosis results from decreased tissue perfusion associated with shock. This acidosis may be exacerbated by the transfusion of older pRBC units with exhausted buffer systems.
Metabolic alkalosis	The metabolism of citrate in pRBC units to bicarbonate results in a metabolic alkalosis.

ongoing acidosis may, on rare occasions, need to be corrected with sodium bicarbonate infusion, especially in the setting of acute renal failure where compensatory mechanisms are lost. This is additionally critical due to the fact that acidosis can exacerbate coagulopathy.

Future directions

Although resuscitation following massive hemorrhage has improved greatly over the past decade, the high incidence of post-transfusion complications and the persistently elevated risks of morbidity and mortality warrant future research. Despite being difficult to organize or conduct, randomized prospective studies to assess the optimum ratios for blood and blood product administration are needed. In addition to these population-based studies, an overall trend towards individualized medicine may also influence massive transfusion practice. A new body of literature and ongoing research studies are assessing goal-directed therapy for coagulopathy by using real-time assessment of coagulation function via rapid thromboelastography (TEG). Rapid TEG has emerged as an individualized approach to coagulation management in trauma, cardiac surgery, transplantation, and other critically ill patients. Guidelines for its use in massive transfusion are on the horizon.

Key references

Boffard KD, Riou B, Warren B, et al. Recombinant factor VIIa as adjunctive therapy for bleeding control in severely injured trauma patients: two parallel randomized, placebo-controlled, double-blind clinical trials. *J Trauma*. 2005;59(1):8–15.

Fenger-Eriksen C, Lindberg-Larsen M, Christensen AQ, et al. Fibrinogen concentrate substitution therapy in patients with massive haemorrhage and low plasma fibrinogen concentrations. *Br J Anaesth*. 2008;101(6):769–773.

Gonzalez EA, Moore FA, Holcomb JB, et al. Fresh frozen plasma should be given earlier to patients requiring massive transfusion. *J Trauma*. 2007;62(1):112–119.

Hauser CJ, Boffard K, Dutton R, et al. Results of the CONTROL trial: efficacy and safety of recombinant activated Factor VII in the management of refractory traumatic hemorrhage. *J Trauma*. 2010;69(3):489–500.

Holcomb JB, Wade CE, Michalek JE, et al. Increased plasma and platelet to red blood cell ratios improves outcome in 466 massively transfused civilian trauma patients. *Ann Surg*. 2008;248(3):447–458.

Holcomb JB, Zarzabal LA, Michalek JE, et al. Increased platelet:RBC ratios are associated with improved survival after massive transfusion. *J Trauma*. 2011;71(2 Suppl 3):S318–S328.

Maegele M, Lefering R, Paffrath T, et al. Red-blood-cell to plasma ratios transfused during massive transfusion are associated with mortality in severe multiple injury: a retrospective analysis from the Trauma Registry of the Deutsche Gesellschaft fur Unfallchirurgie. *Vox Sang*. 2008;95(2):112–119.

McLaughlin DF, Niles SE, Salinas J, et al. A predictive model for massive transfusion in combat casualty patients. *J Trauma*. 2008;64(2 Suppl):S57–S63.

Neal MD, Hoffman MK, Cuschieri J, et al. Crystalloid to packed red blood cell transfusion ratio in the massively transfused patient: when a little goes a long way. *J Trauma Acute Care Surg*. 2012;72(4):892–898.

Nunez TC, Voskresensky IV, Dossett LA, Shinall R, Dutton WD, Cotton BA. Early prediction of massive transfusion in trauma: simple as ABC (assessment of blood consumption)? *J Trauma*. 2009;66(2):346–352.

Perkins JG, Cap AP, Spinella PC, et al. Comparison of platelet transfusion as fresh whole blood versus apheresis platelets for massively transfused combat trauma patients. *Transfusion*. 2011;51:242–252.

Phan HH, Wisner DH. Should we increase the ratio of plasma/platelets to red blood cells in massive transfusion: what is the evidence? *Vox Sang*. 2010;98(3 Pt 2):395–402.

Riskin DJ, Tsai TC, Riskin L, et al. Massive transfusion protocols: the role of aggressive resuscitation versus product ratio in mortality reduction. *J Am Coll Surg*. 2009;209(2):198–205.

Roback JD, Caldwell S, Carson J, et al. Evidence-based practice guidelines for plasma transfusion. Transfusion. 2010;50(6):1227–1239.

Roberts I, Shakur H, Afolabi A, et al. The importance of early treatment with tranexamic acid in bleeding trauma patients: an exploratory analysis of the CRASH-2 randomised controlled trial. *Lancet*. 2011;377(9771):1096–101, 101 e1–2.

Rowell SE, Barbosa RR, Diggs BS, et al. Effect of high product ratio massive transfusion on mortality in blunt and penetrating trauma patients. *J Trauma*. 2011;71(2 Suppl 3): S353–S357.

Scalea TM, Bochicchio KM, Lumpkins K, et al. Early aggressive use of fresh frozen plasma does not improve outcome in critically injured trauma patients. *Ann Surg.* 2008;248(4):578–584.

Shaz BH, Dente CJ, Nicholas J, et al. Increased number of coagulation products in relationship to red blood cell products transfused improves mortality in trauma patients. *Transfusion.* 2010;50(2):493–500.

Sihler KC, Napolitano LM. Complications of massive transfusion. *Chest.* 2010;137(1):209–220.

Snyder CW, Weinberg JA, McGwin G, Jr., et al. The relationship of blood product ratio to mortality: survival benefit or survival bias? *J Trauma.* 2009;66(2):358–362.

Sperry JL, Ochoa JB, Gunn SR, et al. An FFP:PRBC transfusion ratio >/=1:1.5 is associated with a lower risk of mortality after massive transfusion. *J Trauma.* 2008;65(5):986–993.

Stinger HK, Spinella PC, Perkins JG, et al. The ratio of fibrinogen to red cells transfused affects survival in casualties receiving massive transfusions at an army combat support hospital. *J Trauma.* 2008;64(2 Suppl):S79–S85.

Teixeira PG, Inaba K, Shulman I, et al. Impact of plasma transfusion in massively transfused trauma patients. *J Trauma.* 2009;66(3):693–697.

Zink KA, Sambasivan CN, Holcomb JB, et al. A high ratio of plasma and platelets to packed red blood cells in the first 6 hours of massive transfusion improves outcomes in a large multicenter study. *Am J Surg.* 2009;197(5):565–570.

Chapter 8

Ventilator management of trauma patients

Matthew Benns, Babak Sarani, and Alain C. Corcos

General considerations and ventilator-induced lung injury

The indications for mechanical ventilation in the trauma patient falls into three broad categories: shock resulting in metabolic acidosis, insult to the respiratory system resulting in impaired gas exchange, and depressed mental status leading to decreased ability to protect the airway. Once mechanical ventilation has been initiated, the clinician must be cognizant of the possibility of ventilator-induced lung injury. Iatrogenic injury from mechanical ventilation is proposed to occur via three mechanisms: barotrauma, volutrauma, and atelectrauma. Baro- and volu-trauma occur secondary to direct alveolar stress by excessive pressure and volume, respectively. Atelectrauma is a more recently recognized mechanism of lung injury that occurs secondary to shear stresses from the repetitive opening and closing of alveoli. Additionally, it is critical to recall that oxygen exchange is directly proportional to the fraction of inspired oxygen (FiO2) and mean airway pressure (determined most commonly by the positive end-expiratory pressure (PEEP)), while CO_2 exchange is directly proportional to the minute ventilation (determined by the product of the respiratory rate and the tidal volume).

Noninvasive ventilation

Noninvasive ventilation (NIMV) is applied via a face mask, nasal mask, or helmet apparatus. Two forms are commonly used: bilevel intermittent positive airway pressure (BiPAP) and continuous positive airway pressure (CPAP). Both forms deliver positive airway pressure without endotracheal intubation and allow for increased functional residual capacity, decreased work of breathing, and improved oxygenation. NIMV does not provide a definitive airway and requires an awake and cooperative patient for success. It is therefore not appropriate for trauma patients with head injury or other causes of altered mental status for which airway protection is a concern. In addition, it is not a long-term solution to respiratory failure and should only be instituted for patients whose respiratory compromise is thought to be reversible within 48–72 hours. One example seen commonly includes trauma patients with thoracic fractures who develop respiratory compromise from atelectasis and splinting secondary to pain. NIMV can be used to support respiration while aggressive pain control measures (e.g., epidural or paravertebral analgesia) are implemented. The use of NIMV in patients with thoracic trauma has been shown to reduce the incidence of intubation and its associated risks.

Ventilating the intubated trauma patient

Pressure support

Pressure support is a mode of ventilation in which there is no set rate delivered by the ventilator. Instead, spontaneous breathing is augmented by ventilator-supplied pressure during inspiration. The clinician-set variables are FiO_2, amount of pressure support, gas flow rate, amount of PEEP, and the gas flow rate at which the ventilator cycles from inspiration to expiration. The default setting for the ventilator to cycle in most instances is 25% of peak inspiratory flow. The work of breathing required by the patient can vary depending on the level of pressure support delivered, but is never negligible. As such, it is not a common initial mode of ventilation and may not provide adequate support for patients in shock or those with chest injuries or other pulmonary pathology. Because there is no set rate, it is also not appropriate for patients with significantly decreased mental status who do not have a normal respiratory drive. It is therefore most commonly used in the trauma patient as a maintenance weaning mode. The level of pressure support may be gradually decreased as the patient's respiratory mechanics and drive improve. Alternatively, clinicians may test the readiness of a patient for weaning and extubation with a spontaneous breathing trial on "minimal support," typically pressure support of 5 cm H_2O.

Volume control

Volume control is the most common mode of ventilation used in trauma patients. The prototype of volume control on most ventilators is assist control (AC). A set tidal volume is delivered by the ventilator at a set rate. The resulting inspiratory pressure is dependent on the underlying pulmonary compliance. The patient will receive no less than the set number of breaths, but may trigger additional breaths by spontaneous breathing effort. The additional breaths, however, are delivered at the same tidal volume as the set breaths, regardless of patient effort. Thus, in this mode, the majority of the work of breathing is done by the ventilator. Because the delivered tidal volume can be precisely controlled by the clinician, volutrauma can be minimized.

An alternative mode of volume-control ventilation is synchronous intermittent mechanical ventilation (SIMV). In this mode, a set tidal volume is delivered by the ventilator at a set rate. As opposed to AC, however, the tidal volumes associated with additional spontaneous breathing efforts are determined solely by the patient. These spontaneous breaths can be augmented by the addition of pressure support. This mode was created to try and improve patient-ventilator synchrony and possibly to improve ventilator weaning (though trials have not validated this objective). Because this mode of ventilation offers support that varies between the "full support" of AC and spontaneous breathing of pressure support, it tends to be used less frequently.

Regardless of the volume control mode utilized, it is recommended that a tidal volume of 6–8 mL/kg be used in order to minimize ventilator-induced lung injury (VILI). In the setting of acute respiratory distress syndrome (ARDS), the use of a "low stretch" protocol (i.e. tidal volume limit of 4–6 mL/kg) has been shown to decrease mortality when compared to traditional tidal volumes (10–12 mL/kg).

Pressure control

Pressure control methods of ventilation are generally not used as a first-line option in trauma patients, but their use may be required with worsening pulmonary mechanics. Pressure control ventilation delivers a set rate of machine breaths at a set pressure. Spontaneous ventilation is possible, but the patient cannot generate a tidal volume that would result in a peak inspiratory pressure that exceeds the pressure limit set on the machine. The resulting tidal volume is dependent on the underlying pulmonary compliance. This mode is potentially beneficial to minimize barotrauma in patients with poor lung compliance. These patients may develop excessively high peak inspiratory or plateau pressures if ventilated using volume-control methods. Pressure control allows the peak inspiratory pressure to be capped by the ventilator, but possibly at the expense of poor tidal volumes and resulting atelectasis. This can be potentially overcome by the use of increased PEEP. Some modern ventilators also offer additional modes, for example, pressure-regulated volume controlled ventilation, in which the flow rate is continuously varied to allow a set tidal volume, but also a limited pressure.

Inverse ratio ventilation (IRV) is often used when patients manifest severely impaired ability to absorb oxygen. This strategy is frequently used in patients on pressure control mode ventilation. In the normal respiratory cycle, the expiratory phase is two to three times longer than the inspiratory phase. In IRV, this ratio is increased or completely reversed. A longer inspiratory time allows a longer period for gas diffusion as well as the maintenance of alveolar inflation above closing volume. In this manner, mean airway pressure, alveolar recruitment, and oxygenation are increased. The drawbacks to IRV are potentially significant. The decreased expiratory phase may promote air trapping and the development of auto-PEEP, which can impair venous return and decrease cardiac output. In addition, the "nonphysiologic" nature of the imposed respiratory cycle generally requires significant levels of sedation or even paralysis for patient tolerance. Though the use of inverse ratio ventilation techniques has been shown to improve oxygenation, it has not been conclusively shown to improve mortality.

Non-conventional mechanical ventilation: the "open lung" concept

The underlying principle in "open lung" concept (OLC) approaches is to keep the lung uniformly inflated for an extended period of time. This strategy may help to keep more alveoli open and minimize atelectrauma in instances of impaired compliance such as ARDS. Mean airway pressure is also maximized in OLC approaches. These characteristics help to improve oxygenation, but tend to worsen carbon dioxide retention. A strategy of "permissive hypercapnea" is therefore utilized with most OLC approaches. The pCO_2 is allowed to rise as long as the pH remains reasonable (generally > 7.2) for the sake of improved oxygenation. The two most common forms of OLC ventilation are airway pressure release ventilation (APRV) and high frequency oscillator ventilation (HFOV).

Airway pressure release ventilation

Airway pressure release ventilation is a mode of ventilation most commonly used to improve oxygenation in patients with severe ARDS, while limiting barotrauma. It attempts to maximize mean airway pressure and subsequent alveolar recruitment. APRV uses a continuously applied level of positive pressure, or "P high." This is alternated with periods of low pressure, or "P low." The time spent at P high is referred to as "T high," with the time at the lower pressure referred to as "T low." By convention, APRV has a ratio of T high to T low of at least 8:1 (often greater) with T low generally being less than 1 second. Using a very short release time allows for the development of auto-PEEP and increases functional residual capacity. In addition, the patient is able to spontaneously breathe during the P high period. This allows for further gas exchange and should be a more comfortable mode of ventilation for the patient, allowing for decreased sedation compared to other less physiologic modes.

To institute APRV, generally the P high level is set at an appropriate plateau pressure and generally no higher than 30–35 cm H_2O. P low is usually initially set to 0. However, the release time should be set such that full de-recruitment does not occur and auto-PEEP is encouraged. This can be accomplished by setting T low so that expiration ends when expiratory flow equals 50%–75% of peak expiratory flow rate. Most modern ventilators allow visualization of flow versus time graphs to facilitate this setting. Pressures and times can be adjusted based on the patient's oxygenation and ventilation needs.

APRV is generally well-tolerated by the trauma patient, but there are a few relative contraindications to its use. Ideally, patients should breathe spontaneously while on APRV. Patients may still oxygenate adequately without spontaneous breaths on APRV, but minute ventilation will be significantly reduced and hypercarbia may quickly develop. Intravascular volume should also be optimized, as prolonged positive intrathoracic pressure may impact venous return. This does not differ from the effects of high PEEP that may be required to maintain oxygenation using traditional ventilator strategies, but the periodic pressure releases in APRV augment venous return and improve cardiac output. Finally, APRV may be contraindicated in patients with significant obstructive pulmonary conditions such as chronic obstructive pulmonary disease (COPD). The short release times in APRV may be inadequate to obtain sufficient ventilation in these patients and levels of auto-PEEP produced may be excessively high.

Weaning from APRV is most often accomplished using the "drop and stretch" strategy. The level of P high is gradually decreased as well as the number of pressure releases. In this way, the pressure versus time graph will eventually become continuous positive airway pressure with the patient spontaneously breathing. Alternatively, the patient can be switched to a more conventional mode of ventilation once oxygenation has improved.

High-frequency oscillatory ventilation

High-frequency oscillatory ventilation is commonly and successfully used in neo-natology. More recently, it has been found to have potential benefit in improving oxygenation in adult patients with severe ARDS. HFOV utilizes very small tidal volumes delivered at a rapid rate (3–7 breaths per second). The alveoli are maintained open and airway pressure remains relatively constant. In this man-ner, atelectrauma, barotrauma, and ventilation/perfusion mismatch are reduced. Though a mortality benefit has not been shown in the literature, trials have demonstrated the safety of HFOV and the efficacy of improving oxygenation in ARDS patients who are failing traditional mechanical ventilation.

Air flow during HFOV is essentially driven by a piston-type assembly. The piston is driven back and forth at a rapid rate. Movement of the piston in one direction generates the inspiratory phase, while movement back in the other direction creates the expiratory phase. The clinician is able to directly set the frequency of respiration. In addition, the clinician may set the "power" applied to the piston. This setting effects how much the piston will actually move back and forth and therefore the delivered tidal volume. The amplitude of the pres-sure wave generated depends upon the resistance of the piston to movement, which is directly dependent upon airway resistance. Amplitude is also inversely related to the frequency of respiration. For this reason, lower frequencies can potentially lead to high amplitudes and subsequent barotrauma. The increase in amplitude (and therefore tidal volume) is also the reason that ventilation can be improved by *lowering* the frequency of respiration. This may at first be counter-intuitive to clinicians more comfortable with conventional modes of ventilation.

In addition to power and frequency, the clinician may also set the mean air-way pressure, the bias flow, the inspiratory time, and the FiO_2. Inspiratory time can be adjusted, but is generally kept constant at 1/3. Increasing this ratio may put the patient at risk of air trapping and subsequent barotrauma. The bias flow is also generally kept constant at 40 L/min. It may be adjusted to maintain mean

Table 8.1 Initial settings and ranges for High Frequency Oscillator Ventilation (HFOV) in adults	
Frequency	7 Hz (3–7 Hz)
Power (amplitude)	70–90 cm H_2O
Mean airway pressure	5 cm H_2O > last recorded plateau pressure on CV (< 40 cm H_2O)
Bias flow	40 L/min (40–60 L/min)
Inspiratory time	33%
FiO$_2$	100% (35%–100%)

airway pressure in conditions such as significant air leak, but is usually kept below 60 L/min. Mean airway pressure has a direct effect on oxygenation. Current recommendations are that it be set at a level 5 cm H_2O above the last plateau pressure recorded during conventional ventilation and at a level no higher than 40 cm H_2O. Ideally, alveolar recruitment should be maximized prior to the application of the near constant mean airway pressure found in HFOV. Table 8.1 lists some suggested initial settings and associated ranges for HFOV.

HFOV is fundamentally different from other conventional modes of ventilation and has some associated unique aspects that should be considered. Patient-ventilator synchrony generally requires deep sedation. Many centers routinely institute neuromuscular blockade for patients being placed on HFOV. In addition, the ventilator alarms, ventilator mechanics, and physical exam of patients on HFOV are different from conventional ventilation. The unique signs and symptoms of common mechanical ventilation problems for patients on HFOV must be recognizable by clinicians and support staff.

Adjuncts to mechanical ventilation

Occasionally, trauma patients may develop hypoxemia and ARDS that is refractory to both conventional and nonconventional mechanical ventilation strategies. In these circumstances, several adjunctive therapies may be used. The timing, duration, and overall benefit of these therapies have not been decisively defined in the literature, but they are briefly reviewed here.

Pulmonary vasodilators

Nitric oxide and epoprostenol are selective pulmonary vasodilators currently given in a continuous inhaled form that may act to decrease pulmonary vascular resistance as well as right ventricular afterload. Furthermore, they improve ventilation/perfusion (V/Q) matching by selectively dilating the arterioles situated next to aerated alveoli. Selected studies have shown a temporary benefit in oxygenation, but there is insufficient evidence of improvement in duration of mechanical ventilation or mortality. The high cost of these agents limits their widespread usage.

Prone ventilation

Prone positioning in ARDS may act to redistribute gas, recruit alveoli, and redistribute pulmonary blood flow thereby improving ventilation/perfusion mismatch. It can be accomplished via manual positioning by nursing staff, or through the use of mechanically rotating beds. Numerous studies have generally shown improvement in oxygenation with prone positioning, but a mortality benefit has not been consistently found. Its use is limited by concerns regarding the safety of maintaining an airway and other invasive devices in the prone position.

Extracorporeal membrane oxygenation

A detailed discussion of extracorporeal membrane oxygenation (ECMO) is beyond the scope of this chapter, but its utility as a potential rescue therapy in severe ARDS should be noted. The general principle is to exchange oxygen and CO_2 outside of the body and return it such that the lungs are not needed for gas exchange. This is continued until the underlying pathology of the lungs improves. For pure respiratory failure, a veno-venous ECMO circuit can be utilized with less morbidity compared to a veno-arterial ECMO circuit used for combined cardiorespiratory failure. The specific indications, cost effectiveness, and ultimate benefits remain controversial. ECMO in posttraumatic ARDS is generally only utilized at specialized tertiary referral centers.

Mechanical ventilation and specific injuries

A wide variety of injuries may necessitate the need for mechanical ventilation. General principles of limiting the time spent on mechanical ventilation and thereby limiting VILI remain constant regardless of the underlying injury.

Traumatic brain injury

Patients with traumatic brain injury (TBI) commonly require mechanical ventilation secondary to decreased mental status. The prevention of secondary brain injury is paramount in these patients, thus hypoxia and hypotension should be aggressively avoided. Volume control modes are most commonly used to ventilate these patients, as this allows for stricter control of oxygenation and ventilation than in spontaneous breathing modes. Application of PEEP can impair venous return from the head and increase intracranial pressure. Additionally, intracranial pressure will rise with hypercarbia; thus pCO_2 should be kept at 35–40 mm Hg.

Pulmonary contusion

Pulmonary contusion is exceedingly common and results from direct compressive and shear forces applied to the lung parenchyma. Interstitial and alveolar hemorrhage may occur. Additional injury may develop secondary to increased localized inflammation. There is increased capillary permeability and edema, and decreased surfactant production. The end results of pulmonary contusion are ventilation/perfusion mismatch, increased shunt, and decreased pulmonary compliance. The contused lung is prone to atelectasis, but positive-pressure ventilation can be very effective at combating this and maintaining oxygenation. Specific strategies for mechanical ventilation in these patients generally depend upon the severity of the contusion. Minimal contusions can often be managed without mechanical ventilation or with NIMV. Moderate contusions can usually be managed with volume control strategies. Use of increased PEEP can aid in alveolar recruitment and help oxygenation. Severe pulmonary contusions may present with ARDS and significantly decreased compliance. Ventilation strategy in these patients should begin with volume control methods using a limited tidal volume (4–6 mL/kg). Pressure control methods can be useful if high peak airways pressures are noted despite this strategy. If oxygenation is poor, increases in FiO_2 and PEEP are recommended as first-line therapy. If high levels of PEEP are poorly tolerated or ineffective at improving oxygenation, the nonconventional modes of ventilation can be considered.

Rib fractures and flail chest

Patients with rib fractures develop respiratory insufficiency secondary to underlying pulmonary contusion, or from atelectasis caused by splinting and pain. Specific ventilation strategies depend upon the number and severity of the rib fractures as well as underlying patient characteristics and comorbidities. Noninvasive ventilation, pressure support, or volume control ventilation can be used in patients whose rib fractures are resulting in respiratory distress. The presence of a flail segment does not necessarily alter the mechanical ventilation strategy, but it is an independent predictor of respiratory failure and respiratory complications (particularly pneumonia) in trauma patients. Mechanical ventilation is not indicated as a means to splint or stabilize the ribs in patients with flail chest.

Patients with paradoxical motion of the flail segment who fail to wean may be considered for rib fracture repair, provided they have no significant pulmonary contusion or associated injuries, such as TBI, that would preclude operative intervention. Several studies suggest that select patients can benefit from operative repair, citing earlier separation from mechanical ventilation, fewer days in the ICU, and a lower incidence of pneumonia. Some trials also describe improvements in longer-term outcomes, such as vital capacity, pain control, and earlier return to work. Despite these trials, fracture fixation for flail chest is not widely practiced and remains controversial. Centers that do offer repair to select patients typically draw on the knowledge and expertise of trauma, thoracic, and orthopedic surgeons. Although many techniques for repair have been described (wire sutures, intramedullary wires, and various metallic or absorbable plates), dynamic compression osteosynthesis plating with a locking screw design has emerged as the standard.

Pneumothorax and air leak

Pneumothorax is a common injury seen in both blunt and penetrating trauma and is often accompanied by associated thoracic injuries that lead to respiratory failure. The application of positive-pressure mechanical ventilation can rapidly enlarge a preexisting pneumothorax. This is generally not a concern if the patient develops respiratory failure and is treated with tube thoracostomy. However, patients with small pneumothoraces may be observed without chest tube placement. The concern for worsening of the pneumothorax and/or creation of a tension pneumothorax needs to be addressed if these patients are later placed on positive-pressure ventilation, such as in the operating room. A preemptive chest tube should be placed, or the operating room team should be alerted to the possibility of significant pneumothorax and the potential need for chest tube placement.

Patients with an ongoing air leak via chest tube who require mechanical ventilation can present a challenge. The majority of air leaks will seal despite positive-pressure ventilation as the underlying lung heals, as long as the pleural space is adequately drained. If the air leak is significant or prolonged, a strategy of minimizing alveolar distention, mean airway pressure, and the number of positive-pressure breaths is enacted to try and decrease flow through the bronchopleural fistula. Pressure support or low-rate SIMV may be useful to accomplish these goals. PEEP levels and inspiratory time also should be minimized. Although these strategies may be effective at decreasing air leak, they will also worsen oxygenation. Given that additional pulmonary injuries commonly accompany pneumothorax, hypoxemia may be a significant concern. Rarely, the magnitude of air flow through the bronchopleural fistula may be such that adequate gas exchange is not possible using conventional ventilation. In these instances, HFOV may offer an advantage in optimizing oxygenation while stabilizing the lung and minimizing atelectatic trauma so as to encourage the tract to heal.

Unilateral injuries

Occasionally patients may present with injuries predominantly located in one lung. This is especially true in cases of penetrating trauma, but is also seen with some regularity in blunt trauma. In general, strategies for mechanical ventilation in these patients do not differ significantly from other indications. However, techniques of independent lung ventilation have been described in order to deal with severe unilateral injuries. This can be accomplished using single- or double-lumen endotracheal tubes. In cases of significant unilateral pulmonary hemorrhage, the mainstem bronchus on the side opposite the hemorrhage can be directly intubated to limit further aspiration of blood. This technique has also been described in cases of severe ongoing air leak to promote healing. The insertion of a double-lumen tube and the use of dual simultaneous ventilation has also been described. If one lung is severely contused or otherwise injured, it may operate under significantly different pulmonary mechanics than the other side. A single ventilator strategy for both lungs may be inefficient or potentially harmful to the normal lung. In this strategy, the injured lung can be ventilated using a low-stretch protocol while the normal side may receive standard settings of ventilation. Though this strategy has been described with success in the literature, the added complexity and logistical concerns make it rarely indicated.

Spinal cord injury

Patients with spinal cord injury (SCI) may develop respiratory failure and the need for mechanical ventilation. Among the most common are patients with complete SCI above the level of C5, owing to the loss of diaphragm innervation. However, patients with complete and incomplete injuries of the lower cervical and thoracic spine are at increased risk of requiring mechanical ventilation as well, regardless of associated chest injuries. This is in large part secondary to loss of innervation to accessory muscles of breathing and subsequent chest wall rigidity. Positive-pressure ventilation with volume control or pressure support are most often used, but there are reports of patients successfully managed with noninvasive ventilation. Adequate pulmonary hygiene is critical in this cohort due to severely impaired cough and risk of recurrent mucus plugging. Because of this, respiratory failure in this group can be gradual and the decision to terminate mechanical ventilation shortly after the onset of injury should be made with this in mind. In addition, patients with cervical or thoracic spinal cord injuries should be closely monitored for several days for signs of impending respiratory insufficiency following termination of mechanical ventilation.

Key references

Brower RG, Matthay MA, Morris A. Ventilation with lower tidal volumes as compared with traditional tidal volumes for acute lung injury and the acute respiratory distress syndrome. *N Engl J Med.* 2004;342(18):1301–1308.

Gattinoni L, Tognoni G, Pesanti A, et al. Effect of prone positioning on the survival of patients with acute respiratory failure. *NEJM.* 2001;345:568–573.

Habashi N, Andrews P. Ventilator strategies for post-traumatic acute respiratory distress syndrome: airway pressure release ventilation and the role of spontaneous breathing in critically ill patients. *Curr Opin Crit Care.* 2004;10:549–557.

Hernandez G, Fernandez F, Lopez-Reina P, et al. Noninvasive ventilation reduces intubation in chest trauma-related hypoxemia. *Chest.* 2010;137(1):74–80.

Kiraly L, Schreiber M. Management of the crushed chest. *Crit Care Med.* 2010; 38(9):S469–S477.

Nirula R, Diaz JJ, Trunkey DD, Mayberry JC. Rib fracture repair: indications, technical issues, and future directions. *World J Surg.* 2009;33:14–22.

Peek GJ, Mugford M, Tiruvoipati R, et al. Efficacy and economic assessment of conventional ventilator support versus extracorporeal membrane oxygenation for severe adult respiratory failure (CESAR): a multicentre randomised controlled trial. *Lancet.* 2009;374:1351–1363.

Rico FR, Cheng JD, Gestring ML, et al. Mechanical ventilation strategies in massive chest trauma. *Crit Care Clin.* 2007;23:299–315.

Stawicki SP, Goyal M, Sarani B. High-frequency oscillatory ventilation (HFOV) and airway pressure release ventilation (APRV): a practical guide. *J Int Car Med.* 2009;24(4):215–229.

Taylor RW, Zimmerman JL, Dellinger RP, et al. Low-dose inhaled nitric oxide in patients with acute lung injury: A randomized controlled trial. *JAMA.* 2004;291:1603–1609.

Chapter 9

Abdominal trauma

Graciela Bauzá and Andrew B. Peitzman

Introduction

The patient with abdominal injury represents a multitude of challenges to the intensivist. In the trauma patient, the abdomen is defined as the area between the nipples and the symphysis pubis. Understanding injury patterns increases the likelihood of timely diagnosis and treatment of injuries. The corollary is avoidance of missed injury. Missed abdominal injury is a common cause of preventable morbidity and mortality in the trauma patient. The trauma intensivist must understand, recognize, and anticipate potential injury complexes and their complications.

The intent of this chapter is to review the basics of abdominal trauma and emphasize the vital role that the intensivist plays in the care of the trauma patient. The organization of the chapter presents mechanisms of injury followed by specific intra-abdominal organ injury with discussion of diagnosis and management.

Initial assessment

The initial assessment of the trauma patient in the intensive care unit (ICU) begins with reassessment of Airway, Breathing, and Circulation (ABC). The trauma patient arrives to the ICU from the trauma bay, operating room, angiography suite, or emergency department. Based upon patient physiology on emergency department presentation, different levels of detailed examination and attention to life-threatening and non-life-threatening injuries may have occurred. While the primary survey is always performed in the trauma bay, the secondary and tertiary surveys involve detailed physical examination (i.e., extremity injuries, motor/sensory deficits) that, in cases of critically ill patients, may be deferred until the patient is in the ICU. Missed injuries are more common in hemodynamically unstable patients. It is the responsibility of the trauma team, with the help of the ICU team, to complete the patient workup.

Initial resuscitation of the trauma patient with potential abdominal trauma is similar to that of all other trauma patients with important caveats. First, intravenous access should be supradiaphragmatic (i.e., subclavian, internal jugular, or antecubital fossa) given the potential that abdominal vascular injuries such as liver, inferior vena cava (IVC), iliac arteries/veins, or aorta will result in fluid infusion into the abdominal compartment creating further complications and ineffective resuscitation.

Second, critically ill trauma patients who have suffered intra-abdominal hemorrhage are typically cold, coagulopathic, and acidotic, a potentially lethal state referred to as the *triad of death*. As part of the preparation to receive the trauma patient, the ICU room is usually set to 28°C and fluids are warmed and delivered via rapid infuser with a warmer. It is important to keep in mind that trauma patients die from abnormal physiology. One should not focus on defining every anatomic injury in a critically ill trauma patient; for example, an MRI for completion of the cervical spine can wait until homeostasis has been restored.

The most important aspect of patient care, communication, is essential in this setting. Physician-physician and physician-nurse transition-of-care from the trauma team regarding injuries of concern and further potential interventions is essential for good patient care. Lines of communication between the ICU teams and the surgical teams must be established and a relationship of trust nurtured. In addition, the constant presence of the intensivist at the bedside serves as a liaison with critically ill trauma patients and their families.

Blunt trauma

Blunt mechanisms of injury include motor vehicle collision (MVC), motorcycle collision (MCC), pedestrians struck by vehicles, blast and crush injury, and fall from a height. Intra-abdominal injury in these scenarios occurs mostly from compression and shearing forces on the tissues. Solid organ injury is most common: liver, spleen, kidney, or mesentery. In these circumstances, seatbelts not only save lives, but change injury patterns. For instance, intestinal perforation or mesenteric injury is common in the restrained victim of a motor vehicle collision; in fact, it is present in one in four of patients with a lap belt mark.

The initial assessment of the trauma patient with potential abdominal trauma begins with the ABCs. Examination of the abdomen should include observation for ecchymosis, distention (which can be air-filled bowel or hemoperitoneum), tympany or dullness to percussion, and peritoneal signs. The Focused Assessment with Sonography for Trauma (FAST) should be preformed, focusing on the presence or absence of intra-abdominal fluid (presumably blood). In a hemodynamically unstable patient, the presence of fluid may indicate the urgent need for a laparotomy. Conversely, in the stable patient, the FAST may not immediately change management, but it may alert the clinician to potential deterioration and provide baseline findings for later comparison.

Based on the injuries identified externally and radiographically, as well as hemodynamic status, patients typically undergo computed tomography (CT) from head to midthigh, including the abdomen and pelvis. Imaging of the abdominal and pelvic cavities has multiple goals: identify solid organ injury and its severity (Table 9.1), vascular injury, and the presence of free air or free fluid in the pelvis. For these reasons, CT is obtained in an arterial phase and a venous phase.

Table 9.1 Solid organ injury scale			
		Description of Injury	
Grade	**Type of Injury**	**Liver**	**Spleen**
I	Hematoma	Subcapsular, < 10% surface area	Subcapsular, < 10% surface area
	Laceration	Capsular tear, < 1cm parenchymal depth	Capsular tear, < 1 cm parenchymal depth
II	Hematoma	Subcapsular, 10%–50% surface area; intraparenchymal, < 10 cm in diameter	Subcapsular, 10%–50% surface area; intraparenchymal, < 5cm in diameter
	Laceration	Capsular tear 1–3 cm parenchymal depth, < 10cm in length	Capsular tear, 1–3cm depth that does not involve a trabecular vessel
III	Hematoma	Subcapsular, > 50% surface area of ruptured subcapsular or parenchymal hematoma; intraparenchymal hematoma > 10 cm or expanding	Subcapsular, > 50% surface area or expanding; ruptured subcapsular or parenchymal hematoma; intraparenchymal hematoma ≥ 5cm or expanding
	Laceration	> 3 cm parenchymal depth	> 3cm parenchymal depth or involving trabecular vessels
IV	Laceration	Parenchymal disruption involving 25%–75% hepatic lobe or 1–3 Couinaud's segments	Laceration involving segmental or hilar vessels producing major devascularization (> 25% of spleen)
V	Laceration	Parenchymal disruption involving > 75% of hepatic lobe or > 3 Couinaud's segments within a single lobe	Completely shattered spleen
	Vascular	Juxtahepatic venous injuries; for example, involving the retrohepatic vena cava/central major hepatic veins	Hilar vascular injury with devascularized spleen
VI	Vascular	Hepatic avulsion	

Diagnostic peritoneal lavage (DPL) has been supplanted by FAST and CT due to its invasive nature and lack of specificity for organ injury. However, DPL is sensitive for hemoperitoneum and may be appropriate in the unstable patient with a negative or equivocal FAST.

Over the last two decades, a marked shift in paradigm toward nonoperative management of most solid organ (liver, spleen, pancreas, and kidney) injuries in hemodynamically stable patients has occurred. This shift has increased the number of patients admitted to the ICU for close monitoring (hemodynamics, serial abdominal exams, and hemoglobin/hematocrit checks) and increased the responsibility of intensivists to identify failure of nonoperative management.

Liver

Diagnosis of liver injury is generally made by CT or laparotomy. In hemodynamically stable patients, liver injury is managed nonoperatively with serial hemoglobin checks, liver enzymes, and repeat CT at 48 hours for high-grade lacerations (Grade 4–5) or with any unexplained hemodynamic compromise. Although the liver is the most commonly injured abdominal organ, mortality from liver injuries (~10%) has decreased dramatically over the last few decades with the transition to nonoperative management.

As mentioned above, exploratory laparotomy is indicated for hemodynamically unstable patients, not responsive to fluid resuscitation, with positive FAST. Under these circumstances, the conduct of the operation is damage control, that is, the liver and other sites of bleeding are packed, arterial bleeding is managed with ligation or repair, and contamination is controlled. The patient is then taken immediately to the ICU for restoration of homeostasis. High-grade liver lacerations involving injury to the hepatic veins or the retrohepatic IVC carry a high mortality rate. If arterial bleeding is suspected intraoperatively, postoperative angiography/embolization may be necessary. Liver necrosis is not unexpected after significant embolization. This may be complicated by abscess formation.

Biliary injury (extrahepatic bile leak or intrahepatic bile collection) is more likely to occur with high-grade injury; occurring in up to 20% of patients managed nonoperatively. If a bile leak is suspected, a hydroxy iminodiacetic acid (HIDA) scan can be obtained for diagnosis followed by endoscopic retrograde cholangiopancreatography (ERCP) with common bile duct stent and sphincterotomy. This intervention decreases resistance of bile flow, preferentially draining via the common bile duct into the duodenum instead of the hepatic parenchyma or peritoneal cavity. With a large biloma or bile peritonitis, percutaneous drainage of the fluid collection is necessary in addition to ERCP. Uncontrolled bile leakage with peritonitis requires exploration.

Spleen

With the advent of ultrasound, the use of FAST during the initial assessment has become an invaluable tool in hemodynamically unstable patients. Free fluid during FAST, particularly in the splenorenal recess, potentially signifies splenic injury. As discussed above, hemodynamically unstable patients with positive

FAST are taken immediately for laparotomy. Stable patients undergo CT for characterization of injuries (Table 9.1). Splenic injury Grades 1–3 are routinely managed nonoperatively, particularly in children. In the mid-1990s, multiple studies, spurred by the high success rate in children, reported successful nonoperative management of splenic trauma in adults (90%–95%). In 2000, the Eastern Association for the Surgery of Trauma published their multi-institutional study showing that it was safe to observe hemodynamically stable patients with splenic injury Grades 1–3. Over 75% of patients with Grades 4 and 5 required immediate laparotomy with splenectomy or splenorrhaphy. The key criterion for safe observation was hemodynamic stability. Failure of observation was 10%; higher grade splenic injury had greater risk of failure. Sixty percent of patients who failed observation did so within 24 hours; 90% within 72 hours of injury.

Angioembolization is an adjunct for hemodynamically stable patients who are admitted for observation of splenic injuries with arterial extravasation on CT. Careful selection of candidates for angiographic intervention is key, because it does carry risk of serious complications including failure to control bleeding, missed injuries, splenic abscess, iatrogenic injury, and acute kidney injury.

Patients with blunt splenic injures managed nonoperatively are initially monitored in the intensive care unit for hemodynamics, serial abdominal exams and hemoglobin checks. At 48 hours, a follow up CT (arterial and porto-venous phase) should be obtained to evaluate for intrasplenic pseudoaneurysm formation. If not identified, splenic pseudoaneurysms may rupture and cause life-threatening hemorrhage.

Laparotomy or angiography with embolization should be considered in patients who exhibit hemodynamic instability or transfusion requirements during the observation period. Although generally successful in older patients (> 55 years), failure of nonoperative management has a higher failure rate in the elderly when compared to younger counterparts. In addition, failure of nonoperative management is usually associated with higher morbidity and mortality.

Patients who undergo either angiographic embolization or splenectomy should continue to be managed postoperatively in the ICU. Patients who have undergone splenectomy or splenic embolization, or who have a high-grade laceration, should receive immunizations for Neisseria meningitidis, Streptococcus pneumoniae, and Hemophilus influenza by within 2 weeks of surgery or prior to discharge. The incidence of overwhelming postsplenectomy infection (OPSI) after trauma is < 1%; however, OPSI carries a high mortality rate.

Pancreas

Pancreatic injury occurs in 12% of abdominal trauma. Pancreatic injury is difficult to diagnose because it often is not clinically evident. Diagnosis is often delayed, leading to major complications. Early deaths are usually due to associated injuries to adjacent organs or to vascular injury. In 2009, the American Association for the Surgery of Trauma (AAST) conducted a multi-institutional study that found that the sensitivity of 64-slice CT for pancreatic injury and pancreatic duct injury was only 47% and 52%, respectively. Elevated serum amylase and lipase are neither sensitive nor specific. Isolated pancreatic injury does not cause initial hemodynamic instability but can cause a delayed systemic inflammatory response and sepsis. Delayed operative management of pancreatic injury leads to 2–3 times increased morbidity. Mortality from pancreatic injury alone is < 20%. If pancreatic injury is suspected, magnetic resonance cholangiopancreatography (MRCP) can be obtained; however, laparotomy must be performed to confirm diagnosis and treat. Parenchymal contusions are treated by drainage. Injury to the head of the pancreas may often be treated by wide drainage as definitive treatment, but ductal injury in the body or tail of the pancreas generally requires resection in addition to drainage. Complications after pancreatic injury include pancreatitis, peripancreatic abscess, pseudocyst, and pancreatic fistula (7%–35%). The greatest surgical challenge occurs when the head of the pancreas and the nearby duodenum are injured, leading to mortality in ~40%.

Kidney

Approximately 90% of renal injuries result from MVCs. Diagnosis of renal trauma depends upon the patients' hemodynamic status. In stable patients, urinalysis is the first diagnostic step. Hematuria is the most common sign of renal injury, but the degree of hematuria does not correlate with the degree of injury. A positive urinalysis, although not specific, requires further investigation. CT with arterial and porto-venous phase plus delayed imaging is the best diagnostic tool. Intravenous contrast can accurately diagnose renal contusion, laceration, perinephric hematoma, and renal pelvis injury. Delayed imaging is useful in the detection of urinary extravasation. Hemodynamically stable patients warrant a period of observation. Active extravasation of intravenous contrast in stable patients may be managed by angioembolization. Surgical intervention is required in hemodynamically unstable patients with renal pedicle avulsion injuries or expanding perinephric/retroperitoneal hematoma. Urinary extravasation is not a mandatory indication for exploration because most cases resolve spontaneously. If intervention is necessary for persistent urinary extravasation, urinoma, or perinephric abscess, an endoscopic approach with ureteral stenting or percutaneous drainage will suffice.

Hollow viscus (stomach, intestine, bladder)

Hollow viscus injury results from compression that exerts higher than tolerated bursting pressures. Although a rare occurrence (~1%), its diagnosis remains a difficult one. CT (with or without oral contrast) is a poor predictor of small-bowel injury with a false-negative rate up to 15%. Findings suggestive of small-bowel injury include free fluid, free air, and bowel-wall thickening. Eighty-four percent of blunt-trauma patients with free fluid in the abdomen, but no solid organ injury on CT, have some type of intestinal injury, but only 30% of those have full-thickness perforation. Moreover, a negative CT scan does not exclude intestinal perforation. Thus, when there is free fluid in the abdomen without solid organ injury, intestinal/mesenteric injury is present until proven otherwise by surgical exploration. Associated injuries on physical exam include seatbelt or tire marks across the chest or abdomen and abdominal wall contusion or degloving. A Chance fracture (lumbar flexion/compression fracture) secondary to a lap belt has associated intestinal injury in 30% of patients. Delay to operative intervention of hollow-viscus perforation leads to a greater mortality, as well as postoperative incidence of intra-abdominal abscess, sepsis, and wound dehiscence. With delay in diagnosis, overall mortality after small bowel injury can be as high as 19%. Early exploration with control of intestinal contamination reduces morbidity and mortality significantly. The stomach (< 2%) and colon/rectum (2%–5%) are injured less commonly in blunt trauma, but also require prompt diagnosis and exploration. Bladder rupture may be intra- or extra-peritoneal. These can be differentiated by CT or formal cystogram. Extraperitoneal rupture can be managed generally with Foley-catheter bladder decompression for 10–14 days. Intraperitoneal rupture requires laparotomy and repair along with Foley-catheter bladder decompression.

Diaphragm

Diaphragmatic laceration or rupture occurs most commonly after MVCs. Usually located on the left side due to the protective effect of the liver on the right side of the diaphragm, it is difficult to diagnose. It is found on initial CXR only 40% of the time. CT often is not useful unless there is herniation of abdominal contents into the thoracic cavity on presentation. Clinical evidence of diaphragmatic injury includes diminished breath sounds or presence of bowel sounds on the affected side, respiratory distress, or high airway pressures if intubated. If suspected, either clinically or radiographically, laparoscopy or laparotomy should be performed for prompt repair. Diaphragmatic injury is associated with other abdominal injuries in 60%–80% of cases.

Vascular (aorta, IVC, hepatic veins, iliac vessels, mesenteric vessels)

Vascular injury can most commonly be diagnosed by CT arteriography. Patients with compromised circulation to abdominal structures, secondary to intimal flaps, clots, etc., should be placed in the ICU for serial abdominal exams and hemoglobin checks. Pulsatile or expanding hematomas require surgical exploration. Angioembolization can be utilized in selected injuries (e.g., liver, spleen, kidney, internal iliac arteries) in hemodynamically stable patients.

Penetrating trauma

Penetrating trauma mechanisms include gunshot wound (GSW), knife or stab wound (SW), and less commonly, impalement. Unlike blunt injury, most penetrating injuries require exploration. Laparoscopy can be performed in hemodynamically stable patients to confirm penetration of the abdomen by an anterior abdominal wall SW. Transperitoneal GSWs to the abdomen have unpredictable trajectories and require exploration in nearly all cases. If the trajectory is felt to be tangential, CT of the abdomen may be helpful.

Liver

Penetrating injury to the liver results in bleeding and bile leaks. Penetrating injury to the liver can usually be managed as described previously for blunt trauma. A decreasing hematocrit without overt evidence of hemorrhage must clue the clinician to potentially fatal complications such as hemobilia (arterial/venous-biliary fistula) or bleeding from pseudoaneurysms. Angioembolization of the involved hepatic artery branch can be very effective management.

Spleen

Penetrating injuries to the spleen are often the result of GSW to the abdomen. In such cases a splenectomy should usually be performed during exploratory laparotomy. Injury secondary to SW may be managed by splenorrhaphy in the stable patient.

Pancreas

Due to its central location, injury to the pancreas usually involves other organs. The immediate threat to life is associated vascular injury and the late threat is sepsis from pancreatic or hollow-viscus injury. In most cases of significant injury, damage control surgery is performed and final resection and reconstruction is delayed 24–48 hours. If the injury is distal (i.e., left of the superior mesenteric artery), distal pancreatectomy may be performed in hemodynamically stable patients.

Kidney

Penetrating injury, particularly GSW, is more likely than blunt injury to require surgical exploration and nephrectomy. Higher grade injuries carry higher nephrectomy rates. Renal hilum injury, such as avulsion or devascularization, requires nephrectomy as exsanguination is sudden. The diagnosis and management of penetrating injury to the kidneys is similar to that of blunt trauma. However, hemodynamically unstable patients need a laparotomy, not CT imaging; an intravenous pyelogram can be performed in the operating room if needed.

Hollow viscus (stomach, intestine, bladder)

Injury to the stomach (10%–15%), small intestine (5%–15%), or colon/rectum (5%–25%) should be treated by repair, resection, or, at times, diversion. Careful examination is required because multiple injuries can occur from a single SW or GSW, increasing the likelihood of missed injuries. Patients with significant peritoneal contamination are at high risk for sepsis, ileus, bowel repair/anastomotic leak, wound dehiscence, and abdominal compartment syndrome. Hemodynamically unstable patients with multiple abdominal injuries, such as vascular and intestinal injuries, are the typical candidates for damage control surgery. In these cases, the intestines are usually left in discontinuity after contamination is controlled. These patients must remain *nil per os* until intestinal continuity is restored. Bladder injury is managed in a similar fashion in both blunt and penetrating mechanisms of injury.

Diaphragm

Injury to the diaphragm after penetrating trauma tends to be much smaller than after blunt trauma. Clinical or radiographic diagnosis of diaphragmatic laceration after SW or GSW to the upper abdomen or thorax is nearly impossible as the lacerations are usually small and without herniation into the thoracic cavity upon presentation. Exploration of both diaphragms during laparoscopy or laparotomy is crucial to the diagnosis. Missed lacerations result in the development of diaphragmatic hernias, which may present on the same admission or years later with incarcerated bowel.

Vascular (aorta, IVC, hepatic veins, iliac vessels, mesenteric vessels)

Vascular injury secondary to penetrating trauma is challenging as patients often present in extremis. These patients require immediate exploration and ligation, repair, bypass, or temporary shunting of vessels if damage control is performed. Repair or ligation of the vena cava or iliac vessels may result in congestion or ischemia of the buttocks and lower extremities leading to compartment syndrome. The intensivist must be aware of such potential complications in patients who have not undergone prophylactic fasciotomies.

Critical care challenges in the multi-trauma patient

Abdominal compartment syndrome (ACS)

In 2004 and 2007 The World Society of the Abdominal Compartment Syndrome developed consensus definitions, diagnostic criteria, and treatment algorithms based on the best clinical evidence.

- Definitions
    - o Intra-abdominal pressure (IAP): pressure within the abdominal cavity (normal IAP is 5–7 mmHg in ICU population)
    - o Abdominal perfusion pressure (APP): mean arterial pressure—intra-abdominal pressure (APP = MAP – IAP)
    - o Intra-abdominal hypertension (IAH): IAP >= 12 mmHg
    - o Abdominal compartment syndrome (ACS): sustained IAP > 20 mmHg (with or without an APP < 60 mmHg) associated with new organ dysfunction/failure secondary to decreased end-organ perfusion. Intra-abdominal hypertension affects multiple systems in a vicious cycle, which uninterrupted culminates in multiple-system organ dysfunction.

- Classification
  - o *Primary ACS*: associated with injury or pathology within the abdominal cavity (e.g., intra-abdominal hemorrhage, intra-abdominal sepsis, ischemic bowel, ileus, severe pancreatitis, postoperative state)
  - o *Secondary ACS*: associated with conditions that do not originate in the abdominal cavity (e.g., massive fluid resuscitation)
  - o *Recurrent ACS*: ACS that occurs after surgical decompression, prior to or after definitive closure
- Etiology: Common etiologies include major abdominal trauma, massive fluid/colloid resuscitation, burns, ruptured abdominal aortic aneurysm, intra/retroperitoneal hemorrhage, pancreatitis, intestinal ileus/obstruction/edema, and abdominal surgery. Risk factors for the development of ACS include abdominal surgery/trauma, fluid resuscitation > 5L/24h, ileus, pulmonary/renal/liver dysfunction, hypothermia, acidosis, and anemia.
- Clinical manifestations are the best diagnostic tool for abdominal compartment syndrome. Direct end-organ compression combined with decreased cardiac output from abdominal compartment syndrome has a mortality rate of 42%–68% when diagnosed; 100% if left untreated. Physical examination of the abdomen is not a sensitive diagnostic tool for IAH. Pertinent physical exam findings include:
  - o Neurological—potential increase in intracranial pressure secondary to decreased internal jugular venous drainage, important in patients with traumatic brain injury
  - o Pulmonary—high peak airway pressures (> 40 cm H_2O) and decreased functional residual capacity secondary to elevated diaphragm with poor excursion. Ultimately results in hypoxia, hypercapnia, and respiratory acidosis
  - o Cardiovascular—decreased venous return and falsely elevated filling pressures from abdominal hypertension and elevated intrathoracic pressure leads to decreased cardiac output and end-organ perfusion
  - o Gastrointestinal—IAH also leads to splanchnic hypoperfusion, bowel ischemia, and potential bacterial translocation
  - o Renal—oliguria and decreased glomerular filtration rate secondary to renal compression and decreased cardiac output; one of the first signs of ACS
- Diagnosis: The standard method is measurement of bladder pressure via a pressure transducer (Table 9.2). If IAH is suspected, serial bladder pressures are recommended.
- Management: Multiple strategies to decrease intra-abdominal pressure involve medical and surgical approaches. Recommendations for management are listed starting with the strongest available evidence.
  - o Laparotomy with temporary closure: Abdominal decompression is the **only** treatment for ACS once end-organ dysfunction is present.

Table 9.2 Technique for intra-abdominal pressure measurement
1. Place patient in supine position.
2. Zero system at midaxillary line and iliac crest.
3. Clamp Foley catheter distal to aspiration port and instill 25 mL of sterile saline into bladder via Foley catheter.
4. Insert 16-gauge needle and connect to transducer/pressure monitoring device.
5. Measure pressure (mmHg) at end-expiration 30–60 seconds after instillation to allow for detrusor muscle relaxation.
6. Repeat serial measurements as needed.

The intra-abdominal organs are allowed to eviscerate and a temporary closure device is placed on the abdomen (e.g., vacuum-assisted closure [VAC], "Bogota bag," etc.). *Reperfusion syndrome* is a known postoperative complication with its effects ranging from hemodynamic instability to cardiac arrest. The administration of mannitol and bicarbonate prior to decompression may be of benefit. In extreme situations when patients cannot tolerate transport to the operating room, the abdomen may be opened at the bedside in the ICU by surgeons. This may not be a good approach if ACS is secondary to intra-abdominal hemorrhage, as the ICU is not equipped to handle this. As fluid resuscitation continues in patients with temporary or definitive abdominal closures, recurrent ACS can occur. Preemptive "open abdomen" is usually exercised in patients undergoing damage control surgery or in those at high risk for ACS at the time of surgical exploration.

o Abdominal perfusion pressure: Studies suggest increased survival with APP ≥ 50 mmHg. Adequate perfusion pressure varies from patient to patient due to age and comorbidities. Nonetheless, a careful combination of fluids and vasopressors is a prudent strategy to maintain APP in the 50–60 mmHg range.

o Fluid management: Aggressive intravenous resuscitation with isotonic fluids is a major cause of secondary ACS as a result of third-spacing and visceral edema. When massive resuscitation is anticipated, focusing on blood product replacement is recommended, minimizing crystalloids. Restrictive fluid administration should be practiced in patients with IAH or at risk for ACS. There is no evidence for the use of diuretics or intermittent dialysis in hemodynamically stable patients. Nevertheless, fluid removal is key in the medical management of oliguric/anuric patients who may respond to diuretic therapy or continuous renal replacement therapy.

o Additional medical management of IAH includes sedation, analgesia, pharmacologic paralysis, body positioning, intestinal decompression, and percutaneous decompression of the abdomen. Judicious use of neuromuscular blockade in conjunction with adequate sedation and analgesia may help

IAH; however, the benefits must outweigh the risks. Elevation of the head of the bed > 30° in the ICU is standard for prevention of aspiration. When compared to supine positioning, head-of-bed elevation causes proportional increase in IAP. Ileus or bowel obstruction is not an uncommon occurrence in ICU patients at risk for ACS. Decompression of intraluminal intestinal contents via nasogastric or rectal tubes can also reduce intra-abdominal pressure. Percutaneous drainage of intra-abdominal fluid such as ascites or abscesses may also reduce IAP. It is important to remember that these are adjunct measures for the treatment of IAH and prevention of ACS. Close monitoring of urine output and serial (q4–6h) bladder pressures along with these medical strategies may help prevent the transition from IAH without end-organ damage to ACS with renal dysfunction and intestinal ischemia.

Damage control surgery: Damage control is the global approach taken toward the patient in extremis. Life-threatening injuries are addressed first as dictated by the patient's physiologic reserve. Operation of any kind can increase physiologic stress. Damage control is not specific to abdominal catastrophe; it applies to the critically injured multi-trauma patient. Injuries are prioritized and treatment is staged as dictated by physiological state.

- Indications: Multiply injured patients with intra-abdominal injury along with hemodynamic instability, acidosis, hypothermia, massive transfusion or non-surgical bleeding (coagulopathy).
- Procedure: Damage control surgery is a staged operation carried out over the course of 48 hours to several days.
- Goals:
  o Operative control of hemorrhage and contamination (intestinal contents, pus) by packing, temporary shunting of vessels, bowel resection without anastomosis. The abdomen is left open for a second look in 24 to 48 hours.
  o Aggressive resuscitation in the ICU, correction of coagulopathy and acidosis, and core rewarming. Most important in the ICU is the prompt management of hypothermia, coagulopathy, and metabolic acidosis. Hematocrit checks must be accompanied by coagulation panels. Most bleeding is caused by missed injury or technical error, but not all bleeding is surgical. Nonsurgical bleeding (coagulopathy) must be addressed aggressively.
  o Operative re-exploration with more detailed look at injuries, definitive or partial repair of injuries (i.e., bowel anastomosis, pack removal, vessel ligation/bypass) depending upon the patient's reserve, may take more than one operation. The abdomen may be left open or closed depending upon completion of definitive repair.
- Complications of damage control surgery (DCS): While DCS is lifesaving, morbidity is traded for mortality. Important complications include:
  o Intra-abdominal abscess
  o Anastomotic leak
  o Abdominal compartment syndrome

o Gastrointestinal fistula—Abnormal communication between the intestines and the skin surface (i.e., entero-cutaneous fistula) or the atmosphere is not uncommon after DCS—secondary to continued exposure of intestines to open air or artificial materials (e.g., packing), which causes desiccation, abrasion from frequent dressing changes, and suction from vacuum-assisted devices (Figure 9.1).

o Inability to definitively close the abdomen resulting in a ventral hernia necessitating delayed reconstruction.

Open abdomen: The open abdomen is the by-product of damage control surgery and abdominal compartment syndrome. It refers to a patient whose abdominal fascia is left temporarily in discontinuity for the purpose of re-exploration, prevention of ACS in patients who will require massive resuscitation, or as treatment of ACS. In all scenarios, the abdomen is temporarily closed. There are numerous methods of temporary closure. Temporary closure techniques aim to control third-space fluid and allow swelling of intestines during resuscitation. These devices usually consist of a nonadhesive barrier that covers the intestines while allowing excess fluid to be suctioned via superficial drains. Currently, the most common device is the VAC, which uses a sponge as means of suction to collect fluid and pull fascia and skin edges together (Figures 9.2 a–d). Initially, patients with an open

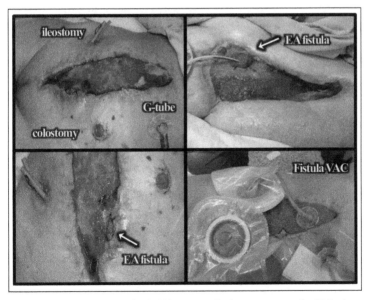

Figure 9.1 Entero-atmospheric fistula. Abbreviations: G-tube=gastrostomy tube; EA fistula= entero-atmospheric fistula; Fistula VAC= fistula vacuum-assisted closure

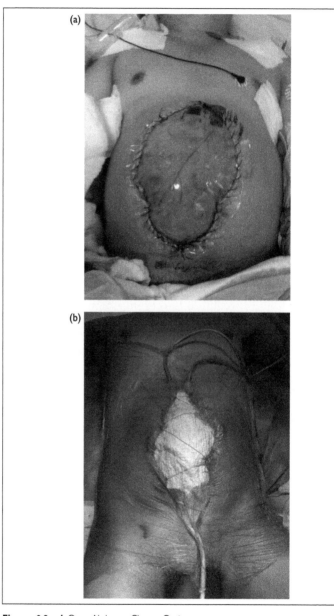

Figures 9.2a–d Open Abdomen Closure Options
a. Bogotá bag
b. Custom drain suction closure device

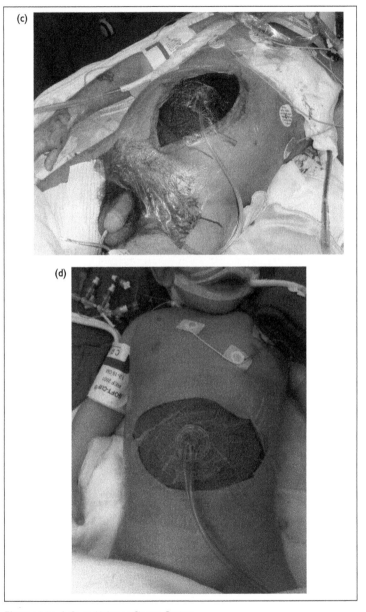

Figures 9.2c–d Open Abdomen Closure Options
c. Vacuum-assisted Closure Device (KCI®)
d. ABThera™ (KCI®)

abdomen are generally managed with adequate sedation and analgesia. Rarely is neuromuscular blockade required. If tolerated, judicious fluid removal may decrease visceral edema and increase the likelihood of primary closure of the abdomen. Timing of closure is key. Ideally, the abdomen is closed within 72 hours prior to the development of visceral edema by reapproximating fascia, leaving the skin open. Primary fascial closure becomes more challenging as edema develops in the intestines and internal organs after 5–7 days and there is loss of abdominal domain. If fascial closure is not possible, skin only closure with future plans to repair the resultant ventral hernia is the next best option. Skin grafting and biologic meshes can be used for closure when fascial or skin-only closure is no longer an option. Subsequent fascial reconstruction can be accomplished when the patient is completely recovered, usually 12 months later.

Summary

Major abdominal injury is rarely isolated. These patients pose a difficult challenge to the trauma surgeon and the intensivist who care for them. Complete evaluation of injuries does not end in the trauma bay. Postoperative and nonoperatively managed patients are in constant evolution and are at risk of serious complications. A high index of suspicion for missed injuries must be present at all times. Close monitoring and correction of temperature derangements, coagulation profile, hematocrit, and metabolic acidosis are essential to patient survival. Any change in hemodynamic status or abdominal exam requires consideration for surgical intervention.

Key references

Cheatham ML, Malbrain MLNG, Kirkpatrick A, et al. Results from the International Conference of Experts on Intra-abdominal Hypertension and Abdominal Compartment Syndrome. II. Recommendations. *Intensive Care Med.* 2007;33:951–962.

EAST guidelines for the diagnosis and management of pancreatic trauma. 2009. Available at: http://www.east.org.

Fakhry SM, Watts DD, Luchette FA, for the EAST Multi-Institutional HVI Research Group. Current diagnostic approaches lack sensitivity in the diagnosis of perforated blunt small bowel injury: analysis from 275,557 trauma admissions from the EAST Multi-Institutional HVI Trial. *J Trauma.* 2003;54:295–306.

Pape HC, Tornetta P 3rd, Tarkin I, et al. Timing of fracture fixation in multitrauma patients: the role of early total care and damage control surgery. *J Am Acad Orthop Surg* 2009;17:541–549.

Peitzman AB, Heil B, Rivera L, et al. Blunt splenic injury in adults: multi-institutional study of the Eastern Association for the Surgery of Trauma. *J Trauma.* 2000;49:177–187.

Peitzman AB, Rhodes M, Schwab CW, Yealy DM. *The Trauma Manual: Trauma and Acute Care Surgery.* 3rd ed. Lippincott Williams and Wilkins, Philadelphia, 2007.

Peitzman AB, Richardson JD. Surgical treatment of injuries to the solid abdominal organs: A 50-year perspective from the *Journal of Trauma*. *J Trauma*. 2010;69:1011–1021.

Phelan HA, Velmahos GC, Jurkovich GJ, et al. An evaluation of multidetector computer tomography in detecting pancreatic injury: results of a multicenter AAST study. *J Trauma*. 2009;66:641–646.

Santucci RA, Wessells H, Bartsch G, et al. Evaluation and management of renal injuries: consensus statement of the renal trauma subcommittee. *BJU International*. 2004;93:937–954.

Chapter 10

Soft tissue trauma and rhabdomyolysis

Paula Ferrada

Introduction

Rhabdomyolysis is the breakdown of muscle fibers with leakage of intracellular contents into the systemic circulation. The result of this extracellular rush of intracellular contents is multi-systemic. One of the devastating consequences of this disease is renal failure. This is due to decreased renal perfusion, cast formation with tubular obstruction, and the direct toxic effects of myoglobin on the renal tubules. Trauma, particularly crush injury, is the most common predisposing factor for this disease.

Traditionally the teaching is that muscle pain is a landmark of developing rhabdomyolysis. However, as a consequence of blunt trauma, it is almost impossible to distinguish pain from this disease from the pain of contusion. In one study in adults, Gabow found that only 50% of patients initially complained of muscle pain and only a minority of patients reported dark discoloration of the urine.

Because the clinical symptoms of this disease are subtle until the repercussions are irreversible, it is imperative to have a high level of suspicion to be able to make the diagnosis.

Any patient with crush injury or/and a large amount of muscle compromise from soft tissue injury must be treated for rhabdomyolysis until proven otherwise.

Crush syndrome

After muscle compression is relieved or vascular interruption is corrected, the cellular contents of the affected muscle tissue are released into the circulation. Large volumes of intravascular fluid also can be sequestered in the involved extremities because of increased capillary permeability. The systemic manifestations of rhabdomyolysis, caused by hypovolemia and toxin exposure, are the components of the crush syndrome.

Diagnosis

As mentioned previously, the diagnosis of rhabdomyolysis requires a high index of suspicion. Definitive diagnosis is made by laboratory evaluation. The most useful measurement is serum creatine kinase (CK). This assay is widely available and 100% sensitive. Rhabdomyolysis has been previously defined as total CK levels 5–10 times above normal. Total CK elevation is a sensitive but nonspecific marker for rhabdomyolysis. Levels of less than 5000 U/liter are typically not associated with a risk for acute kidney injury. The CK level may increase from the initial values with reperfusion of the muscle; repeat total CK levels should be drawn serially until a peak level is established. Patients with other disorders, such as acute myocardial infarction and acute stroke, may have high CK levels. Serum CK levels peak within 24 hours and should decrease after the initial insult. Persistent elevation suggests continuing muscle injury or development of a compartment syndrome.

Lactate dehydrogenase (LDH) and aspartate aminotransferase (AST) are nonspecific enzyme markers that also are elevated in patients with rhabdomyolysis. Elevations of cardiac troponin have also been reported. In such circumstances, electrocardiography (ECG), and possibly echocardiography, should be considered to rule out a cardiac source.

Hyperkalemia occurs in 10%–40% of cases. ECG may reveal changes of acute hyperkalemia, including peaked T waves, prolongation of the PR and QRS intervals, loss of the P wave or a "sine wave" appearance. High potassium can cause life-threatening dysrhythmias and death, especially in the setting of acute kidney injury, which can develop in up to 40% of the cases.

It is important to make sure the patient with rhabdomyolysis does not have any underlying reason to have a coagulopathy, because thromboplastin released from injured myocytes can cause disseminated intravascular coagulation.

Compartment syndrome is usually a preventable complication of a crush injury or ischemia/reperfusion. Though compartment syndrome is a clinical diagnosis, many trauma patients with multiple injuries can't specify tenderness in specific areas. It is therefore important to measure the pressures in any suspicious compartments in patients with trauma and rhabdomyolysis. Pressures above 25–30 mm Hg, particularly when sustained, are concerning.

Treatment

Intravenous fluid hydration with isotonic crystalloid is the most important step in the therapy for rhabdomyolysis. Retrospective studies of patients with severe crush injuries resulting in rhabdomyolysis suggest that the prognosis is better when prehospital personnel provide fluid resuscitation. Support of the intravascular volume increases the glomerular filtration rate (GFR) and oxygen delivery. Intravenous fluids dilute myoglobin and other renal tubular toxins. However, there may be a fine line between adequate resuscitation and fluid overload, particularly if acute kidney injury ensues. Some type of invasive or functional hemodynamic monitoring, such as use of central venous pressure measurements, pulse contour cardiac output devices, or echocardiography with inferior vena cava measurements can guide fluid resuscitation.

In one review, predictors for the development of renal failure included peak CK level more than 6000 IU/L, dehydration (hematocrit > 50, serum sodium level > 150 mEq/L, orthostasis, pulmonary wedge pressure < 5 mm Hg, urinary fractional excretion of sodium < 1%), sepsis, hyperkalemia or hyperphosphatemia on admission, and the presence of hypoalbuminemia. Acute kidney injury has occasionally developed in severely dehydrated patients with peak CK level as low as 2000 IU/L.

To prevent renal failure, some advocate urine alkalinization, mannitol, and loop diuretics in addition to aggressive hydration. Urinary alkalinization to prevent the development of acute renal failure in patients with rhabdomyolysis has been supported by animal studies and small, retrospective human studies; prospective randomized human studies are lacking. Urinary alkalinization may be considered for patients with rhabdomyolysis and CK levels in excess of 6000 IU/L. Alkalinization should be considered earlier in patients with acidemia, dehydration, or underlying renal disease.

Only after establishing adequate intravascular volume should diuretic therapy be considered. Mannitol may be administered to enhance renal perfusion. Loop diuretics may be used to enhance urinary output in oliguric patients, despite adequate intravascular volume. Similar to alkalinization, the use of mannitol or loop diuretics cannot be strongly recommended due to a lack of good prospective studies.

Treatment of hyperkalemia consists of intravenous sodium bicarbonate, glucose, and insulin, as well as hemodialysis. Administration of intravenous calcium is recommended for patients who have ECG changes secondary to hyperkalemia.

Indications for hemodialysis include hyperkalemia that is persistent despite therapy, severe acid-base disturbances, refractory pulmonary edema, and progressive renal failure. There is a limited efficacy and prognostic impact of extracorporeal myoglobin removal by standard blood-purification techniques.

Summary

1. Suspect rhabdomyolysis in any patient with large soft tissue injury, history of crush injury, and/or abrupt interruption of blood flow.
2. CK is very sensitive but not specific, and will peak at 24 hours. Recheck periodically.
3. Watch for hyperkalemia.
4. Resuscitate appropriately with isotonic fluids. The key is prevention of renal failure, keeping in mind that these patients are typically hypovolemic. Alkalinization may be of benefit.

5. Use diuresis *only when the patient has been adequately resuscitated.*
6. Use hemodialysis for the treatment of fluid overload, hyperkalemia, acid-base disturbances, and progressive renal failure.

Key references

Bosch X, Poch E, Grau JM. Rhabdomyolysis and acute kidney injury. *N Engl J Med.* 2009;361(1):62–72.

Fernandez WG, Hung O, Bruno GR, Galea S, Chiang WK. Factors predictive of acute renal failure and need for hemodialysis among ED patients with rhabdomyolysis. *Am J Emerg Med.* 2005;23(1):1–7.

Ferrada P, Murthi S, Anand RJ, Bochicchio G, Scalea T. Transthoracic focused rapid echocardiographic examination (free): real-time evaluation of fluid status in critically ill trauma patients. *J Trauma.* 2011;70(1):56–62.

Gabow PA, Kaehny WD, Kelleher SP. The spectrum of rhabdomyolysis. *Medicine.* 1982;61(3):141–152.

Li SF, Zapata J, Tillem E. The prevalence of false-positive cardiac troponin I in ED patients with rhabdomyolysis. *Am J Emerg Med.* 2005;23(7):860–863.

Malinoski DJ, Slater MS, Mullins RJ. Crush injury and rhabdomyolysis. *Crit Care Clin.* 2004;20(1):171–192.

Minnema BJ, Neligan PC, Quraishi NA, Fehlings MG, Prakash S. A case of occult compartment syndrome and nonresolving rhabdomyolysis. *J Gen Intern Med.* 2008;23(6):871–874.

Chapter 11

Orthopedic trauma

Boris A. Zelle, Peter A. Siska, and Ivan S. Tarkin

General principles of fractures and dislocations

A significant number of trauma patients sustain musculoskeletal injuries. As compared to major head, thoracic, abdominal, and vascular injuries, most musculoskeletal injuries are not immediately life threatening. However, the long-term functional outcomes of polytrauma patients are often predicated on their orthopedic injuries. Thus, thoughtful and timely treatment of fractures and dislocations plays a major role in the management protocol of the severely injured patient.

Clinical signs of fractures include pain, deformity, and loss of limb function. Appropriate description of the specific fracture includes the location (proximal vs. middle vs. distal portion of the involved bone; extra-articular vs. intra-articular), fracture pattern (transverse vs. oblique vs. spiral), and the fracture morphology (two-part vs. comminuted; displaced vs. nondisplaced; angulated vs. nonangulated). These parameters provide important information on the injury mechanism and the energy imparted at the time of injury. Further, accurate fracture classification facilitates communication among treating physicians.

Additional characterization of the fracture is provided by the degree of associated soft tissue trauma. The degree of soft tissue injury is indicative of the risk of compartment syndrome and the risk of postoperative infection following fracture fixation. Fractures are further classified into closed (surrounding skin intact) and open (fracture communicating with external environment). Open fractures represent an orthopedic emergency and require timely surgical irrigation and debridement in an effort to minimize septic complication.

Dislocations are characterized by loss of contact between the mating joint surfaces. The pathophysiology of joint dislocation includes ligamentous and/or capsular disruptions. Further, joint dislocation can occur with associated periarticular fracture (fracture/dislocation). Clinical signs of dislocation include pain, swelling, deformity, and loss of limb function. Dislocations are described according to the direction of the distal part of the joint relative to the proximal segment. Joint dislocations are prone to significant compromise of the surrounding soft tissues and have a high risk of neurovascular injuries. Thus, timely reduction of dislocated joints should be performed at the time of presentation.

Clinical evaluation of fractures and dislocations

In severely traumatized patients, the initial evaluation is typically focused on major life- and limb-threatening injuries. The so-called "minor" orthopedic injuries are all too frequently overlooked during the initial evaluation phase. Despite improvements in trauma protocols up to 15%–20% of "minor" fractures (i.e., hand, foot) are missed during the initial evaluation. However, in many patients, the functional recovery is limited by their orthopedic injuries. For example, functionality of foot and ankle trauma is a major predictor for long-term functionality in the multi-system trauma patient. Thus, careful evaluation for orthopedic injuries, both major and minor, is crucial in multiply injured patients.

The patient's history plays an important role in the orthopedic evaluation. Relevant data include patient complaints, injury mechanism, and the preexisting medical morbidities. The orthopedic physical examination includes a careful inspection of all extremities with particular attention to asymmetries, deformities, swelling, and breaks in the skin. As part of a complete orthopedic examination, the trauma patient needs to be turned onto a lateral decubitus position to appropriately evaluate for spinal and pelvic injuries. All extremities should be palpated and fully examined for focal tenderness, crepitus, firmness of the muscle compartments, and decreased range of motion. A careful neurovascular examination records the quality of peripheral pulses, sensation in all nerve distributions and motor function of all key muscles. If the clinical evaluation of lower extremity pulses is suspicious for injury, the Ankle-Brachial Index (ABI) should be obtained and documented.

Motor strength should be documented according to the Medical Research Council system into grades from 0 to 5 as follows:

5—Complete range of motion against gravity with full resistance
4—Complete range of motion against gravity with some resistance
3—Complete range of motion against gravity
2—Complete range of motion with gravity eliminated
1—Evidence of slight contractility, no joint motion
0—No evidence of contractility

Vigilance in detecting occult orthopedic injuries is of paramount importance. A crucial part of the clinical examination is the repeat evaluation at 24–48 hours after the injury to diagnose potential injuries that were missed during the initial evaluation. At this point, the severely injured patient may be more responsive and able to provide more detailed information on potential areas of musculoskeletal trauma. In addition, swelling and ecchymosis may be more apparent. The examiner may be less distracted as presumably the major injuries have been diagnosed. For this reason, the repeat evaluation should be thorough and complete, including a full evaluation of all body regions.

Radiographic evaluation

As directed by history and physical exam, all musculoskeletal regions that are deemed traumatized deserve an imaging study. Radiographs should always include at least two views at right angles, typically an anteroposterior view and a lateral view. In fractured long-bones it is mandatory to obtain radiographs of the joint above and below the fracture to evaluate for associated joint dislocations and articular extension of the fracture. In some particular situations, stress views may be necessary to assess for joint stability.

Advanced imaging studies, such as computer tomography (CT) scans, magnetic resonance imaging (MRI), or angiograms may be required in some circumstances to complement existing medical data. CT scans are helpful in the assessment of articular injuries, as well as pelvic and acetabular fractures. As CT scans of the head, cervical spine, chest, and abdomen are frequently obtained as part of Advanced Trauma Life Support protocols, the CT scans required for the evaluation of orthopedic injuries should be obtained at the same time in the stable patient. It is important to recognize that appropriate CT evaluation of pelvic and acetabular fractures requires 2.5 mm fine cuts through the pelvis as opposed to 5 mm cuts that are frequently obtained to evaluate for pelvic hemorrhage.

MRI studies are a valuable resource to assess for soft tissue injuries, such as ligament and tendon ruptures. This expensive exam should be ordered by the orthopedic surgeon only when indicated.

Angiograms are an important tool for the evaluation of vascular injuries and should be obtained whenever there is suspicion for a vascular injury. This should be done in consultation with the vascular or trauma surgeon. Certain orthopedic injuries, such as knee dislocations or talus dislocations (Figure 11.1a and 11.1b), are associated with a high risk of vascular injuries, making angiograms an integral part of the workup in these patients.

Acute musculoskeletal management

The initial management of fractures and dislocations in the emergency department serves to stabilize the injured extremity temporarily until definitive treatment can be rendered. Reduction and splinting are the primary treatment modalities on presentation. Reduction is intended to improve the alignment of the affected region. Splinting maintains the alignment after fracture or joint manipulation.

Fractures with significant displacement should be reduced and splinted at the time of presentation under local anesthesia and/or conscious sedation. These maneuvers "stop the cycle of injury." Neglected displaced fractures cause irreversible damage to the surrounding soft tissues. Further, displaced bone spikes can cause secondary neurovascular injuries, or may even broach the skin causing open fractures.

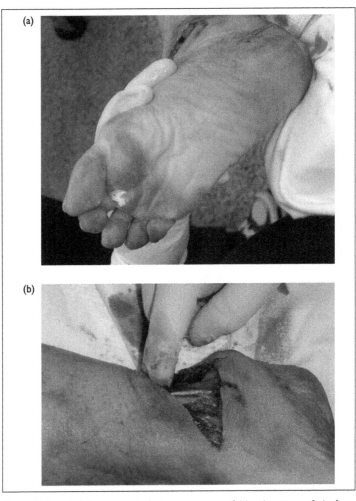

Figure 11.1a and 11.1b Dysvascular foot as consequence of delayed treatment of talar fracture/dislocation (Figure 11.1a). Dislocated talus tenting the neurovascular bundle at the level of the ankle joint (Figure 11.1b)

A well-padded splint should be applied to the reduced fracture. The splint maintains skeletal alignment. Immobilization of the injury is effective for pain control. When applying a splint, it is important to be aware that the sedated and intubated trauma patient has no protective sensation and is at high risk for developing skin compromise. For this reason, the applied splint should be well-padded, particularly over the bony prominences. Further, plaster produces heat when it is curing. Thus, thickness of the plaster should be limited and plaster alone should not directly touch the patient's skin.

Just like fractures with significant displacement, the initial management of dislocated joints typically requires immediate reduction/splinting under local anesthesia or conscious sedation. Significant compromise of the joint surfaces, surrounding soft tissues, and neurovascular structures mandate that dislocated joints be reduced as soon as possible. Irreducible fracture-dislocations typically require immediate surgical treatment to achieve reduction and stabilization.

Open fractures

Open fractures are characterized by bone exposure with the outside environment through a laceration in the skin (Figure 11.2). These injuries are infamous for complications, including nonunion and infection. The Gustilo-Anderson system is the most widely used classification scheme for these injuries (Table 11.1). The increasing open fracture grade suggests a more extensive zone of injury with increasing risk for complications, especially infection.

Immediate tetanus prophylaxis and administration of intravenous antibiotics at the time of diagnosis is mandatory for all open fractures. Delaying administration of antibiotics for more than 3 hours after injury may increase the infection risk. The choice of antibiotics remains controversial. Most protocols suggest a first-generation cephalosporin for 48–72 hours in all grade 1 and grade 2 open fractures. For grade 3 open fractures, most protocols suggest adding an aminoglycoside. For patients with farm injuries and injuries with vascular compromise, penicillin should be added to prevent anaerobic infections, such as clostridial myonecrosis.

Although antibiotic management is a successful adjunct for open fracture care, surgical debridement is essential to prevent limb-threatening infection. Fracture debridement is considered an orthopedic emergency and should be performed in a timely fashion. Debridement should be comprehensive in nature. Gross

Table 11.1 Gustilo-anderson classification of open fractures	
Type	Description
Type I	Wound < 1 cm, clean
Type II	Wound > 1 cm without extensive soft tissue damage
Type III	Extensive soft tissue damage (gunshot wound, farm injury, vascular injury, segmental fracture)
Type IIIA	Extensive soft tissue laceration, adequate soft tissue coverage, irrespective of wound size
Type IIIB	Extensive soft tissue injury, periosteal stripping, bone exposure, massive contamination, inadequate coverage
Type IIIC	Arterial injury requiring repair

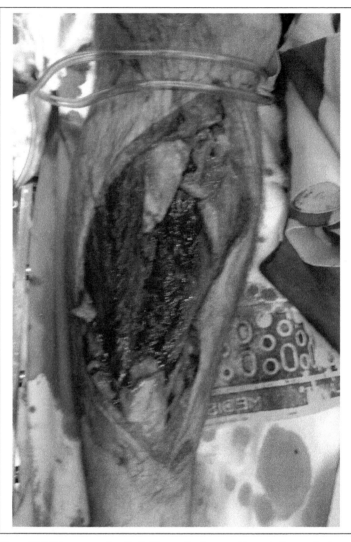

Figure 11.2 Polytrauma patient Grade 3B open tibia fracture with massive bone and soft tissue injury

contamination (i.e., dirt, grass, gravel) should be removed from the wound. All necrotic soft tissues (skin, fat, fascia, muscle) are sequentially debrided. Further, devascularized bone devoid of soft tissue attachment is excised. Any nonviable tissue may become a nidus for infection. After debridement, the wound and bone is cleansed with a mechanical irrigator. Many surgeons choose to add antibiotics, such as bacitracin, polymyxin, or gentamycin, to the irrigation solution.

Open-fracture wounds, which are not amenable to primary closure, are optimally treated with a negative pressure dressing. These dressings prime the wound for healing by secondary attention or with plastics closure procedure. Further, contamination to patient and hospital personnel is minimized when using this technology for open-fracture wound care.

Gunshot wounds

Evaluation of open fractures from gunshot wounds includes a thorough clinical and radiographic evaluation. The clinical evaluation should include a careful inspection for bullet entrance and exit wounds. The associated soft tissue injury should be thoroughly assessed. Because bullets may be deflected, their paths through the human body become fairly unpredictable. For this reason, all gunshot victims need to be fully exposed and all body areas should be carefully inspected for signs of injuries. A thorough documentation of the neurovascular status is mandatory. Radiographic studies should include standard radiographs, including the joints above and below the fracture. In addition, angiographic studies may be useful in the assessment for possible vascular injuries based upon physical examination findings suggesting vascular injury.

Fractures from gunshot wounds are frequently unstable and require operative fixation. The soft tissue management in gunshot wounds follows modified principles of open fracture treatment based on weapon velocity.

Firearm wounds are widely divided into three types: (1) low velocity pistol and rifle wounds (< 2,000 ft/sec); (2) high velocity rifle wounds (> 2,000 ft/sec); and (3) close range shotgun wounds. Low velocity gunshot wounds usually cause minimal soft tissue damage and do not require extensive surgical debridement. Treatment includes tetanus prophylaxis, appropriate fixation of the fracture, irrigation, and local debridement of the skin edges. The duration of antibiotics remains controversial, with recommendations ranging from 24 hours to 7 days of systemic antibiotics. There is a decreased risk of infection in low velocity gunshot wounds as compared to high velocity weapon wounds.

High velocity gunshot wounds and close range shotgun wounds should be treated similar to type 3 open fractures. The soft tissue damage in these injuries typically extends over a large zone and is associated with significant loss of viable soft tissue. Thorough irrigation and debridement should be performed on an urgent basis. Planned repeat surgical debridements may become necessary at 48 to 72 hour intervals until a clean and healthy wound bed is achieved. As with any open fractures, it is paramount to carefully debride any necrotic tissue and devascularized bone fragments to minimize the risk of infection. In many circumstances, wounds from high velocity gunshot injuries result in significant skin and soft tissue loss and require further coverage procedures such as skin grafts or muscle flaps.

Compartment syndrome

Compartment syndromes represent a limb- and life-threatening disorder. The consequences of delay or missed diagnosis may be devastating.

The pathophysiology of compartment syndromes is a vicious cycle that is initiated by swelling within a muscle compartment. When the intracompartmental pressure exceeds the venous capillary pressure, venous obstruction occurs at the capillary level. With continued arterial inflow, the intracompartmental pressure further increases resulting in decreased tissue perfusion and tissue oxygenation. This, in turn, causes further cell death with subsequent edema and an ultimate increase in compartment pressures.

It is important to be aware that any fracture or any soft tissue trauma may result in a compartment syndrome. Overall, tibia fractures represent the most common causes of compartment syndrome (36%). In contrast to common belief, compartment syndromes may not only occur with closed fractures, but are also common with open fractures. Younger patients sustaining long-bone fractures are at higher risk for developing compartment syndrome than are elderly patients, possibly because they have thicker fascia and more abundant muscle tissue.

The most important aspect in the management of compartment syndromes is immediate recognition and diagnosis of this disorder followed by prompt surgical fasciotomy (Figure 11.3). It has been well-documented that increased compartment pressures for more than 8 hours result in irreversible death of the involved muscles. Early signs of compartment syndrome include pain out of proportion to physical exam findings, increased need for narcotics, and firmness of the compartments. Paresthesias in the involved extremity

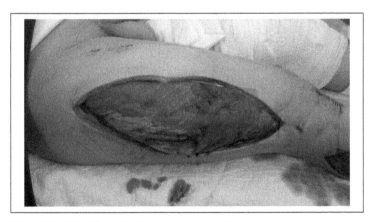

Figure 11.3 Right thigh after fasciotomy for compartment syndrome

represent an early sign of nerve compression. Dense sensory findings, motor weakness, and arterial occlusion are usually seen in later stages if the disorder is left untreated.

Although compartment syndrome is usually a clinical diagnosis, objective testing can be used as an adjunct. Measurement of compartment pressures can be performed using an 18-gauge needle catheter or commercially available hand-held intracompartmental pressure monitors. A compartment pressure within 30 mmHg of the diastolic blood pressure is widely considered to be an indicator of compartment syndrome.

Definitive fracture management

The goal of fracture treatment is to achieve optimal alignment, union, and restoration of limb function. The options to achieve these goals include closed management, external fixation, percutaneous fixation methods, and open reconstruction. The method of treatment needs to be tailored to the type and location of the fracture, the associated injuries, the patient's medical comorbidities, and the patient's expectations.

Closed treatment of fractures can be considered if appropriate fracture reduction can be achieved and maintained until fracture union. Closed treatment of fracture is desirable because it avoids the associated risks of surgery. However, "cast disease" including the formation of stiff adjacent joints is a concern for the adult patient population. Further, patient satisfaction and compliance with this treatment strategy can sometimes be suboptimal.

Several fractures can be considered for conservative care with activity restriction, cast, cast brace, or sling. Selected fracture variants of the shoulder girdle, including the clavicle and scapula body, are examples of injuries that can be treated simply with a sling and an early-motion protocol. Functional bracing can be instituted for stable isolated fractures of the humeral shaft. Casts or cast braces can be applied for certain ankle fractures and forefoot injuries. Activity restriction can be prescribed for stable pelvic and acetabular injuries.

This conservative approach, however, may not be optimal for the multiply injured patient. In this patient population, a more aggressive treatment algorithm is typically prescribed. Patients with multiple extremity fractures frequently benefit from operative fixation of their injuries because this allows earlier patient mobilization, reducing the risk of pulmonary complications, thromboembolic events, and pressure sores. For example, operative fixation may be indicated for injuries that would otherwise be treated nonoperatively (e.g., humeral shaft fractures).

External fixators have a diverse utility for fracture care. They can be used for definitive fracture stabilization. More often, however, these devices serve as a temporary means of obtaining skeletal alignment. Definitive use of an external fixator is often hampered by pin-site infection and patient dissatisfaction.

The external fixator is an invaluable tool for staged fracture treatment of the polytrauma patient. The multiply injured patient may be too unstable to tolerate the burden of acute total care. Thus, a damage control approach is prescribed. In contrast to splints, external fixators allow for inspection of the skin, soft tissue, and muscle compartments. Also, bone apposition achieved after reduction tamponades ongoing blood loss from the fracture. In contrast to skeletal traction, external fixators allow for easy patient mobilization. Safe conversion from external fixation to definitive fracture fixation is a safe procedure if performed within the 2-week interval.

The external fixator is also invaluable for temporary skeletal stabilization of fracture when adjacent soft tissue injury precludes early internal fixation. Use of an external fixator is common prior to definitive internal fixation of grossly contaminated open fractures. Serial debridements are preformed prior to the placement of internal appliances. Further, the fixator is commonly employed in the staged treatment of high-energy closed periarticular injuries with associated massive soft tissue damage. The fixator is used until soft tissue injury resolution. This is followed by formal open reconstruction. Typical examples are periarticular fracture of the tibial plateau and plafond.

Percutaneous reduction/fixation techniques are desirable as they are associated with minimal disruption to the soft tissue environment. Also, minimal blood loss is typically realized. These techniques are employed when closed manipulation can achieve fracture/joint reduction. This technique is commonly used for stabilization of the posterior pelvic ring. Sacroiliac screws are placed after closed manipulation produces reduction of the sacrum-iliac bone relationship (Figures 11.4a and 11.4b).

Open surgical reconstruction is the mainstay of treatment for the adult patient with significant bone or joint injury. Open reduction and internal fixation techniques have become widely available since the 1960s and have been popularized by the Arbeitsgemeinschaft für Osteosynthesefragen (AO) from Switzerland. The goals of open reduction and internal fixation were defined by the AO as follows: (1) fracture reduction to restore anatomical relationships; (2) stability by fixation; (3) preservation of blood supply; and (4) early and safe mobilization. Plating and nailing are the typical implants used to maintain fracture alignment until bone union. Plating is performed for periarticular fracture of the upper and lower extremity such as proximal humerus, elbow, and distal radius, as well as knee and ankle (Figure 11.5). Plates and screws can be employed to directly appose the fracture. Also, these implants can be placed to "bridge" a comminuted fracture zone. Plates are applied either through formal exposures or via minimally invasive (submuscular) techniques (Figure 11.6).

Intramedullary nailing is commonly used for diaphyseal and some selected metaphyseal long-bone fractures. Intramedullary nailing can be considered standard-of-care for most femoral and tibial shaft fractures and is also frequently performed in humeral shaft fractures. The intramedullary nail or rod is typically inserted remote to the fracture site into the intramedullary cavity, thus preserving fracture biology. Prior to nail insertion, the intramedullary cavity is reamed to accommodate the implant. Interlocking screws are inserted into the nail proximal and distal to the fracture site to limit translation and rotation of the fracture.

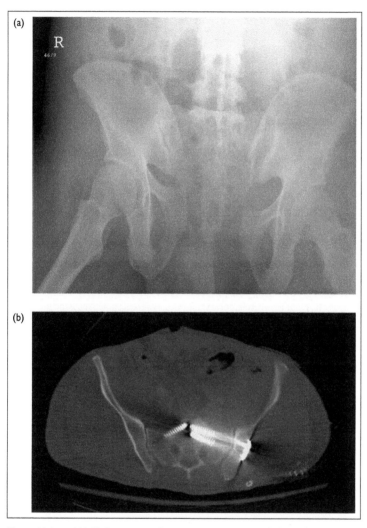

Figure 11.4a and 11.4b Percutaneous fixation is commonly employed for fixation of posterior pelvic ring injuries (Figure 11.4a). Axial CT scan of the pelvis following bilateral sacroiliac screw fixation (Figure 11.4b)

The implant functions as an internal splint of the long-bone fracture. Thus, the intramedullary nail is sharing compressive, bending, and rotational loads with the surrounding bone.

The systemic clinical effects of the reaming process are controversial. The main concern of intramedullary reaming is embolization of marrow contents.

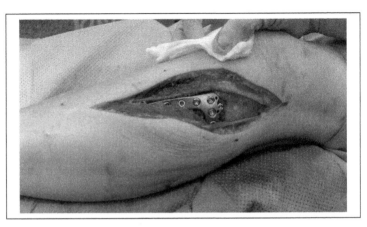

Figure 11.5 Open reduction and internal plate fixation of right tibial plateau fracture

While some studies suggested significant pulmonary compromise through reaming of femoral shaft fractures, other studies did not find any significant increase of pulmonary emboli, adult respiratory distress syndrome (ARDS), multiple organ failure (MOF), or death in femoral shaft fractures treated with reamed intramedullary nailing versus non-reamed intramedullary nailing. At this juncture, reamed

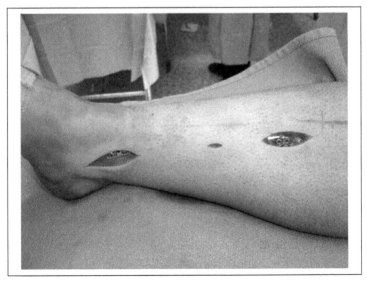

Figure 11.6 Minimal invasive plate fixation of the tibia performed through small incisions and sliding of the plate

intramedullary nailing of femoral and tibial shaft fractures remains the standard procedure at most trauma centers in North America.

Timing of fracture care in polytrauma patients

The timing of fracture fixation in patients with isolated musculoskeletal injury is primarily determined by local soft tissue conditions surrounding the involved bone or joint as well as the health status of the patient. However, the decision for operation in the patient with multiple injuries remains controversial. Delayed fixation increases the risk of complications such as pneumonia, thromboembolic events, and decubitus ulceration. Early total care and definitive fixation of long-bone fractures within the first days after the injury can improve outcomes and decrease rates of ARDS. Optimal technique, however, remains unclear, because intramedullary femoral nailing with reaming may increase the risk of respiratory compromise compared to nailing without reaming.

The term "damage control" in the general trauma literature refers to a treatment approach in which the only major life-threatening injuries are addressed acutely in the operating room. Definitive, lengthy repairs of visceral injuries are performed after adequate resuscitation has been achieved in the intensive care unit. This treatment approach has also been introduced in the orthopedic literature as "damage control orthopedics" (DCO). In polytrauma patients with multiple orthopedic injuries, the DCO approach includes immediate application of external fixators to stabilize the patient's long-bone fractures (Figure 11.7). Patients return to the operating room for definitive fracture fixation at several

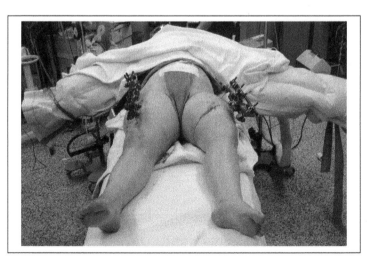

Figure 11.7 Bilateral femur fractures in multiply injured patient treated with temporary external fixation of both femurs

days after their injury when their physiologic parameters have improved. DCO appears to be a reasonable treatment approach for a subset of patients who are at risk of ARDS and MOF, but clearly defining this high-risk group has been problematic. It must be emphasized that as of today, early total care remains the standard of care at most trauma centers in North America. Early definitive fixation should be pursued in the majority of patients with multiple long-bone injuries.

Key references

Bhandari M, Zlowodzki M, Tornetta P III, Schmidt A, Templeman DC. Intramedullary nailing following external fixation in femoral and tibial shaft fractures. *J Orthop Trauma.* 2005;19:140–144.

Bosse MJ, MacKenzie EJ, Riemer BL, et al. Adult respiratory distress syndrome, pneumonia, and mortality following thoracic injury and a femoral fracture treated either with intramedullary nailing with reaming or with a plate: a comparative study. *J Bone Joint Surg Am.* 1997;79:799–809.

Pape HC, Tornetta P III, Tarkin I, Tzioupis C, Sabeson V, Olson SA. Timing of fracture fixation in multitrauma patients: the role of early total care and damage control surgery. *J Am Acad Orthop Surg.* 2009;17:541–549.

Park S, Ahn J, Gee AO, Kuntz AF, Esterhai JL. Compartment syndrome in tibial fractures. *J Orthop Trauma.* 2009;23:514–518.

Scalea TM, Boswell SA, Scott JD, Mitchell KA, Kramer ME, Pollak AN. External fixation as a bridge to intramedullary nailing for patients with multiple injuries and with femur fractures: damage control orthopedics. *J Trauma.* 2000;48:613–621.

Tarkin IS, Clare MP, Marcantonio A, Pape HC. An update on the management of high-energy pilon fractures. *Injury.* 2008;39:142–154.

Tarkin IS. The versatility of negative pressure wound therapy with reticulated open cell foam for soft tissue management after severe musculoskeletal trauma. *J Orthop Trauma.* 2008;22(suppl 10):S146–151.

Werner CM, Pierpont Y, Pollak AN. The urgency of surgical débridement in the management of open fractures. *J Am Acad Orthop Surg.* 2008;16:369–375.

Zelle BA, Brown SR, Panzica M, et al. The impact of injuries below the knee joint on the long-term functional outcome following polytrauma. *Injury.* 2005;36:169–177.

Chapter 12

Traumatic brain injury: assessment, pathophysiology, and management

Ramesh Grandhi and David O. Okonkwo

Traumatic brain injury (TBI) is the most common cause of death among individuals under 45 years of age in the Western World. Each year, roughly 1.7 million people in the United States sustain head injuries, most of which are concussions or mild TBI. However, brain trauma has a significant impact in the United States, as underscored by the approximately 52,000 deaths and 275,000 hospitalizations per year, as well as the considerable financial burden placed on the healthcare system in terms of direct medical expenditures, including long-term care to patients with disabilities from TBI, and indirect costs related to loss of productivity.

Neurologic assessment

Glasgow Coma Scale

The Glasgow Coma Scale (GCS) is the most commonly used scheme to determine the neurologic status of a patient following a head injury (Table 12.1). The GCS serves as a readily reproducible, objective measure of ascertaining a patient's level of consciousness by assessing three factors:

- Eye opening
- Verbal response
- Motor response

Severe TBI is classified by GCS scores of 3 to 8, while moderate and mild TBI are classified by GCS scores from 9 to 12 and 13 to 15, respectively. A patient's initial GCS score correlates significantly with outcome; however, factors such as age, pupil reactivity, head computed tomography (CT) scan findings, and extent of trauma-related extracranial injuries also serve as key predictors of patient outcome following severe TBI.

Primary and secondary traumatic brain injury

Primary brain injury

Primary brain injury refers to damage suffered as a *direct* result of the initial traumatic event and may be caused by penetrating, blunt, and blast trauma. Primary

Table 12.1 Glasgow Coma Scale (GCS)
Eye opening (E)
Spontaneous 4
To speech 3
To pain 2
Not open 1
Verbal response (V)
Conversant 5
Confused 4
Nonsense 3
Sounds 2
Silence 1
Intubated 1T
Motor response (M)
To command 6
To pain:
Localizing 5
Withdrawal 4
Arm flexion 3
Arm extension 2
No response 1
GCS Score = E + V + M (range, 3 or 3T–15)

From: Teasdale G, Jennett B. Assessment of coma and impaired consciousness: A practical scale. *Lancet.* 1974;2:81–84.

brain injury can be broadly divided into focal and diffuse injuries. Focal injuries include traumatic intracranial hematomas and contusions. Diffuse injuries, which encompass a wide range of injury patterns including diffuse axonal injury (DAI), are more common and constitute upwards of 60% of severe TBI.

Secondary brain injury

Secondary brain injury is attributable to local phenomena within the skull or systemic factors that cause damage following the initial insult. Preventing secondary brain injury is of fundamental importance in the management of patients following severe head trauma. Research has shown that the reduced mortality rate over the past 30 years—from 50% to less than 25%—in patients with severe TBI is a function of avoiding and treating factors known to precipitate secondary brain injury. The endpoint of these key factors—hypotension, hypoxia, inadequate cerebral perfusion pressure, and intracranial hypertension—is cerebral ischemia, the avoidance of which lies at the very foundation of modern evidence-based severe TBI management protocols.

Understanding the pathophysiology behind cerebral ischemia and intracranial hypertension, the reasons for invasive monitoring of both systemic and brain-related physiologic parameters, and the available treatments employed in the management of patients with severe TBI are important concepts to grasp in modern-day critical care medicine.

Posttraumatic cerebral ischemia

Pathophysiology

Cerebral ischemia occurs when there is insufficient cerebral blood flow (CBF) to meet its metabolic demands. The brain is unique among our organs due to its near complete dependency on blood flow to provide substrates for metabolism. Up to 95% of the brain's metabolism is oxidative and it lacks a capacity for significant oxygen storage. It also has minimal glucose and glycogen reserves. In turn, cerebrovascular physiology is predicated on prevention of cerebral ischemia and various mechanisms exist to ensure homeostasis. A metabolic autoregulatory mechanism exists through which cerebral blood flow is coupled to the cerebral metabolic rate of oxygen, thus assuring that, under physiologic conditions, the brain parenchyma receives adequate perfusion to support its metabolic needs.

A separate autoregulatory mechanism, termed pressure autoregulation, is also present. Under the principle of pressure autoregulation, CBF is kept relatively constant over a range of cerebral perfusion pressures (CPP), which similarly allows for a constant supply of oxygen and products needed for metabolism. Through a dynamic system of arteriolar vasoconstriction and dilation, CBF is maintained despite CPPs that may range from between 50 mm Hg and 150 mm Hg (Figure 12.1).

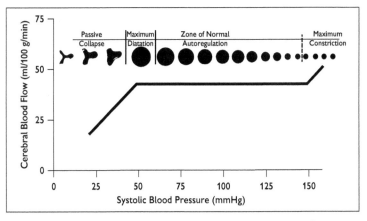

Figure 12.1 Cerebral blood flow (CBF) is kept relatively constant over a range of cerebral perfusion pressures via a dynamic system of arteriolar vasoconstriction and dilation. From: White H, Venkatesh B. Cerebral perfusion pressure in neurotrauma: a review. *Anesth Analg.* 2008;107:979–988

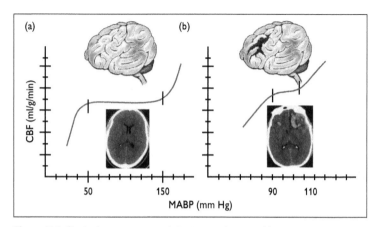

Figure 12.2 Cerebral pressure autoregulation in normal patients (a) versus in patients with traumatic brain injury (b). From: Rangel-Castilla L, Gasco J, Nauta HJ, Okonkwo DO, Robertson CS. Cerebral pressure autoregulation in traumatic brain injury. *Neurosurg Focus.* 2008;25:1–8

Intuitively, CBF can't be maintained under conditions in which CPPs are outside of the autoregulatory threshold.

Low CPP in the setting of TBI is linked to higher mortality rates and increased morbidity, especially when systemic hypotension occurs concomitantly. Another important consideration is that pressure autoregulation is frequently absent or impaired in patients following severe TBI. Thus, there are significant implications when aberrant pressure autoregulation occurs at a range outside normal physiologic parameters. For example, shifting the lower threshold for autoregulation from 50 mm Hg to 70 mm Hg would result in cerebral ischemia (Figure 12.2), which is especially important in light of the fact that upwards of 60% of patients with severe brain injury experience a reduction in CBF during the first few hours following their trauma.

On the other hand, if autoregulation occurred at a lower range of cerebral perfusion pressures than typical, it could precipitate malignant hyperemia or lead to secondary hemorrhages as a consequence of damage to microvasculature.

Other risk factors for cerebral ischemia: hypotension and hypoxia

Systemic hypotension (systolic blood pressure < 90 mm Hg) and hypoxia (oxygen saturations of < 60%) lead to worse patient outcomes after severe TBI because they decrease oxygen delivery to the brain, increasing patient mortality and morbidity in proportion to the number and duration of hypotensive or hypoxic events. Establishing an airway early in the postinjury period is a key method of preventing hypoxia; in fact, early intubation improves outcomes in patients with severe head injuries.

Principles underlying monitoring for cerebral ischemia

As previously mentioned, CPP serves to gauge the adequacy of CBF and, hence, must be monitored and maintained in patients with severe TBI. CPP is calculated by subtracting the patient's intracranial pressure (ICP) from their mean arterial pressure (MAP); in turn, direct transduction of systemic blood pressure via an indwelling arterial line and ICP via an intracranial pressure monitor are needed. Monitoring the patient's systemic arterial oxygen saturation and hematocrit, as is standard practice in trauma critical care, are also necessary to preventing secondary brain injury from decreased cerebral oxygenation.

Brain oxygen monitoring

Brain oxygen monitoring allows for the adequacy of oxygen delivery to brain tissue to be directly assessed. Two commonly used methods are jugular venous oxygenation sampling via an internal jugular vein catheter directed toward the jugular bulb and direct brain tissue oxygen monitoring by a fiberoptic catheter. Studies have shown that episodes of jugular venous oxygen desaturation ($S_{jv}O_2$ < 50%) are associated with increased mortality and worse outcomes in patients after severe TBI. Low values of $P_{bt}O_2$ (< 10–15 mm Hg) and the extent of their duration (> 30 min) are also associated with high rates of mortality.

Management principles

The current guidelines of severe TBI management advocate treatment thresholds for CPP at 60 mm Hg and jugular venous oxygen saturation and brain tissue oxygen tension at 50% and 15 mm Hg, respectively. Of note, maintaining CPPs above 70 mm Hg with use of vasopressors and volume expansion has been shown to carry a significantly increased risk of developing acute respiratory distress syndrome. Consequently, overly aggressive treatment of CPPs should be avoided.

In patients with inadequate CPP, systemic causes of hypotension such as cardiac or spinal shock, tension pneumothorax, and bleeding must be ruled out. Intravascular volume must be assessed via central venous pressure (CVP) monitoring or other methods of functional hemodynamic monitoring. Isotonic fluids should be administered as needed. In cases of low CPP refractory to fluid boluses, vasopressors need to be used.

Because the delivery of oxygen to brain tissue is predicated on the oxygen content of the blood, in addition to insufficient cerebral blood flow, hypoxemia or anemia can precipitate secondary brain injury. Arterial oxygen saturations should be maintained above 90%. No consensus exists delineating a particular transfusion threshold; however, low hematocrit is associated with increased mortality and morbidity in patients with severe TBI. Current data offers little support for aggressively transfusing packed red blood cells to correct for anemia. Some studies have noted increasingly negative neurologic outcomes in patients with severe TBI who underwent transfusion, while others have shown no difference in mortality rates among patients treated under an aggressive transfusion protocol as opposed to those treated along a more restrictive one. Taking into account all the evidence for and against transfusing blood in patients with severe

TBI, and given that brain tissue oxygen delivery does start to decline at a hematocrit less than 33%, we recommend a transfusion threshold of 30%.

Intracranial hypertension

Pathophysiology

Intracranial contents include blood, brain, and cerebrospinal fluid (CSF), all of which are enclosed within the rigid, nonexpansile skull. Based on the fundamental concept that the total volume available to intracranial contents is fixed, ICP is determined by the dynamic interplay among the individual components, as noted by the Monro-Kellie doctrine. Therefore, an increase in one component—as seen with posttraumatic cerebral edema—will result in a concomitant decrease in another. The same concept holds true when an additional component is added to the intracranial space, as when a mass lesion is present. Interestingly, ICP may actually remain within normal limits through compensations of the intracranial vascular volume, CSF volume, and brain parenchyma. However, an uncompensated increase in one or more existing compartments or the acute development of a new component will result in an ICP higher than the normal range of 5 to 15 mm Hg (Figure 12.3).

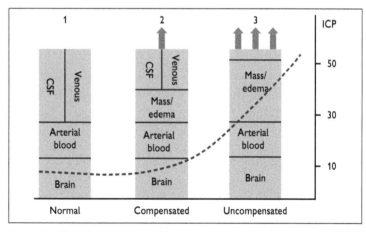

Figure 12.3 The rigid, nonexpansile skull (represented by the rectangle) contains blood, brain, and cerebrospinal fluid (CSF). Because the total volume available to intracranial contents is fixed, ICP is determined by the dynamic interplay among the individual components (1). The presence of an additional component within the intracranial space, as seen with posttraumatic cerebral edema or when a mass lesion is present, will result in a concomitant decrease in another. ICP may actually remain within normal limits through compensations of the intracranial vascular volume, CSF volume, and brain parenchyma (2). However, an uncompensated increase in one or more existing compartments or the acute development of a new component will result in an ICP higher than the normal range of 5 to 15 mm Hg (3). From: Exo J, Smith C, Bell MJ. Emergency treatment options for pediatric traumatic brain injury. *Pediatric Health.* 2009;3:533–541

Elevated ICP, termed intracranial hypertension, leads to brain herniation and a decrement in the CPP (given that CPP is defined as MAP–ICP).

Principles underlying monitoring for intracranial hypertension

Uncontrolled intracranial hypertension leads to worse patient outcomes after severe TBI. Consequently, the treatment of elevated ICPs in this population is a cornerstone of patient management in neurocritical care.

Intracranial pressure monitoring devices, indications and techniques of usage

Per the protocol at our institution, all patients with severe head injuries (GCS < 8) undergo placement of an external ventricular drain (EVD), or ventriculostomy, for purposes of ICP monitoring. The EVD also allows for CSF diversion and is useful for patients believed to be at risk for development of intracranial hypertension or hydrocephalus. Thus, EVD placement has a dual utility in that it serves to guide therapies and interventions to decrease ICP in the setting of intracranial hypertension, and also is a key therapeutic modality in and of itself by allowing for the sustained reduction of ICP due to its ability to divert CSF.

Other ICP monitoring devices are frequently used, sometimes as an adjunctive means of monitoring ICP when they are placed in tandem with an EVD, and, at other times, when slit-like ventricles preclude EVD placement. These devices measure ICP by means of a microtip strain gauge transducer, fiberoptic transducer, or coupling to a pneumatic transducer, and may be positioned within the brain parenchyma, or the subdural, subarachnoid, or epidural space.

Management principles

Based on evidence showing worse morbidity and mortality in severely brain-injured patients associated with ICPs in excess of 20 mm Hg, the most recent guidelines published by the Brain Trauma Foundation recommend an ICP treatment threshold of 20 mm Hg. The rationale behind treating intracranial hypertension is two-fold: (1) it ensures adequacy of CPP and thus avoids the occurrence of cerebral ischemia; (2) it prevents brain herniation.

There are a number of basic maneuvers that should be used to prevent patients from developing intracranial hypertension. Should a patient experience elevated ICPs, one must confirm that these fundamental factors have been addressed:

• Patient positioning—head should be in a neutral position with the head of the bed at 30 degrees
• Cervical spine clearance—following a negative helical CT scan of the cervical spine, cervical spine precautions must be discontinued and cervical collars removed
• Normocapnea (P_aCO_2 between 35–40 mm Hg) should be maintained
• Sedation with appropriate pharmacologic agents should be provided

With regards to patient positioning, elevation of the head in a neutral position serves to reduce the intracranial blood volume by maximizing venous return from the brain, while concomitantly preserving CPP and CBF. In terms of cervical collar removal, the policy at our institution is that in severe TBI patients who have no evidence of neurologic deficit that can be ascribed to spinal cord injury, cervical spine precautions are discontinued following a negative helical CT of the cervical spine. We feel that a cervical MRI is unnecessary, given that numerous recently published studies have highlighted the efficacy of negative cervical CT scans in obtaining cervical spine clearance in this particular patient population. In turn, expedient removal of external cervical collars, which are known to cause a significant and sustained elevation in baseline ICP, is important for treating and preventing elevations in ICP.

Finally, a number of different pharmacologic agents are used in patients with severe TBI with the goal of treating pain and agitation and minimizing the effect of a multitude of noxious stimuli that may contribute to elevations in blood pressure, body temperature, ICP, and resistance to controlled ventilation. In addition to using sedative agents in these patients, one often needs to determine their efficacy and titrate accordingly. Bispectral index monitoring may be a useful tool to accomplish this, because it can provide objective information regarding the degree of sedation in these critically injured patients.

Hyperosmolar therapy

After utilizing the methods described previously, there are many other interventions that can be used to decrease ICP. Hyperosmolar agents form the cornerstone of such therapies.

Mannitol

Intravenous administration of mannitol has been used for decades to reduce ICP. Moreover, it also has been shown to improve MAP, CPP, and CBF. The mechanism by which mannitol reduces ICP is thought to be attributable to two separate phenomena. The rheologic properties of mannitol involve its capacity to achieve an expansion in plasma volume and bring about a reduction in hematocrit and an increase in red blood cell deformability. In turn, the decreased blood viscosity leads to an increase in CBF and a subsequent decrease in ICP due to arteriolar vasoconstriction (via the principle of pressure autoregulation). The second means by which mannitol leads to an ICP reduction is through its osmotic effect. Mannitol creates an osmotic gradient between the intravascular compartment and the brain parenchyma, which leads to water diffusing from the parenchyma into the vasculature. Current guidelines support the administration of mannitol via bolus dosing of 0.25 g/kg to 1 g/kg of body weight.

One important potential side effect of mannitol administration is its capacity to cause acute renal insufficiency from acute tubular necrosis, which has an increased likelihood of occurring when serum osmolarity increases to greater than 320 mOsm. Also, one must pay close attention to a patient's intravascular volume status and electrolyte concentrations when mannitol is given. Finally, prolonged administration may result in a reversal of the osmotic gradient because it can cross the blood-brain barrier and be taken up into edematous brain tissue.

Hypertonic saline

Hypertonic saline solutions similarly treat intracranial hypertension through exerting both a rheological and an osmotic effect. They have been shown to be effective in achieving a reduction in ICP when given as boluses to brain-injured patients with intracranial hypertension refractory to mannitol administration. Interestingly, studies have demonstrated hypertonic saline to be more efficacious in comparison to mannitol in achieving a more profound ICP reduction; in addition, more patients respond to it as an ICP-lowering agent. Another advantage of using hypertonic saline is that it is believed that the blood-brain barrier is less permeable to hypertonic saline than it is to mannitol. Therefore, there is less of a risk of rebound intracranial hypertension from the paradoxical reversal of the osmotic gradient that sometimes occurs when mannitol is taken up into brain parenchyma.

When administering hypertonic saline to patients, one must be acutely attentive to not raising serum sodium concentrations too quickly, for fear of causing central pontine myelinolysis, especially in patients with preexisting chronic hyponatremia. Other potential complications associated with hypertonic saline use are electrolyte abnormalities; seizures; pulmonary edema, in patients with a history of cardiac or pulmonary disease; coagulopathy; and phlebitis.

Intracranial hypertension refractory to first-line treatment modalities: second-line treatments

In up to 25% of all patients with severe TBI, ICP will be refractory to the first-line treatments noted above, thus necessitating second-line treatment. While helpful in achieving a reduction in ICP, all of these second-line treatments can potentially result in significant morbidity.

Neuromuscular blockade

Neuromuscular blockade causes a decrement in intrathoracic pressure, which improves venous outflow from the brain and, in turn, results in reduced ICPs. However, early, routine, and long-term use of paralytic agents does not improve outcomes in severe TBI patients and should only be used when patients have intracranial hypertension refractory to other treatment modalities. Complications of neuromuscular paralysis include:

- Longer ICU stays
- Higher rates of infection (pneumonia, sepsis)

If a paralytic must be utilized, agents with a short half-life (e.g., vecuronium) are preferable because longer-lasting paralytics interfere with the patient's neurologic examination.

Hyperventilation

Based on the phenomenon of CO_2 reactivity, arteriolar smooth muscle in the cerebral vasculature responds to changes in arterial CO_2 by dilating and constricting. Hence, CBF changes 2%–3% for each mm Hg change in P_aCO_2: hypercarbia from hypoventilation causes reactive vasodilation and increased CBF, whereas hypocarbia from hyperventilation results in vasoconstriction and a decrement in CBF with a subsequent reduction in ICP. Despite the fact that pressure and metabolic autoregulation may be impaired after traumatic brain injury, CO_2 reactivity often remains intact.

Hyperventilation carries with it the risk of causing iatrogenic secondary brain injury due to cerebral ischemia. Severe TBI patients have a high risk of cerebral ischemia at baseline, as evidenced by studies showing a reduced CBF in the first 24 hours after injury and confirmed by postmortem histologic analysis. In fact, worse clinical outcomes have been seen in severely head-injured patients subjected to prophylactic hyperventilation during the first 5 days postinjury. Thus, as a principle, hyperventilation should be avoided during the critical initial 24-hour postinjury period and should not be used routinely in the management of intracranial hypertension in patients with severe TBI. However, it may serve as an important maneuver to reduce ICP in the event of acute neurologic deterioration and impending herniation, while more definitive measures are taken.

Barbiturate-induced burst suppression

The means by which barbiturates lower ICP is not completely known, but is thought to involve causing:

- Cerebral vasoconstriction
- Decreased cerebral metabolism
- Prevention of excitatory neurotoxic cascades

In general, barbiturates are administered in the presence of continuous EEG monitoring. Maximal reduction in CBF and cerebral metabolism is achieved when electrographic burst-suppression of cerebral activity occurs. Prophylactic use of barbiturates has no clinical benefit, but, in the setting of intractable intracranial hypertension, patients whose ICPs are responsive to barbiturate therapy have a reduced mortality.

Barbiturates, however, often precipitate systemic hypotension—a known risk factor for poor neurologic outcomes in patients with severe TBI. Hence, care should be taken to carefully monitor and treat any hemodynamic effects. Current guidelines note that high-dose barbiturate therapy should only be initiated in cases of intracranial hypertension refractory to all other medical and surgical alternatives.

Decompressive craniectomy

Surgical intervention via removing a portion of the cranial vault is a highly effective method of reducing intracranial pressure and is an important higher level treatment strategy for patients with medically refractory intracranial hypertension. Based on the Monro-Kellie doctrine, performing a decompressive craniectomy removes the volumetric constraint provided by the rigid, nonexpansile skull and provides a means of decreasing ICP when an uncompensated state exists.

Therapies to avoid in the management of intracranial hypertension
Steroids

There is no role for the use of steroids in severe TBI. The administration of steroids is associated with increased mortality, and potentially dangerous complications including gastrointestinal bleeding and hyperglycemia.

Systemic medical management

Given the fact that a severe head injury has a profound effect on numerous organ systems, a systems-based approach is crucial in optimizing the neurocritical care of severe TBI patients.

Fluid balance and electrolytes

Up to 60% of patients with TBI develop some sort of electrolyte abnormality. Alterations in serum sodium concentration are most frequently seen and also carry the most important consequences. Posttraumatic hyponatremia is associated with worse outcomes and longer hospital stays and occurs due to:

- Syndrome of inappropriate antidiuretic hormone (SIADH)
- Cerebral salt wasting

Patients with SIADH should be fluid restricted while those with cerebral salt wasting require sodium supplementation. Volume status represents a key differentiating feature distinguishing the two entities: SIADH results in euvolemia or hypervolemia, while cerebral salt wasting causes hypovolemia.

Hypernatremia after TBI is generally attributable to central diabetes insipidus from pituitary stalk dysfunction. It is seen with increased severity of brain injury and has significant implications on mortality. Management of hypernatremia may involve administration of hypotonic fluids, desmopressin (DDAVP), and free-water boluses.

After initial resuscitation, normal saline (0.9% NaCl) is the standard maintenance fluid used for patients with head injuries. Fluids with dextrose are not administered because of concern for inducing or exacerbating hyperglycemia, which is associated with a worse prognosis in patients with TBI. Hypotonic fluids are not given since they may worsen cerebral edema.

Of note, fluid and electrolyte management in patients with severe TBI requires monitoring of cardiovascular parameters with central venous lines and indwelling arterial catheters. Frequent serum sodium concentration checks in the first 48 hours postinjury may also be helpful in avoiding grossly aberrant serum sodiums and help guide therapeutic interventions.

Glycemic control

Patients with severe head injuries commonly have supranormal glucose levels, which likely occurs due to upregulation of the sympathetic nervous system and increased catecholamine release from the adrenal glands. Hyperglycemia, both early and persistent, in patients with severe TBI is associated with poor outcomes. Frequent glucose checks and aggressive glycemic control by subcutaneous administration of insulin according to a sliding scale help maintain blood glucose levels below 130 mg/dL.

Hyperpyrexia

Fever increases cerebral metabolism and is a positive predictor for mortality in patients with head injury. Antipyretics and cooling blankets are often employed in fever management. Therapeutic temperature management, utilizing servo-controlled surface cooling or specialized intravascular catheters, can help prevent fever. When appropriate, an infectious workup should be pursued aggressively.

Altered endocrine function

Dysfunction of the neuroendocrine axis is not uncommon during the acute post-TBI period. At our institution, a neuroendocrine panel testing for the hormones noted below is drawn on posttrauma days 3 and 7 in severe TBI patients:

- Cortisol
- Insulin-like Growth Factor-1
- Free T4
- Thyroid Stimulating Hormone
- Estradiol and prolactin levels in females
- Testosterone levels

Of particular concern is adrenal insufficiency—manifesting as hyponatremia, hypotension, and hypoglycemia—because of its potential to have life-threatening consequences in the critically ill patient population. Dramatic responses have been reported subsequent to glucocorticoid replacement in these individuals. Early posttraumatic hypopituitarism resolves in most patients, generally by 6 months postinjury.

Nutrition

Polytrauma and severe TBI induce a systemic hypermetabolic state. Nutritional support via the enteral route (unless there is an absolute contraindication) must be established as soon as possible and patients should attain full caloric replacement by postinjury day 7. Severe malnutrition during the first 2 weeks after injury is associated with significantly increased mortality rates as compared to when full caloric replacement is achieved by postinjury day 7. Early initiation of feeding seems to lead to decreased rates of infection and complications.

Orogastric tubes are preferred to nasogastric tubes in the presence of skull-base fractures or sinus disease. Altered function of the lower esophageal sphincter and slowed gastric emptying are seen in patients with severe TBI and must be considered with gastric feeding, especially since this increases the risk of aspiration. Long-term feeding may require placement of a percutaneous endoscopic gastrostomy tube or jejunal tube. While enteral nutrition is preferred due to the reduced risk of bacteremia and sepsis, parenteral nutrition may used for temporary nutritional support.

Infections

Higher rates of systemic infection are seen with increased severity of brain trauma as well as in patients with concomitant multiple trauma. Pneumonia is an important source of increased morbidity and mortality in the severe TBI population, especially given that up to 70% of mechanically ventilated patients can develop pneumonia. Interestingly, studies in which tracheostomy was performed within a week of brain injury did not lead to a decrease in the rate of ventilator-associated pneumonia, nor did it reduce patient mortality. There has been a suggestion of a decrease in ventilator days. Another key infectious risk factor in the severe TBI population comes from the placement of invasive cerebral ICP monitoring devices. Of note, bacterial colonization of intraparenchymal ICP monitors occurs more readily than with external ventricular drains.

The key to avoiding infections in these patients lies with hand washing and using proper sterile technique when placing lines and hardware. Furthermore, if infections do develop, prolonged therapy with broad-spectrum antibiotics should be avoided in order to prevent selection of highly resistant bacterial species.

Prophylaxis

GI prophylaxis

The formation of gastric ulcers is often seen in patients after severe TBI and carries with it a high mortality rate. Histamine type 2 (H2) antagonists or proton pump inhibitors (PPIs) are the most commonly used agents for GI prophylaxis, with both medications having a similar efficacy in preventing upper GI tract bleeding among mechanically ventilated patients. Early enteral feeding and aggressive fluid resuscitation also help decrease this complication.

Anticonvulsants

Early posttraumatic seizures (PTS)—those occurring within 7 days of injury—occur in between 4% and 25% of patients; and late posttraumatic seizures—those occurring after postinjury day 7—occur in 9% to 42% of patients. PTS are more likely to occur in patients with:

- Cortical contusions
- Depressed skull fractures
- Subdural, epidural, or intracranial hematomas
- Penetrating injuries
- Initial seizures occurring within 24 hours of injury
- Initial GCS < 10

Seizures have a profound effect on the brain because they cause an increase in ICP and cerebral metabolic rate for O_2, alterations in blood pressure, cerebral blood flow, and oxygen delivery, as well as contribute to excess neurotransmitter release. Prophylactic phenytoin administration decreases the incidence of early PTS but not late PTS. Anticonvulsants should only be administered for 1 week postinjury due to the potential for side effects such as fevers and behavioral changes, and because antiseizure prophylaxis does not influence the likelihood of developing late PTS.

Prevention of venous thromboembolism (VTE)

The risk of deep venous thrombosis (DVT) among severe TBI patients may be as high as 20% in the absence of mechanical and pharmacologic prophylaxis. DVTs that specifically involve the proximal leg veins result in an increased risk of pulmonary embolism (PE), which occurs in 0.38% of TBI patients during their acute hospital stay. Hence, preventing the development of VTE is crucial, because it not only has a significant effect on patients' morbidity and mortality, but also on patient management issues because of intracranial bleeding risks associated with institution of anticoagulation.

Administration of low-dose heparin or low-molecular weight heparin is an effective means of preventing VTE. These agents are significantly more efficacious than mechanical modalities (e.g., pneumatic compression devices) alone. Because pharmacologic prophylaxis carries an increased risk of progression of intracranial bleeding, at our institution we do not start these agents until 48 hours after either a CT scan demonstrates stable imaging findings or an operative intervention occurs.

Placing a retrievable inferior vena cava filter would prevent PEs from lower extremity DVTs and may spare the risk of anticoagulating patients with DVTs; however, because of extremely low rates of successful filter retrieval and long-term risks of filters, there is no clear indication for their use in the management of patients with severe TBI.

Key references

Aarabi B, Hesdorffer DC, Ahn ES, Aresco C, Scalea TM, Eisenberg HM. Outcome following decompressive craniectomy for malignant swelling due to severe head injury. *J Neurosurg.* 2006;104:469–479.

Andrews PJ, Sleeman DH, Statham PF, et al. Predicting recovery in patients suffering from traumatic brain injury by using admission variables and physiological data: a comparison between decision tree analysis and logistic regression. *J Neurosurg.* 2002;97:326–336.

Bouderka MA, Fakhir B, Bouaggad A, Hmamouchi B, Hamoudi D, Harti A. Early tracheostomy versus prolonged endotracheal intubation in severe head injury. *J Trauma.* 2004;57:251–254.

Deogaonkar A, Gupta R, DeGeorgia M, et al. Bispectral Index monitoring correlates with sedation scales in brain-injured patients. *Crit Care Med.* 2004;32:2403–2406.

McIntyre LA, Fergusson DA, Hutchison JS, et al. Effect of a liberal versus restrictive transfusion strategy on mortality in patients with moderate to severe head injury. *Neurocrit Care.* 2006;5:4–9.

Moro N, Katayama Y, Igarashi T, Mori T, Kawamata T, Kojima J. Hyponatremia in patients with traumatic brain injury: incidence, mechanism, and response to sodium supplementation or retention therapy with hydrocortisone. *Surg Neurol.* 2007;68:387–393.

Ogden AT, Mayer SA, Connolly ES Jr. Hyperosmolar agents in neurosurgical practice: the evolving role of hypertonic saline. *Neurosurgery.* 2005;57:207–215.

Roberts I, Sydenham E. Barbiturates for acute traumatic brain injury. *Cochrane Database of Systematic Reviews* 1999; Issue 3. Art. No.: CD000033. DOI:10.1002/14651858. CD000033.

Struchen MA, Hannay HJ, Contant CF, Robertson CS. The relation between acute physiological variables and outcome on the Glasgow Outcome Scale and Disability Rating Scale following severe traumatic brain injury. *J Neurotrauma.* 2001;18:115–125.

Taylor SJ, Fettes SB, Jewkes C, Nelson RJ. Prospective, randomized, controlled trial to determine the effect of early enhanced enteral nutrition on clinical outcome in mechanically ventilated patients suffering head injury. *Crit Care Med.* 1999;27:2525–2531.

The Brain Trauma Foundation. The American Association of Neurological Surgeons and Congress of Neurological Surgeons. AANS/CNS Joint Section on Neurotrauma and Critical Care: Guidelines for the management of severe traumatic brain injury. 3rd ed. *J Neurotrauma*. 2007;24(suppl 1):S14–S21, S59–S86, S91–S95.

Timofeev I, Dahyot-Fizelier C, Keong N, et al. Ventriculostomy for control of raised ICP in acute traumatic brain injury. *Acta Neurochir*. 2008;102(suppl):99–104.

Tomycz ND, Chew BG, Chang YF, et al. MRI is unnecessary to clear the cervical spine in obtunded/comatose trauma patients: the four-year experience of a level I trauma center. *J Trauma*. 2008;64:1258–1263.

Winchel RJ, Hoyt DB. Endotracheal intubation in the field improves survival in patients with severe head injury. *Arch Surg*. 1997;132:592–597.

Chapter 13

Management of the brain-dead organ donor

Kai Singbartl

Introduction

The shortage of transplantable organs has amounted to a public health crisis in the United States and worldwide. There are currently more than 110,000 patients in the United States awaiting organ transplantation, but far fewer transplantable organs are available, causing nearly 7% of transplant candidates to die while on the waiting list. Use of marginal, high-risk donors and the extension of criteria for donation have attenuated the shortage to a small degree. In addition, several administrative and clinical measures, such as the institution of in-house organ procurement coordinators, have also been introduced to address this problem. Unfortunately, these measures by themselves are insufficient to alleviate the shortage of transplantable organs. Therefore, the accurate and careful management of brain-dead organ donors becomes of utmost importance in our attempts to further maximize the number of organs that can be retrieved for transplantation and, the number of other recipient lives that can subsequently be saved.

In this chapter, we will discuss the management of brain-dead organ donors in detail. We will focus on the organization of donor management as well as medical aspects, in particular hemodynamic and pulmonary management.

Organization of donor management

In the United States, the United Anatomic Gift Act regulates organ donation. A patient who has been declared brain dead, and for whom organ donation is considered, becomes a patient of the local organ procurement organization (OPO). From this time on, the donor and all are related issues are managed by organ procurement coordinators (OPC). OPCs approach the next of kin to discuss organ donation and possibly obtain consent. Individual states and OPOs handle the issues of prospective consent (e.g., through driver's licenses), and who is designated to request consent, in different ways. This clear separation between the team caring for the patient prior to brain death and the organ donation team is intended to avoid any (perceived) conflict of interest.

However, this separation also has some serious disadvantages. Organ procurement coordinators, who often lack a critical care background, cannot perform all aspects of donor care themselves but rather have to rely on the (often voluntary) support of randomly available physicians. In addition to the delay in care caused by the need to search for a qualified and willing physician, this situation is also prone to miscommunication and inconsistencies in the donor care, ultimately giving rise to suboptimal management of the donor.

The University of Pittsburgh Department of Critical Care Medicine and the Center for Organ Recovery and Education have therefore implemented a so-called organ donor support team that consists of an OPC and a dedicated attending intensivist with substantial expertise in neurocritical care. Organ donor support is provided with 24/7 on-call coverage without any other clinical obligations for the intensivist, thereby avoiding any potential conflict of interest as described above. This approach has significantly increased the chances for successful organ donation, in particular lungs (increased by ~200%) and kidneys (by ~50%).

In some countries, on the other hand, the original patient-care team performs both duties: declaration/notification of brain death and discussion of organ donation. Although sound data are lacking, proponents of this approach claim a higher conversion rate of potential to actual donors.

Regardless of local regulations or systems, optimal organ donor management requires a team approach for which dedicated, experienced personnel have to be readily available and standard operating procedures have to be in place.

Medical management

Brain-dead donors represent a special population that differs greatly from patients usually encountered in the intensive care unit (ICU). Successful donor management and therefore transplantation outcome strongly depend on a detailed understanding of the pathophysiology of brain death.

Immediately prior to brain death, a sympathetic storm leads to an overwhelming release of catecholamines resulting in an increase in systemic vascular resistance, hypertension, cardiac dysfunction, arrhythmias, and pulmonary edema. Brain death and subsequent herniation, in contrast, result in spinal cord infarction and loss of sympathetic tone, aggravating preexisting hemodynamic instability. Another crucial consequence of brain death is the cessation of hormonal secretion from the pituitary gland causing a pan-hypopituitary state. Low plasma concentrations of cortisone, T3, T4, insulin, and anti-diuretic hormone (ADH) are frequently encountered in this situation.

Brain death also leads to a massive inflammatory response with substantially elevated plasma concentrations of proinflammatory cytokines, such as interleukin-6 (IL-6) and tumor necrosis factor. The degree of inflammatory response after brain death correlates well with the immunogenicity of the graft and subsequent allograft dysfunction.

Pulmonary management

Because the disparity between supply and demand for transplantable organs is the greatest for lungs, pulmonary management of the brain-dead organ donor deserves special attention. The clinical observation that, despite the great demand for transplantable lungs, almost no potential lung donors receive specific ventilator adjustments during the pretransplantation period further highlights this need.

In addition to neurogenic pulmonary edema, as discussed above, the lungs of a brain-dead and potential organ donor are also at higher risk for ventilator-induced lung injury, diminishing the chances for successful donations. Recent clinical studies have shown that lung-protective ventilation not only reduces the risk of ventilator-induced lung injury in brain-dead organ donors but also doubles the number of lungs available for transplantation. Lung-protective ventilation under these circumstances consists of a low tidal-volume strategy (6–8 ml/kg of predicted body weight), mild to moderate positive end-expiratory pressure (8–10 cm H_2O), and apnea test performed in a closed circuit with continuous positive pressure application. Measures to prevent aspiration, such as 30° head-of-bed elevation, and recruitment maneuvers (for P_aO_2/F_iO_2 ratios < 300 or radiographic findings of atelectasis) have a positive effect on the number of lungs eligible for transplantation. There is also some evidence from retrospective data analyses that the application of high-dose steroids may improve oxygenation and procurement rates for lungs.

The need for, and the potential benefits of, a dedicated organ donor support team, as outlined above, become particularly evident in the context of pulmonary management. Early, timely bronchoscopy; close and appropriate ventilator management; and prudent fluid management are only three examples of crucial interventions that are best performed by a well-connected and experienced team. Figure 13.1 summarizes the key points for pulmonary management of brain-dead organ donors.

✦ **Lung protective ventilation !!!**

⮑ Low-tidal volume 6–8ml/kg, PEEP 8–10 cmH$_2$O

✦ **Standardized ventilator management !!!**

⮑ Ventilator recruitment maneuvers (if P_aO_2/F_iO_2 < 300)

⮑ Techniques to prevent aspiration (e.g., 30° head-of-bed elevation)

✦ **Methylprednisolone! ?**

⮑ 15mg/kg q24h, can improve potential for lung donation

Figure 13.1 Crucial aspects of pulmonary management of the brain-dead donor. Whereas there are strong clinical data for the top two points, the recommendation for high-dose steroids to improve the potential for lung donation is only based on retrospective data analyses

Hemodynamic management

Nearly 50% of all brain-dead donors become hemodynamically unstable at one time or another during the pretransplantation process. As already indicated above, hemodynamic instability in organ donors is multi-factorial. Autonomic dysfunction, hypovolemia, cardiac dysfunction, release of vasoactive proinflammatory molecules, and pan-hypopituitarism all may contribute to this problem. Hemodynamic instability not only leads to organ ischemia/hypoperfusion, but it also further aggravates the inflammatory response, maintaining a vicious, deleterious cycle. Optimization of donor resuscitation is therefore of utmost importance. A recent observational study found that nearly 50% of all brain-dead donors were preload responsive (pulse pressure variation > 13%), that is, they were not adequately fluid resuscitated. Preload responsiveness was associated with a greater degree of inflammation, as measured by plasma IL-6 concentrations, and ultimately a significantly lower organ yield for transplantation.

Although it is well known among experts that donor resuscitation is crucial for the transplantation outcome, clear data regarding optimal monitoring of the brain-dead organ donor are missing. However, considering the frequent need for hemodynamic stabilization and administration of vasoactive substances in this population, invasive blood pressure monitoring and central venous access appear mandatory as minimal monitoring. Moreover, the detection of preload responsiveness itself is much more important than the actual device used. The type of fluid used also remains a matter of personal preference. Following general ICU practice, hemoglobin > 7 mg/dL appears desirable.

If the brain-dead organ donor remains hemodynamically unstable despite sufficient fluid resuscitation, the need for vasoactive agents arises. The choice of vasoactive agents and the order in which they are administered should ideally differ from what is used for "standard" ICU patients, considering the special pathophysiology and needs of a brain-dead organ donor (Figure 13.2). Failure to recognize the special needs and to manage the donor appropriately will result in persistent hemodynamic instability and adverse donation outcome.

Considering the brain-dead donor's hormonal deficiencies, vasopressin (up to 6 U/h) represents a logical first choice for persistent hypotension or diabetes insipidus. Well-accepted goals are (1) mean arterial blood pressure > 65 mm Hg; (2) heart rate < 100 beats per minute; (3) urine output of 0.5–3 mL/kg/h. Desmopressin (DDAVP) is a widely considered alternative but has a few important disadvantages when compared to vasopressin. DDAVP is less convenient to titrate and also inferior with respect to hemodynamic stabilization.

Thyroxine replacement should also be considered early on, especially when the donor's heart is considered for transplantation, or when inotropic support is needed. Thyroxine administration, usually as a bolus followed by a continuous infusion, has to be preceded by insulin and dextrose 50% injections to prevent severe hyperkalemia following the thyroxine bolus. As thyroxine can also cause severe tachycardia, hypertension, and arrhythmias, it should not automatically be given in all donors.

1. **Respect and follow the underlying pathophysiology.**

2. **Assess fluid responsiveness, restore euvolemia.**

3. **Hypotension or (suspected) diabetes insipidus**

⮱ Hormone replacement with vasopressin (0.5-6 U/h i.v.)

⮱ MAP >65mmHg, HR <100 bpm, Urine output 0.5-3ml/kg/h,

serum Na+ 135-145mM

⮱ Desmopressin less convenient (titration) and limited hemodynamic support

4. **Improve cardiovascular stability (persisting hypotension)**

⮱ 50ml Dextrose 50% i.v. plus 10IU insulin i.v.

⮱ 20µg Thyroxine T4 i.v. (positive inotrope, mild vasopressor, hyperkalemia)

⮱ 10µg/hThyroxine T4 i.v.

5. **Persisting hypotension, hemodynamic instability**

⮱ "Conventional" vasopressors and inotropes

Figure 13.2 Algorithm for hemodynamic stabilization of the brain-dead organ donor

It is only after hormone replacement therapy has been started that the application of "conventional" vasoactive agents, such as norepinephrine or dobutamine, should be considered.

Studies showing benefits of hormone replacement therapy in brain-dead organ donors, with respect to the number of eligible organs, graft survival, and recipient survival, are limited by their design and sample size. Nonetheless, there are no studies showing superiority of "conventional" vasoactive substances in this setting, making them less desirable as primary choices for the hemodynamic stabilization of brain-dead organ donors.

Summary

Successful management of the brain-dead organ donor requires a team-based, proactive approach that includes early notification of the organ donor management team. Medical management has to respect the special pathophysiology of a brain-dead donor and treat accordingly, including fluid lung protective ventilation, pulmonary recruitment and toilet, fluid resuscitation, invasive hemodynamic monitoring, and timely hormonal replacement therapy.

Key references

Chen JM, Cullinane S, Spanier TB, et al. Vasopressin deficiency and pressor hypersensitivity in hemodynamically unstable organ donors. *Circulation*. 1999;100(suppl 19):II244–II246.

Kurtz SF, Strong CW, Gerasimow D. The 2006 Revised Uniform Anatomical Gift Act—A Law to Save Lives. *Health Law Analysis.* Feb, 2007, pp 44–49.

Mascia L, Bosma K, Pasero D, Galli T, Cortese G, Donadio P, Bosco R. Ventilatory and hemodynamic management of potential organ donors: an observational survey. *Crit Care Med.* 2006;34(2):321–327.

Mascia L, Pasero D, Slutsky AS, et al. Effect of a lung protective strategy for organ donors on eligibility and availability of lungs for transplantation. *JAMA.* 2010;304(23):2620.

Murugan R, Venkataraman R, Wahed AS, et al. Increased plasma interleukin-6 in donors is associated with lower recipient hospital-free survival after cadaveric organ transplantation. *Crit Care Med.* 2008;36(6):1810–1816.

Murugan R, Venkataraman R, Wahed AS, Elder M, Carter M, Madden NJ, Kellum JA. Preload responsiveness is associated with increased interleukin-6 and lower organ yield from brain-dead donors. *Crit Care Medicine.* 2009;37(8):2387–2393.

Novitzky D, Cooper DK, Rosendale JD, Kauffman HM. Hormonal therapy of the brain-dead organ donor: experimental and clinical studies. *Transplantation.* 2006;82(11):1396–401.

Singbartl K, Murugan R, Kaynar AM, Crippen DW, Tisherman SA, Shutterly K, et al. Intensivist-Led Management of Brain-Dead Donors Is Associated with an Increase in Organ Recovery for Transplantation [Internet]. *American Journal of Transplantation.* 2011; dx.doi.org/10.1111/j.1600–6143.2011.03485.

Chapter 14

Management of traumatic spinal cord injury

David M. Panczykowski, David O. Okonkwo, and Richard M. Spiro

Epidemiology

In the United States, the annual incidence of traumatic spinal cord injury (SCI) ranges from 25 to 58 per million people. The average age at time of injury is 32, with a 4:1 male to female ratio. Traumatic brain injury (TBI) occurs in 25% to 50% of patients with SCI, conversely 5% to 10% of TBI patients sustain SCI. The highest mortality is within the first 3 months of injury (~20%); however, the average life expectancy of a complete paraplegic SCI patient is only 16% shorter than that of an uninjured peer, and only 8% shorter for patients with incomplete SCI.

Pathophysiology

Primary Injury is defined as neuronal death or dysfunction as a consequence of initial impact, transient or persistent compression, distraction, and laceration/transection. Secondary Injury involves progressive ischemic, inflammatory, and cytotoxic processes initiated or potentiated by systemic and/or local insults. The prophylaxis and/or correction of systemic insults such as hypotension, decreased oxygen content, and hyperthermia are the central goals of management to prevent secondary injury.

Diagnosis

Clinical assessment

Initial assessment should be in accordance with Advanced Trauma Life-Support recommendations, beginning with an evaluation of airway, breathing, and circulatory function; 20%–60% of SCI patients also sustain concomitant injuries to other organ systems.

The American Spinal Injury Association (ASIA) Classification System is the most widely used, rapid, and reproducible method of neurologic classification of SCI, specifically injury level and degree of impairment. (Figure 14.1). The motor

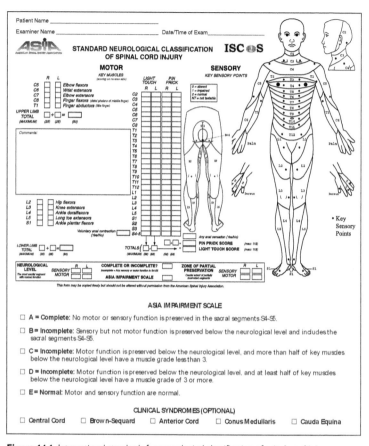

Figure 14.1 International standards for neurological classification of spinal cord injury

score grades strength (0–5) in 10 bilateral motor segments (C5-T1 & L2-S1); a level is considered intact if the motor grade ≥ 3. The sensory level is determined at 28 bilateral dermatome points assessed for pinprick and light touch. The neurologic level is defined as the most caudal segment of the spinal cord with normal bilateral motor (≥ 3/5) and sensory (light touch and pinprick) function. The degree of impairment is categorized as complete (e.g., no voluntary anal contraction, no S4–5 sensation, and no deep anal pressure sensed) or incomplete (e.g., presence of sacral sparing).

Early neurologic findings (24–72 hours) may be confounded by spinal shock, that is, transient loss of all neurologic function below the level of injury demonstrated by flaccid paralysis and areflexia. The resolution of spinal shock is often heralded by return of anal-cutaneous and/or bulbocavernosus reflexes. This syndrome should not be confused with neurogenic shock, which is characterized by bradycardia, hypotension, and priapism caused by loss of sympathetic tone.

Complete SCI involves complete loss of any motor, sensory, or sphincter control below lesion, often associated with neurogenic shock. A number of incomplete SCI syndromes have been described. The central cord syndrome involves disproportionate weakness of the upper extremities (especially distal motor groups) compared to the lower extremities, with signs of myelopathy (usually urinary retention) and variable sensory disturbances (hyperpathia, hypesthesia, etc). Fifty percent recover the ability to ambulate, most recover bladder control. The anterior cord syndrome involves dissociated sensory loss (no pain or temperature sensation, preserved proprioception, vibratory sense, and deep pressure) with either paraplegia or quadriplegia (if above C7). Prognosis for recovery is poor. The posterior cord syndrome, which is relatively rare, includes pain and paresthesias (burning sensations) of the neck, upper arms, and torso with mild paresis of upper extremities. Hemisection of the spinal cord (secondary to penetrating injury) results in the Brown-Sequard syndrome with ipsilateral motor paralysis and loss of proprioception and vibratory sense with contralateral loss of pain and temperature sensation. The conus medullaris syndrome consists of bilateral sacral sensory deficit ("saddle anesthesia"), pronounced autonomic dysfunction (especially urinary retention), and symmetric paraparesis.

Radiographic assessment

Imaging should be obtained in all trauma patients with one or more key risk factors for spine or cord injury, including (1) neck or back pain/tenderness; (2) neurologic deficits; (3) impaired level of consciousness; (4) intoxication; and (5) painful distracting injuries. Multi-slice helical computed tomography (CT) with slice thickness ≤ 3 mm is the screening modality of choice for osseous injury, while magnetic resonance imaging (MRI) is the primary modality for characterizing acute spinal cord and ligamentous injury.

Imaging modalities should be evaluated for markers of spinal column stability. Lateral spine radiographs and/or CT reconstructions should demonstrate smooth, uninterrupted planes along the anterior vertebral body, posterior vertebral body, and spinolaminar lines. Spinal canal diameter should exceed 13 mm at every vertebral level. Instability is suggested by subluxation of > 3.5 mm or > 20% listhesis, angulations exceeding 11° cervical or 20° thoracolumbar, and/or loss of > 50% anterior compared with posterior vertebral body height.

Cervical spine clearance

Cervical collars should be removed as soon as it is safe to do so. They have been associated with skin breakdown, increased ICU stays, and elevated intracranial pressure. Cervical collars may be removed in patients who are awake, alert, and without neurologic deficit or distracting injury; who have no neck pain/tenderness; and who have full range of motion of the cervical spine without the need for imaging. Meta-analysis of the current literature demonstrates that multi-slice helical CT alone is sufficient to detect unstable cervical spine injuries in trauma patients unable to be clinically cleared, thus permitting the removal of the cervical collar from obtunded or intubated trauma patients if a modern CT is negative for acute injury.

Treatment

Patients with acute traumatic SCI should be managed at a Level I trauma center because these centers have demonstrated better outcomes. Patients suffering SCI, regardless of severity, frequently experience cardiovascular instability and pulmonary insufficiency necessitating vigilant monitoring. Management in an ICU has been shown to improve neurologic outcome and reduce cardiopulmonary related morbidity and mortality.

Respiratory management

Endotracheal intubation is frequently indicated in the setting of airway compromise, respiratory failure (P_aO_2 < 60 mm Hg or P_aCO_2 > 60 mm Hg), and/or associated severe TBI (GCS ≤ 8). Care should be taken to avoid spinal movement during intubation. Options include awake fiberoptic guidance or direct laryngoscopy with manual in-line spine stabilization.

Ventilatory dysfunction correlates with level and completeness of injury. Ventilation typically worsens between postinjury days 2 and 5, improving thereafter with mean duration of mechanical ventilation being 22 days in C5–8 SCI and 12 days in thoracic SCI.

Pulmonary complications are the leading cause of death and morbidity in the SCI population; atelectasis, pneumonia, aspiration pneumonitis, pulmonary edema, and pulmonary embolism occur in > 60% of patients with cervical and upper thoracic SCI. Additionally, SCI patients frequently suffer from comorbid traumatic injuries further predisposing them to acute lung injury and acute respiratory distress syndrome (ARDS).

Management strategies advocate lung protective ventilation utilizing low tidal volumes (6–8 mL/kg predicted body weight) with steps to enhance alveolar recruitment (positive end-expiratory pressure). Early conversion to tracheostomy should be considered in patients anticipated to require > 2 weeks ventilatory support. Early tracheostomy has been associated with better subjective tolerance, improved ventilation, reduced airway resistance, shorter ventilator weaning, and shorter ICU stays.

Cardiovascular management

Neurogenic shock, which may occur in 90% of patients suffering complete cervical SCI (compared to 50% of patients with incomplete SCI and 30% with SCI below T1) is caused by sympathetic denervation leading to arteriolar dilation and hypotension (SBP ≤ 80 mm Hg) with relative hypovolemia (venous pooling).

Interruption of cardiac sympathetic innervation leads to unopposed parasympathetic drive (bradycardia and decreased contractility).

Management should be tailored to the etiology of hemodynamic disturbance while optimizing cord perfusion and avoiding injury to other organ systems. Potential causes include neurogenic shock, bleeding, tension pneumothorax, myocardial injury or tamponade, and sepsis. Hemodynamic instability secondary to neurogenic shock may be corrected by judicious volume resuscitation, avoiding pulmonary edema, followed by norepinephrine infusion (increases systemic vascular resistance and has inotropic properties) as needed.

Optimal blood pressure management in patients with SCI is largely inferred from data on cerebral autoregulation and perfusion pressure goals with TBI. Class II and III evidence suggests hemodynamic augmentation in SCI with a goal of maintaining mean arterial pressure (MAP) > 80–85 mm Hg for at least 7 days is safe and may be associated with improved neurologic outcomes in SCI. Hypotension should be aggressively avoided.

Venous thromboembolism

Patients suffering SCI have the highest risk of venous thromboembolic disease of any hospitalized patients, with risk being highest during the first 3 months. Untreated, 40%–100% will develop deep venous thrombosis (DVT). Even with adequate prophylaxis (unfractionated heparin and pneumatic compression stockings or low molecular weight heparin alone) 12%–16% will develop major venous thromboemboli. Although the necessity of DVT/PE prophylaxis has been established, the optimal treatment strategy remains elusive. Systematic reviews and evidence-based consensus conferences have recommended low molecular weight heparin alone, adjusted-dose unfractionated heparin, or unfractionated heparin combined with a nonpharmacologic device; treatment should begin no later than 24–72 hours postinjury.

Other critical care concerns

Infectious complications most frequently involve the respiratory or urinary tract and are a leading cause of death and morbidity following SCI. Fever or leukocytosis not explained by an infectious source should prompt investigation of acute abdominal processes (e.g., pancreatitis, cholecystitis, bowel obstruction/ischemia/perforation) that may be occult with SCI.

Gastrointestinal stress ulceration is a known complication in trauma, with SCI conferring independent risk. Either H2-blockers or proton pump inhibitors are indicated, and should be started at admission and continued for at least 4 weeks.

Autonomic dysreflexia is characterized by symptoms of paroxysmal hypertension, cutaneous flushing, blurred vision, and nausea in response to a stimulus (hollow viscera distention or surgical procedures) below the level of the cord lesion. If untreated, this may result in encephalopathy, seizures, stroke, myocardial infarction, arrhythmias, and death. Management priorities are removal of stimulus and correction of hypertension.

Surgical management

Surgical intervention plays a role in the management of spine trauma regardless of whether SCI exists. Surgery is performed with two goals in mind: (1) to decompress neural elements in those with neurologic deficit; and (2) to reestablish spinal alignment and stability in order to prevent further cord injury and facilitate early mobilization. Early surgical intervention is not associated with increased complication rates and may improve neurologic outcome.

Neuroprotective strategies and future research

Research in SCI over the past several decades has elucidated many of the mechanisms at play in secondary injury. Pharmacologic therapies investigated to date in large multi-center prospective randomized controlled trials have included methylprednisolone and the related compound tirilizad mesylate, GM-1 ganglioside, thyroid releasing hormone, gacyclidine, naloxone, and nimodipine. None of these therapies has yet been shown in a randomized control trial to definitively improve neurologic outcome.

Early studies with methylprednisolone demonstrated modest motor score benefits. Subsequent studies and analyses, however, have demonstrated higher rates of severe pneumonia, severe sepsis, and death. The American Association of Neurological Surgeons/Congress of Neurological Surgeons systematic review of this literature in 2002 concluded that "treatment with methylprednisolone for either 24 or 48 hours is recommended as an option in the treatment of patients with acute spinal cord injuries that should be undertaken only with the knowledge that the evidence suggesting harmful side effects is more consistent than any suggestion of clinical benefit."

There is much ongoing clinical research in both pharmacologic as well as non-pharmacologic interventions for SCI. This include trials on the optimal timing of surgical decompression, therapeutic hypothermia, cerebrospinal fluid drainage, cellular transplantation (e.g., Schwann cells, stem cells, etc), as well as targeting specific cellular inhibitors of regeneration.

Key references

Casha S, Christie S. A systematic review of intensive cardiopulmonary management after spinal cord injury. *J Neurotrauma.* 2011;28(8):1479–1495.

Chiodo AE, Scelza WM, Kirshblum SC, Wuermser LA, Ho CH, Priebe MM. Spinal cord injury medicine. 5. Long-term medical issues and health maintenance. *Arch Phys Med Rehabil.* 2007;88(3)(suppl 1):S76–S83.

Consortium for Spinal Cord Medicine. Respiratory management following spinal cord injury: a clinical practice guideline for health-care professionals. *J Spinal Cord Med.* 2005;28(3):259–93.

Hawryluk GW, Rowland J, Kwon BK, Fehlings MG. Protection and repair of the injured spinal cord: a review of completed, ongoing, and planned clinical trials for acute spinal cord injury. *Neurosurg Focus.* 2008;25(5):E14.

Kirshblum SC, Priebe MM, Ho CH, Scelza WM, Chiodo AE, Wuermser LA. Spinal cord injury medicine. 3. Rehabilitation phase after acute spinal cord injury. *Arch Phys Med Rehabil.* 2007;88(3) (suppl 1):S62–S70.

Krassioukov A, Warburton DE, Teasell R, Eng JJ. A systematic review of the management of autonomic dysreflexia after spinal cord injury. *Arch Phys Med Rehabil.* 2009;90(4):682–695.

Marino RJ, Barros T, Biering-Sorensen F, et al. International standards for neurological classification of spinal cord injury. *J Spinal Cord Med.* 2003;26(suppl 1):S50–S56.

Panczykowski DM, Tomycz ND, Okonkwo DO. Comparative effectiveness of using computed tomography alone to exclude cervical spine injuries in obtunded or intubated patients: meta-analysis of 14,327 patients with blunt trauma. *J Neurosurg.* 2011;115(3):541–549.

Paralyzed Veterans of America., Consortium for Spinal Cord Medicine. Early acute management in adults with spinal cord injury: a clinical practice guideline for health-care providers. Washington, DC: Consortium for Spinal Cord Medicine; 2008.

Chapter 15

Burn care

Jennifer Ziembicki

Thermal burns

More than one million burn injuries requiring medical attention occur annually in the United States. Although improvements in both legislation and critical care management have helped to advance care for these patients, more than 50,000 will require hospitalization, and 4,500 individuals will die annually from burn injury. The morbidity and mortality of thermal injury depend largely upon patient age, preexisting comorbidities, the presence of inhalational injury, and the extent of the cutaneous burn, described as the total body surface area or TBSA. Proper critical care management of the severely burned patient begins with airway assessment for adequate ventilation and oxygenation, as well as fluid administration for the prevention of burn shock. Ultimately, surgical debridement and wound closure are required for definitive care of the patient, which may only be accomplished with proper nutritional support.

Thermal injury evokes an inflammatory response in the patient unlike that seen in any other field of medicine. This response is directly proportional to the extent of injury or TBSA burn and will continue until surgical closure of the wound is complete. In the first 24 to 48 hours following burn injury, the capillary membrane integrity is significantly compromised resulting in a profound leak of the plasma volume into the interstitial space. This loss of capillary membrane integrity combined with an initial decrease in the cardiac output will ultimately lead to fatal burn shock if left untreated. With proper fluid administration, shock is prevented and the patient will then elicit a hypermetabolic response. This response is largely driven by the β-adrenergic system and influenced by cortisol, glucagon, and thyroid hormone, as well as various cytokines and chemokines. During this phase, the patient will demonstrate significantly increased cardiac output, low systemic vascular resistance, elevated temperature, and increased white blood cell counts. Clinically, this may be indistinguishable from the systemic inflammatory response, seen in other areas of medicine. Patients unable to mount such a response in the face of severe injury, secondary to preexisting cardiac disease are at particular risk for fatal burn shock and may require invasive monitoring and inotropic support during the resuscitative phase.

The pathophysiology of a burn wound may be described by three zones of injury that evolve during the first 72 hours following the initial insult (Figure 15.1).

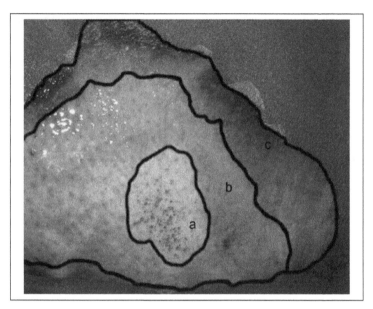

Figure 15.1 Burn wound demonstrating the 3 zones of injury related to a burn wound. In the center is the zone of coagulation, containing irreversible injury. Surrounding this is the zone of stasis which may include vasoconstriction and ischemia, putting the wound at risk for worsening. Farthest from the center of the wound is the zone of hyperemia

In the center of this three-dimensional area is the zone of coagulation, which is considered to contain irreversible injury. Surrounding this is the zone of stasis, where vasoconstriction and ischemia may cause the wound to deepen if there is inadequate fluid administration during the resuscitative phase of the patient's care. Outside the zone of stasis lies the zone of hyperemia, which is created by blood vessel dilation and typically heals without surgery.

Initial evaluation and resuscitation

Airway

Initial evaluation of the burn patient begins with an assessment of the patient's airway. An adequate history remains essential, followed by determination of the patient's symptoms and physical findings. Immediate intubation will be required for those who are unconscious, in obvious respiratory distress, or experiencing hemodynamic instability. Additional "hard signs" of impending airway obstruction include dyspnea, chest tightness, tachypnea, stridor, accessory muscle use, and swelling of the tongue and oropharynx. As a rule, early intervention is preferred in order to prevent airway obstruction necessitating surgical intervention.

Inhalational injuries may complicate nearly one-third of all major burns and may double the mortality predicted by the cutaneous burn alone. Although one should suspect an inhalational injury in the presence of facial burns and singed facial hair, more important is a history of exposure to smoke in an enclosed space and evidence of oropharangeal carbon deposits and carbonaceous sputum. Inhalational injury may be thought of as having three distinct components— carbon monoxide poisoning, upper airway thermal burns, and lower airway chemical injuries—each of which may exist in a single patient.

Carbon monoxide is produced by the combustion of organic material and acts as a systemic poison, inhibiting the transport and mitochondrial use of oxygen. Carbon monoxide will bind hemoglobin with two hundred times greater affinity than oxygen, displacing the oxygen-hemoglobin dissociation curve to the left, and prohibiting oxygen unloading at the cellular level. It is important to remember that the pulse oximeter will give a falsely high reading for oxygen saturation. A carboxyhemoglobin level should be obtained by arterial blood gas upon the patient's arrival. Carboxyhemoglobin levels of up to 5% may be normal, whereas levels of 15%–20% may cause headache and confusion. Increasing levels of carboxyhemoglobin may cause hallucinations, combativeness, and coma with a mortality rate of more than 50% for carboxyhemoglobin levels greater than 60%.

The mainstay of treating carbon monoxide poisoning remains prompt administration of 100% inspired oxygen. Treatment should begin at the scene and continue until carboxyhemoglobin levels are less than 10% (approximately 30 to 40 minutes). While hyperbaric oxygen may decrease the half-life of carboxyhemoglobin even further, several randomized controlled trials have failed to show a significant decrease in mortality.

The body's capability to cool inspired air leaves the upper airway susceptible to direct thermal injury, while the tracheobronchial tree and lower airway are more likely to succumb to chemical injury. Supraglottic injury can be diagnosed by direct laryngoscopy and may manifest as swelling, sloughing and carbonaceous sputum. Maximal airway swelling will occur at 12–24 hours with severe edema developing quickly. When severe edema is suspected, prophylactic intubation is indicated. Given the lower airway's more efficient heat-carrying capacity, injury to it secondary to the toxic elements of smoke or inhaled steam results in atelectasis, decreased ciliary action, pooling of secretions, bronchorrhea, and bronchospasm (Figure 15.2). When lower airway injury is a concern, fiberoptic bronchoscopy should be performed, with an appropriate-sized endotracheal tube placed over the scope to ensure intubation of the airway when indicated.

The care of patients with inhalational injuries requires strict attention to pulmonary hygiene with techniques aimed to mobilize pulmonary secretions. Frequent bronchoscopy along with chest physiotherapy and percussion are essential. For patients who meet the criteria for acute lung injury/acute respiratory distress syndrome, low tidal-volume ventilation with 6 mL/kg predicted body weight and maintenance of plateau pressure less than 30 cm is recommended. Additionally, high-frequency percussive ventilation may have a role in

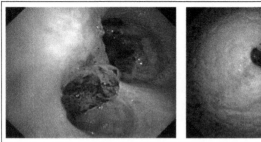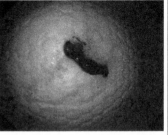

Figure 15.2 Bronchscopic evaluation of a patient with inhalation injury demonstrating thick, carbonaceous secretions

loosening airway exudate and casts, which may be beneficial for inhalational injuries. Scheduled aerosol administration using heparin 5000 U/3mL, acetylcysteine 3 mL of a 20% solution, and albuterol sulfate will also help inhibit fibrin clot formation, minimize hemorrhagic casts, and promote mucolysis.

Breathing

After ensuring an adequate airway, the patient's breathing must be assessed. Of utmost importance is to always evaluate the patient for coexisting trauma, such as pneumothorax, pulmonary contusions, head injuries, and spinal injuries, which otherwise may be initially overlooked in the presence of large cutaneous burns. Once trauma has been assessed, the patient's chest wall should be evaluated for the degree and severity of burn injury. Full-thickness circumferential burns to the chest may limit chest wall expansion, decrease pulmonary compliance, and increase peak airway pressures. Although not typically a problem upon initial presentation, this full-thickness burn, or eschar, forms a constrictive band as the patient undergoes volume resuscitation. When present, chest wall escharotomy should be performed by creating bilateral incisions through the eschar in the anterior axillary, infraclavicular, and subcostal lines.

Resuscitation and fluid management

The optimal means of fluid resuscitation in the severely burned patient remains an area of controversy. The goal of such resuscitation is to restore adequate tissue perfusion with the least amount of fluid possible in order to avoid complications that coincide with the massive administration of fluid. Initial calculations should be based on the admission weight of the patient and the size of the burn, including only areas of partial and full-thickness dermal injury. To estimate the size of the burn, the "Rule of Nines" may be used where the head and each upper extremity constitute 9% of the TBSA of the patient, while each leg, the anterior trunk, and the posterior trunk account for 18% TBSA each. This works well for adults, but may underestimate the head size in children. Charts that adjust for changes in surface area with age are important for younger age groups.

An initial estimate of the patient's fluid needs may be calculated using the American Burn Association's Consensus formula. The total volume of fluid to be administered may be calculated by multiplying 2 mL lactated Ringer's solution per kilogram of body weight by the percentage of TBSA burn. Half of the total calculated volume should be administered in the first 8 hours, while the second half of fluid should be given over the ensuing 16 hours. It must be recognized, of course, that this is only an estimate of the patient's needs and that each patient must be monitored hourly to adjust fluid needs. Fluid administration must ensure hemodynamic stability. In addition, in the hemodynamically stable patient, urinary output remains the primary indicator of adequate tissue perfusion. In adults, the goal is a urinary output of 0.5 to 1.0 mL/kg/hr. Children, however, have a greater ratio of surface area to volume, and therefore require 1.0 to 1.5 mL/kg/hr urinary output. For most, fluid may be administered through two large-bore peripheral intravenous lines, but in the case of preexisting cardiovascular or renal disease, consideration should be given to the placement of a central venous line or pulmonary artery catheter. Fluid adjustments should be made on an hourly basis, either increasing or decreasing the rate by 15% to 20% of the total volume.

Several factors may significantly increase the volume of fluid required for adequate resuscitation. These factors include delayed resuscitation, high-voltage electrical injuries, hyperglycemia, alcohol intoxication, and inhalational injuries. Additionally, particularly in the hemodynamically unstable patient, associated trauma should be assessed, if not previously done. Rhabdomyolysis should be suspected in patients with deep burns, electrical burns, and those with evidence of compartment syndrome. When present, the urine output should be maintained at a minimum of 100mL/hr. Alkalinization of the urine as well as mannitol administration are sometimes used with significant rhabdomyolysis, but data supporting their use are controversial.

No single perfect formula exists to adequately resuscitate patients sustaining large burn injuries. Adverse consequences of fluid administration include poor tissue perfusion, pulmonary edema, pleural effusion, and the development of extremity and abdominal compartment syndromes. Severely burned patients, therefore, require constant monitoring of their response to resuscitation, and the potential for complications should continually be assessed.

Metabolic support and nutrition

Optimal nutritional support remains essential for the severely burned patient. The metabolic response seen in such patients is one of profound hypermetabolism displaying the highest resting energy expenditures seen in any field of medicine. Epinephrine, cortisol, and glucagon interact, producing an overall catabolic state. The body will enter a state of accelerated gluconeogenesis, glycogenolysis, and muscle proteolysis. Unlike other states of starvation, the burn patient has a reduced ability to utilize fat; skeletal muscle, therefore, becomes the major obligatory fuel.

Several formulas exist to determine the caloric needs of the burn patient, including the Harris-Benedict and Curreri equations. Although these may provide an overall estimate of the patient's requirements, indirect calorimetry remains more accurate.

Nutritional support should be implemented within the first 24 hours of the patient's arrival to the hospital. Enteral nutrition is preferred with the tube placed in a postpyloric position when possible. Interruptions in feeding should be kept to a minimum, and feeding throughout the operative course is desired. Carbohydrates provide the major energy source for the burn patient, while the optimal dose and composition of lipids remain controversial. In general, lipid composition should be kept to less than 30% of nonprotein calories. Because burn patients use skeletal muscle as a fuel, leading to rapid loss of lean body mass, their protein needs approach 1.5 to 2.0 gm/kg/day, with children displaying even greater needs. Vitamins A, C, D, and E as well as zinc are added to the enteral feeds to further promote wound healing. Additionally, adjuncts such as recombinant human growth hormone and oxandrolone, an anabolic steroid, may be employed to assist in promoting protein synthesis.

Wound management

Treatment of the burn wound begins with inspection of the wound and determination of the depth of the burn. Superficial partial-thickness burns, in which only the outer layers of dermis are affected, require topical antimicrobials to promote spontaneous wound healing, whereas deeper partial-thickness and full-thickness burns will require topicals designed to penetrate the devitalized and avascular eschar in order to delay wound colonization and prevent infection. Systemic antibiotics are not routinely indicated unless there is surrounding cellulitis or invasive burn-wound infection.

Several choices exist for the selection of topical antimicrobials. Silver sulfadiazine (Silvadene®) is a soothing cream that provides excellent gram-positive and gram-negative coverage as well as coverage for candida species. Patch testing should be performed for those patients with sulfa allergies. While neutropenia has been reported, this generally improves with discontinuation of therapy. There are also a variety of dressings that contain silver, which may be left in place for up to 7 days, making these a popular choice for smaller burns in children. Mafenadine acetate (Sulfamylon®) is formulated as both a cream and solution, and has the ability to penetrate the burn eschar. Mafenadine acetate is a potent carbonic anhydrase inhibitor; patients must, therefore, be monitored for the development of metabolic acidosis. Although mafenadine acetate has good gram-positive and gram-negative coverage, it does not cover candida, making other topicals necessary for those patients requiring extended use.

Early excision and grafting is required for patients with deep partial-thickness and full-thickness burns. Even with the use of topicals, necrotic tissue carries the potential for the development of infection and burn-wound sepsis. Early excision and grafting improves patient survival, reduces burn-wound infection rates, shortens hospital stays, and decreases scarring. Ideally, for those patients with severe burns, resuscitation is complete by 48 hours postburn, with excision beginning as early as postburn day 3. For those patients with extensive burns, serial operations placed several days apart may be performed.

There are two main methods of surgical excision: fascial excision and tangential excision. Fascial excision, where the full-thickness of skin and subcutaneous tissue is removed en masse, may be performed with electrocautery and produces little blood loss. The resulting wound, however, may be cosmetically unpleasing, as the body's natural contour may be lost. Tangential excision utilizes a large scalpel to serially remove necrotic tissue until healthy, bleeding tissue is identified. This type of excision has the potential for far greater blood loss, with some reporting as much as 100 mL to 200 mL blood loss per percent total body surface area excised. In extensive burn injury, the goal is to perform the excision swiftly, as the patient may develop significant hypothermia, owing not only to the loss of skin integrity, but also secondary to the infusion of crystalloids and blood products throughout the procedure.

Autograft remains the best choice for replacement of lost skin. Depth of graft is chosen as either full-thickness or partial-thickness. Thicker grafts contract less and should be placed over areas of function when there is sufficient donor skin. Grafts are applied as a sheet (unmeshed) or meshed. Although meshing has the advantage of minimizing hematoma and seroma formation, sheet grafts are more aesthetic and contract less. Sheet grafts are also preferred for areas of function including the hands, face, and neck. When the body area to be excised is larger than can be covered by autografts it becomes necessary to employ biological dressings and skin substitutes. Choices in the case of insufficient autograft include cadaver allograft, porcine xenograft, amniotic membranes, and cultured epithelial autografts. Additionally, in the case of full-thickness burns, dermal replacement may be necessary, for which several options exist.

Chemical burns

Chemical injury may occur in the household or industrial setting. All chemical injury results in the denaturation of proteins, though the specifics may vary with the agent. Acids produce coagulative necrosis, whereas alkalis produce liquifactive necrosis, often resulting in deeper injury. The treatment of chemical injury follows essentially the same principles as the treatment of thermal injury. Treatment begins with removal of the chemical from the patient while protecting oneself from additional injury. Dry chemicals should be brushed from the skin followed by copious lavage of all wounds. Neutralizing agents should be avoided because they may generate heat via exothermic reactions. Material Safety Data Sheets and regional poison control centers provide valuable information on a variety of chemical exposures.

Electrical injury

Electrical injury may be divided into low-voltage (less than 1000 volts) and high-voltage (greater than 1000 volts) injury. Indoor burns are more likely to be low-voltage and localized to areas of contact. In high-voltage injuries, electrical current flow causes significant destruction of deep tissue including muscle and bone. All patients sustaining electrical injury should undergo cardiac monitoring because the development of virtually any cardiac arrhythmia is possible. Fluid resuscitation may be initiated with the Consensus formula; however, it is imperative to recognize that the cutaneous burn may not fully express the degree of deeper injury. Calculated fluid needs are often in excess of those determined by the Consensus formula. Patients should be monitored for the development of the extremity compartment syndrome. When myoglobinuria is diagnosed, fluid administration should be increased to maintain a urine output greater than 100 mL/hour. Alkalinization of the urine as well as mannitol administration may be considered.

Summary

Severe burn injury evokes a significant inflammatory response in the patient proportional to the size of the cutaneous injury. Early mortality may be attributed to inability to control the airway as well as failures of initial resuscitation. Early excision and grafting is essential to halt the ensuing inflammatory response and improve patient survival.

Key references

Herndon DN. *Total Burn Care*. 4th ed. Saunders; Philadelphia, PA, 2012.

Hyakusoku H, Orgill DP. *Color Atlas of Burn Reconstructive Surgery*. Springer, Philadelphia, PA, 2010.

Sheridan RL. *Burns: A Practical Approach*. Manson Publishing; London, UK, 2011.

Wolf SE. *Burn Care*. Landes Bioscience; Austin, TX, 1999.

Chapter 16

Acute kidney injury

Greta L. Piper and Lewis J. Kaplan

Epidemiology

The epidemiology of acute kidney injury (AKI) and acute renal failure (ARF) is deceptively complex. Not only are the available data dependent on the various populations of patients studied, the epidemiology is also related to the diverse definitions and classifications for AKI and ARF. In contrast, the epidemiology of End Stage Renal Disease (ESRD) is more easily described with ongoing analysis by the United States Renal Data System (USRDS), which collects and analyzes trends in the incidence, prevalence, treatment, morbidity, and mortality associated with ESRD.

Worldwide prevalence of renal failure is difficult to determine in part because studies from most non-Western and developing nations are often small and not widely published. In developed countries, the reported incidence of ARF in critically ill patients ranges widely from 1%–25%. Although no national database yet exists for AKI, several studies have attempted to define the epidemiology of acute kidney injury, primarily in single centers.

The Program to Improve Care in Acute Renal Disease (PICARD) was a prospective, observational, cohort study of 618 ICU patients in five academic centers in the United States. Patients with a Scr increase ≥ 0.5 mg/dL in those with a baseline Scr ≤ 1.5 mg/dL or a Scr increase of ≥ 1.0 mg/dL in those with a baseline Scr between 1.6 and 4.9 mg/dL who warranted a nephrology consult were included. Although the most common cause of AKI in each center was acute tubular necrosis, the in-house mortality broadly ranged between 24% and 62%. The largest AKI cohort study is the Beginning and Ending Supportive Therapy for the Kidney (BEST Kidney) investigation. Inclusion criteria for patients in the 54 involved ICUs in 23 countries was severe AKI defined by treatment with renal replacement therapy, oliguria, or blood urea nitrogen (BUN) > 84 mg/dL. AKI incidence was 5.7%, and the most common etiology was septic shock. In-house mortality varied across centers between 50.5% and 76.8% with an overall mortality of 60.2%.

These studies highlight the lack of consensus in the incidence, prevalence, and outcomes related to acute kidney injury, even among institutions in the same study. In addition, the need for a common definition is clear as underlying physiology leading to AKI is common across each of these studies, but the detection and analysis is rather disparate.

Definition

The term "ARF" has been commonly applied to any amount or type of acute renal dysfunction, and has been further confused by such common terms as "acute renal insufficiency." The earliest descriptions involved only a decrease or absence of urine output. More recently, ARF has been defined as an abrupt and sustained decline in glomerular filtration rate (GFR) that leads to the plasma accumulation of urea and other substances that are normally cleared by renal processing, filtration, and excretion. A lack of universally accepted definitions has limited progress in the understanding and management of AKI.

The Acute Dialysis Quality Initiative (ADQI) group in conjunction with representatives from the American Society of Nephrology, the International Society of Nephrology, the National Kidney Foundation, and the European Society of Intensive Care Medicine defined a classification system for renal dysfunction known by the acronym RIFLE (Risk, Injury, Failure, Loss of kidney function, and End-stage kidney disease) (Table 16.1). Each of these stages is accompanied by precise criteria that encompass changes in Scr, urine output (Uop) as well as GFR. RIFLE classification system includes criteria for both GFR/Scr and Uop. Although patients can qualify through a change in either set of criteria, the criteria that lead to the most severe classification are used. Advantages of this system include its consideration of change from the patient's baseline, classification of acute or chronic disease, and generalizability to different populations and disease processes. One limitation of the RIFLE classification is that diuretic use decreases the sensitivity and specificity of the Uop criteria. The balance of the Uop criteria to the GFR/Scr criteria has also been questioned. Hoste et al (2006) noted that patients with RIFLE-F by GFR/Scr criteria have a higher mortality than patients with RIFLE-F by Uop criteria, further supporting an imbalance in patient allocation between the two arms of the ADQI classification system. Another

Table 16.1 RIFLE classification

Class	Creatinine/GFR Criteria	Urine Output Criteria
Risk	Serum creatinine × 1.5 / GFR decrease > 25%	< 0.5 mL/kg/hour × 6 hours
Injury	Serum creatinine × 2 / GFR decrease > 50%	< 0.5 mL/kg/hour × 12 hours
Failure	Serum creatinine × 3 / GFR decrease > 75%, or Serum creatinine ≥ 4 mg/dL with an increase > 0.5 mg/dL	< 0.3 mL/kg/hour × 24 hours, or anuria × 12 hours
Loss	Persistent ARF with loss of kidney function > 4 weeks	
End-stage kidney disease	Complete loss of kidney function > 3 months	

Table 16.2 AKIN classification		
Stage	**Creatinine Criteria**	**Urine Output Criteria**
1	Serum creatinine increase of ≥ 0.3 mg/dL or Serum creatinine 1.5 – 2 x baseline	< 0.5 mL/kg/hour x 6 hours
2	Serum creatinine > 2 or 3 x baseline	< 0.5 mL/kg/hour x 12 hours
3	Serum creatinine ≥ 4 mg/dL with an increase > 0.5 mg/dL or Serum creatinine > 3 x baseline	< 0.3 mL/kg/hour x 24 hours, or anuria x 12 hours

disadvantage is the need for a baseline Scr, though the ADQI has allowed for estimation when the actual value is unavailable. Nonetheless, utilizing a classification scheme that may be broadly applied and readily implemented serves to create a platform in which therapeutic strategies may be equitably evaluated.

The Acute Kidney Injury Network (AKIN) recently proposed a modification of the RIFLE classification for AKI (Table 16.2). The AKIN criteria define AKI as an abrupt (within 48 hours) reduction in renal function that includes an increase in Scr ≥ 0.3 mg/dL or ≥ 1.5-fold from baseline, or a reduction in Uop for > 6 hours. The three stages of AKI according to the AKIN classification correlate with the Risk, Injury, and Failure classes of the RIFLE system. Stage 3 also includes patients who require renal replacement therapy; Loss and End-stage kidney disease are not included in the AKIN scheme. The AKIN classification does not require a baseline Scr, although two values within 48 hours of one another are needed. In a comparison of the RIFLE and AKIN classification systems, AKIN criteria demonstrated improved diagnostic sensitivity, but unaltered ability to predict in-house mortality for critically ill patients.

The RIFLE classification system is becoming the most widely used definition of AKI in critical care and nephrology literature. It is simple, uses commonly and regularly obtained clinical data, and fulfills the purpose of stratifying renal dysfunction severity and broadly correlating with mortality. As more randomized studies are performed, it will likely become even more useful as an outcome predictor.

Underlying causes

The causes of acute kidney dysfunction have been traditionally characterized by the affected structure of renal anatomy or the antecedent systemic etiology. Classification of the cause as prerenal, renal, or postrenal simplifies discussions and may help determine the next step in management. Prerenal dysfunction, or renal hypoperfusion, is the result of absolute or relative hypovolemia or hypotension and is related to inadequate oxygen delivery as well as restoration of oxygenated reflow with the generation of toxic oxygen metabolites. Etiologies such as hemorrhage, dehydration, sepsis, as well as cardiovascular pathologies such as heart failure, thromboembolism, or vasculitis are often implicated. Renal disorders encompass acute glomerular, tubular, and interstitial diseases including allergic and autoimmune interstitial nephritides. Postrenal or obstructive uropathy involves the impedance of urine flow anywhere from the renal pelvis to the urethra. Common etiologies of AKI in the critically ill may affect multiple areas of the kidney, and it is therefore important to identify the source whenever possible in order to guide initial therapy.

Specific etiologies

Contrast media–induced nephropathy (CIN; radiocontrast nephropathy) describes AKI that occurs after parenteral administration of iodinated contrast media in the absence of any other cause—although contrast delivery without clinical illness is relatively infrequent in hospitalized patients. The incidence of CIN varies from 1%–50%, again depending on the definition of AKI as well as the population studied, but it is implicated as a frequent cause of hospital-acquired renal dysfunction. The mechanisms of radiocontrast AKI induction are not yet completely understood. Several factors have been elucidated including impaired renal circulation and medullary oxygenation from vasoconstriction, as well as direct cytotoxicity from the contrast media. Hypovolemia, preexisting renal impairment, and diabetes mellitus are the most significant well-established risk factors, although age > 75 years, heart failure, liver cirrhosis, diuretic administration, and concurrent nephrotoxic medication administration are cited as predisposing conditions.

Accordingly, the most important means of mitigating against CIN is restoration or maintenance of appropriate circulating volume. The role of bicarbonated fluid remains controversial although no risk is incurred in patients receiving bicarbonate anion instead of chloride anion as the mate to cationic sodium. Additional radiocontrast administration within 72 hours of a prior dose also increases AKI risk. N-acetyl cysteine (NAC) administration remains similarly controversial and is likely inferior to volume therapy; NAC may, however, have a role in patients who cannot receive an adequate amount of intravenous fluids prior to radiocontrast administration (e.g., emergency cardiac catheterization). CIN is usually nonoliguric with an increase in Scr within 48 hours that peaks at 4 to 5 days and then normalizes in 7 to 10 days following exposure. More than 75% of patients completely recover, but up to 10% become dialysis dependent, and in-house mortality risk is increased. The introduction of low- and iso-osmolar contrast media agents has reduced the frequency and severity of AKI, but does not eliminate the risk, especially in patients with predisposing conditions.

Sepsis can lead to multi-system organ failure (MSOF) in critically ill patients. Septic AKI has been identified as an entity distinct from nonseptic AKI, and complicates almost 12% of ICU admissions. Clinical characteristics include a greater acuity of illness, greater hemodynamic instability, and greater severity of AKI by RIFLE criteria. When compared to patients with nonseptic AKI, septic AKI is associated with greater ICU and overall in-hospital mortality. The mechanisms underpinning septic AKI are thought to be multifactorial. In the earliest phases of the disease, the systemic inflammatory response involves a cytokine

Table 16.3 Medications associated with rhabdomyolysis

Salicylates
Fibric acid derivatives (e.g., gemfibrozil, fenofibrate)
Neuroleptics
Anesthetic and neuromuscular blocking agents (via malignant hyperthermia induction)
Quinine
Corticosteroids
Statins
Theophylline
Tricyclic antidepressants
Selective serotonin uptake inhibitors
ε-Aminocaproic acid
Phenylpropanolamine
Propofol

release that leads to systemic vasodilation and hypotension followed by renal vasoconstriction. Activation of the coagulation cascade causes disseminated microthrombi that result in ischemic injury and tubular necrosis. In addition, the systemic inflammatory response is due in part to the interaction of endotoxin with Toll-like receptor 4 (TLR4) on immune effector cells. TLR4 has recently been identified on renal tubular and vascular cells, suggesting that a direct renal cytotoxic effect is exerted by endotoxin signaling of these cells.

Rhabdomyolysis is a potentially life-threatening condition that occurs when skeletal muscle is broken down, leading to release of intracellular contents, such as creatine kinase, lactate dehydrogenase, myoglobin, uric acid, potassium, and phosphates into the systemic circulation. It can occur after severe blunt trauma, crush injuries, high voltage electrical injuries, and burns. It may also result when recreational substance abuse leads to prolonged immobilization or direct muscular cytotoxicity as well as from sustained tetanic contraction. Prescription medications can also cause rhabdomyolysis (Table 16.3).

AKI occurs in rhabdomyolysis through a combination of mechanisms. Hypovolemia causes renal hypoperfusion via renal vasoconstriction. In the presence of acidic urine (pH < 5.6), myoglobin and uric acid may precipitate to form obstructing casts. Iron released from myoglobin breakdown reacts with oxygen via the Fenton and Haber-Weiss reactions to generate toxic oxygen metabolites (TOM). Lipid peroxidation results from the interaction of TOM and tubular epithelium cell phospholipids. The net result of oxidant damage is acute tubular necrosis (ATN).

Rhabdomyolysis-induced AKI may present with (most common) or without oliguria. The need for renal support therapies, management of serum potassium and calcium, and mortality rates appear to be similar for rhabdomyolysis-induced and nonrhabdomyolysis-induced AKI. Patients with rhabdomyolysis-induced

AKI, however, generally have higher serum uric acid levels. Hyperkalemia is a potentially life-threatening complication of rhabdomyolysis especially when associated with AKI and hypocalcemia. Treatment should be initiated to prevent cardiac dysrhythmia and diastolic arrest.

Nephrotoxins are an under-recognized cause of AKI in the intensive care unit. Antibiotics, especially aminoglycosides and amphotericin B, as well as nonsteroidal anti-inflammatory medications are the most common culprits.

Aminoglycosides have excellent efficacy in the treatment of severe gram-negative infections and continue to be used despite the well-known nephrotoxicity. The incidence of aminoglycoside-related nephrotoxicity has increased from 2%–3% in 1969 to 20% in the past decade. Risk factors include hypovolemia, male gender, advanced age, concomitant use of other nephrotoxins, preexisting renal impairment, and prolonged duration of treatment. Extended daily-dosing of aminoglycosides is one effective strategy that may reduce the identified nephrotoxicity associated with this class of antimicrobials. The mechanism of aminoglycoside-associated AKI is proximal tubular necrosis. The most common presentation is nonoliguric renal dysfunction, and the initial sign is increased Scr and enzymuria as the brush border sloughs. The rise in Scr is slower than in other causes of AKI, often occurring 7–10 days after treatment initiation. In more than half of cases, the renal injury does not become clinically evident until after therapy has been completed. Recovery time is also longer, requiring 4–6 weeks to return to baseline if no other insults are incurred.

Amphotericin B is important for the treatment of severe systemic fungal infections, but it is also potentially nephrotoxic. Early after the initiation of therapy, despite adequate systolic and pulse pressures, medication associated renal vasoconstriction leads to a significant rise in Scr and decrease in Uop. Amphotericin B also induces direct tubular injury leading to hypokalemia and hypomagnesemia. It then causes a local release of adenosine in the distal tubules leading to afferent vasoconstriction. In individuals treated with high doses for prolonged periods, loss of functioning nephrons leads to significant renal impairment and the need for renal support therapy. Risk factors for nephrotoxicity include male gender, average daily dose ≥ 35 mg/day, body weight > 90 kg, concomitant use of other nephrotoxic agents, and abnormal baseline renal function. The increasing incidence of nephrotoxicity with increasing number of risk factors suggests that alternative therapy may be more appropriate in patients with two or more risk factors. Controversy exists regarding the use of slower continuous infusions as well as liposomal encapsulation or lipid emulsified formulations of amphotericin B rather than larger doses over shorter time periods as a means of decreasing both the degree of nephrotoxicity and the associated mortality rates.

Nonsteroidal anti-inflammatory medications (NSAIDs) are commonly used analgesics and antipyretics in the ICU. They block the normal prostaglandin-induced vasodilation of afferent vessels and result in undesirable vasoconstriction and renal hypoperfusion. These vascular alterations induce a functional prerenal state that, if sustained, may progress to ATN. NSAIDS also cause acute interstitial nephritis (AIN), a hypersensitivity reaction resulting in inflammatory cell infiltration and cytokine activation, subsequently causing renal tubular injury and dysfunction. Both mechanisms are usually reversible with discontinuation of the culpable medication.

Abdominal compartment syndrome (ACS) leads to acute kidney injury when intra-abdominal hypertension (IAH) compromises venous return, decreasing cardiac output and renal inflow. IAH may also reduce renal perfusion pressure by compressing the renal vein. Because the vein is thinner walled than the renal artery, venous compression exceeds arterial inflow reduction. Impeded outflow may lead to renal edema within a tightly bounded renal capsule and Gerota's fascia. A renal compartment syndrome may therefore theoretically occur. In addition, concomitant nonrenal visceral edema may establish extrinsic kidney compression and worsen renal hypoperfusion. The expected renal response to inadequate oxygen delivery is the activation of the renin-angiotensin-aldosterone pathway and increased antidiuretic hormone (ADH) production. These protective mechanisms cannot overcome the resulting ATN and cellular damage if abdominal decompression and relief of the compartment syndrome does not quickly occur.

The kidneys are vulnerable to both blunt and penetrating injury. In general, unilateral renal injury may be symptomatic, with resulting anemia, pain, and hematuria, but it is rarely enough to meet criteria for AKI if the contralateral kidney has normal function. The most common reasons for AKI related to injury are acute hemorrhage and hypovolemia leading to decreased renal perfusion. Although not described or easily evaluated, it is also possible that a perirenal or retroperitoneal hematoma from blunt trauma may result in a local compartment syndrome that impairs renal function. Blunt injury evaluation also commonly employs radiocontrast for CT scanning and as such may compound hypovolemia with CIN. Because their time frames are disparate and sequential, hypovolemia-induced AKI may mask CIN-associated renal injury. Rarely, renal vascular injury can lead to renal ischemia and AKI.

Obstructive uropathy can impair the flow of urine anywhere from the renal pelvis to the urethra and generally does not require renal support. AKI or ARF from obstructive uropathy requires bilateral flow obstruction most commonly as a result of prostate disease, neurogenic bladder, or metastatic cancer; bilateral surgical injury has been described as well. Large volume urinary retention leads to progressive upper urinary tract dilation and decreased GFR. Obstructive uropathy is also associated with interstitial nephritis. Diagnosis involves imaging to confirm hydronephrosis. In addition to directly treating the source of the obstruction with surgery or medication, obstructive uropathy may be acutely relieved with bilateral nephrostomy tube placement.

Workup

The investigation of renal dysfunction has traditionally been based on determining whether the insult is due to a prerenal (reduced renal perfusion), renal (glomerular, tubular or interstitial), or postrenal (obstructive) cause. Although this paradigm still has some utility in focusing diagnostic efforts, the more relevant goal should be to determine whether acute kidney injury exists, the likely cause(s), and the severity of impairment. Therapies can then be focused on minimizing further insult, monitoring progress, and determining the prognosis for renal recovery.

As in all diagnostic endeavors, the initial evaluation starts with a history and physical examination whenever possible, understanding that this may not be as complete or specific in the critically ill ICU patient as desired. Past medical history should include prior renal disease, infections, recent contrast administration, medications with nephrotoxic potential, diuretics, pressors, heart disease, diabetes mellitus, hepatic dysfunction, and other organ failure. Past surgical history, known allergies, substance misuse, and family history of renal and other organ dysfunction are also relevant. In certain circumstances, a travel history is also appropriate.

The physical exam should focus on signs and symptoms of hypovolemia or hypervolemia taking into account trends in the patient's vital signs, mental status, mucous membranes, respiratory dynamics, peripheral edema, and Foley catheter presence, as well as urine volume and color. A measured decrease in Uop over time is important in characterizing the severity of AKI by RIFLE criteria.

Basic laboratory data including the current BUN and Scr, electrolytes, and hemoglobin are helpful; knowledge of a patient's baseline values can be invaluable. Though not perfect, an estimation of GFR using the Cockroft-Gault and the Modification of Diet in Renal Disease equations provides a useful working estimate of renal function; more precise determination is optimally obtained only by a 24-hour collection for assessment of creatinine clearance. Serum osmolality (SerumOsm) as well as urinary sodium (UNa) may help to elucidate a patient's true volume status as well.

Urinalysis with microscopic examination can reveal otherwise undetectable renal dysfunction. Although the results do not fulfill any RIFLE criteria, they can help to determine the etiology if acute kidney injury is present.

The fractional excretion of sodium (FENa) has long been used to distinguish prerenal kidney dysfunction from ATN. Values less than 1% indicated renal hypoperfusion while values greater than 2% demonstrated ATN. Unfortunately the use of diuretics or any other sodium affecting medication renders this value inaccurate. More recently, the fractional excretion of urea (FEUrea) has been employed by some investigators to clarify renal hypoperfusion.

Ultrasound is a noninvasive method to evaluate for significant postrenal obstructive nephropathy by looking for hydronephrosis, change in kidney size, or perirenal fluid or hematoma. It can also evaluate changes in renal blood flow using Doppler techniques. The use of ultrasound for the evaluation of acute renal failure has recently come under scrutiny. The nephrology group at Yale has decried its use as a routine workup tool, documenting that in vanishingly few patients does the renal ultrasound return data that prompts clinicians to initiate or change therapy.

A renal biopsy is not routinely performed for AKI in the intensive care unit, as it rarely alters therapy. In severe cases where acute interstitial nephritis (AIN) is strongly suspected, biopsy can confirm the diagnosis prior to steroid administration. It is also useful to detect rejection in the transplanted kidney.

Prevention

Clinical trials focused on potential preventive methods (including volume expansion, diuretics, vasoactive drugs, and antioxidants) have demonstrated up to a 90% reduction in the incidence of AKI, but as a whole these studies are flawed and underpowered. Nonetheless, prevention and avoidance of AKI remains the best way to prevent progression to ARF requiring renal replacement therapy. Several specific preventive measures have been evaluated, although not in relation to the RIFLE criteria for diagnosis.

Volume expansion using fluid such as hetastarch, albumin, and plasma has been undertaken as a means of preventing renal hypoperfusion and therefore decreasing AKI. Hetastarches do not appear to have any specifically beneficial effect on the prevention of AKI, and, in fact, may have deleterious effects. Albumin is also not recommended for large volume resuscitation. It is expensive and the molecule is small enough (60kDa) to readily egress from capillary beds when capillary leak syndrome exists. Instead, a molecule would need to have a molecular weight of > 108 kDa to have its size exceed that of the typical capillary gap. Plasma carries additional risks with regard to allosensitization, transfusion-related acute lung injury (TRALI), and increased infection and organ failure risk. As such, it is not recommended as a plasma-volume expanding agent except in certain circumstances, such as massive transfusion or the management of a correctable coagulopathy prior to an intervention or to stem coagulopathy-associated hemorrhage.

The so-called low-dose dopamine, infused at rates of 3 mcg/kg/min or less was historically thought to improve outcomes from renal dysfunction by increasing renal perfusion and preventing oliguria. Instead dopamine shows no protective benefit compared to placebo in terms of renal recovery and mortality.

Renal replacement therapy

The current treatment for AKI is supportive therapy and reduction or elimination of injury inciting factors. Since the development of dialysis techniques in the 1950s, classic indications of therapy have included severe volume overload refractory to diuretics, hyperkalemia, metabolic acidosis, uremia, and azotemia. However, the specific values that define these conditions are subjective, leading to varied clinical practices.

Optimal timing for RRT remains unclear. A more recent meta-analysis of the early institution of continuous renal replacement therapy (CRRT) resulted in mortality benefit but no improvement in renal recovery.

A commonly used threshold is a predialysis BUN of 75 mg/dL in otherwise asymptomatic patients. However, the use of urea as a marker for treatment initiation is less than ideal because it may not indicate a true change in GFR, especially in the setting of increased protein-intake during critical illness. Changes in urea may reflect nonrenal conditions such as gastrointestinal (GI) bleeding, poor nutrition with associate catabolic state, systemic inflammatory response, rhabdomyolysis, or multi-organ failure. Likewise, oliguria should be evaluated with caution as it can vary with a variety of factors that do not reflect intrinsic renal function.

For those whose renal function is judged to be inadequate, renal support using intermittent or continuous techniques is appropriate. Nonetheless, RRT is not without risks, including bleeding, hypotension, arrhythmia, and infection. Potential advantages for CRRT over intermittent renal replacement therapy (IRRT) include hemodynamic stability, predictable solute clearance, easier fluid management, improved gas exchange, unlimited ability to provide nutritional support volume, and more stable intracranial pressure. Despite the predictable nature of CRRT and its predictable effects on a host of parameters, a recent Cochrane Database Review compared continuous with intermittent hemodialysis, and identified no significant differences in mortality or dialysis dependence. Peritoneal dialysis is uncommonly used in the ICU because it is less precise and effective in solute and fluid management compared with extracorporeal techniques, may impede diaphragmatic excursion in those with reduced pulmonary compliance, and is associated with a higher mortality in patients with ARF.

Special populations

Pregnancy—Physiologic changes of pregnancy include a total body-water increase of 6–8 liters and an increased GFR and creatinine clearance. AKI during pregnancy is rare, with an estimated frequency of < 1 in 20,000 pregnancies. When AKI occurs during the second trimester, it usually relates to septic abortion or prerenal azotemia due to hyperemesis gravidarium. It is more common for AKI to occur after gestational week 35 as a result of preeclampsia and hemorrhage. Preeclampsia associated with hypertension, elevated liver enzymes, and low platelets (HELLP) syndrome can be accompanied by significant renal dysfunction. ATN induced by hypovolemia or nephrotoxins is uncommon. AKI therapy during gestation is similar to that of nongravid patients with few special considerations. Urea, creatinine, and other metabolites of uremia cross the placenta. Thus, dialysis should be instituted earlier to maintain BUN < 50 mg/dL. Rapid and large-volume fluid removal may induce hemodynamic instability, decreased fetal perfusion, and premature labor. Peritoneal dialysis can be considered as an option that is more gradual than hemodialysis but is often limited by the size of the gravid uterus.

Burn patients—AKI is common in critically ill burn patients and is associated with high morbidity and mortality. Palmieri et al (2010) demonstrated a 53.3% incidence of AKI in patients with burns > 20% total body surface area. Those patients who developed AKI had a 34.4% mortality rate while those who did not enjoyed uniform survival. Progression to higher RIFLE class was associated with sepsis, nephrotoxic antibiotic administration, increasing total fluid balance, and greater number of operative procedures. Strong evidence supports that early aggressive fluid resuscitation improves clinical outcomes in burn patients, but the optimal fluid remains elusive. A Cochrane Database Review demonstrates that compared to resuscitation with crystalloids, resuscitation with colloids does not reduce the risk of death in critically ill trauma and burn patients.

Elderly patients—Elderly populations present a unique challenge in managing AKI. Immunosenescence, decreased cardiac output, aging vessels, and multiple comorbidities managed with an increased number of potentially nephrotoxic medications make it common for renal dysfunction to exist prior to acute illness and hospitalization. Renal blood flow may decrease by 10% per decade of life, and an exaggerated response to sympathetic mediated vasoconstriction, decreased nitric oxide production, and poor response to vasodilators such as atrial natriuretic peptide and prostacyclin lead to increased renal vascular resistance. This inflow limitation creates an impaired adaptation to hypovolemia. Absolute Scr, a product of creatinine generation, volume of distribution, and renal elimination, is difficult to interpret in the elderly patient with decreased muscle mass. Impairment may exist with a "normal" serum creatinine because the pre-illness baseline Scr may be at the low end of normal; small increases that remain within the normal range may represent AKI in the elderly. The RIFLE criteria account for such a situation in that small rises in creatinine coupled with a period of oliguria will identify AKI. Importantly, the RIFLE criteria have been validated in several large studies including elderly patients with a mean age > 60 years.

Therapies for AKI in this population are essentially the same as those in nonelderly populations. Meticulous care must be taken to appropriately dose medications for renal function and to manage drug interactions. Elderly patients are more vulnerable to hemodynamic instability, bleeding, infection, and neurologic changes, but RRT is generally well-tolerated when warranted.

Obesity—Clinically severe obesity is generally defined as a body mass index (BMI) > 40. As the obese population continues to increase, so, too, does the proportion of critically ill patients with clinically severe obesity. In the nonobese population a history of chronic renal insufficiency is an independent risk factor for AKI, and obese patients are at increased risk for chronic renal disease. Prerenal azotemia and ATN are likely the most common causes of AKI in the clinically severely obese ICU patient, although this has not been well-analyzed. It is worth noting that obese surgical patients are at higher risk of pressure-induced rhabdomyolysis and AKI. This increased risk correlates with higher BMIs as well as longer operative times, and myonecrosis is most frequently found in the sacral area, a challenging area to assess and examine. Vascular access for volume administration, flow-based monitoring, as well as dialysis access devices may be difficult to obtain. Weight-based dosing of RRT and medications is problematic due to the discrepancy between actual body weight and ideal body weight. Generally, some estimate of "adjusted" body weight is utilized and may be approximated by the following formula:

Adjusted BW = IBW + 1/3 (Actual BW − IBW)
where IBW is ideal body weight

Underexplored domains

The traditional biomarkers for AKI, including Scr, urea, and Uop fail to detect injury until after the insult has occurred. Early identification of AKI prior to oliguria and a rise in Scr would be ideal to minimize the impact of AKI on patient outcome and resource utilization. The use of a single biomarker versus a panel of biomarkers is yet to be determined. Many urinary biomarkers have shown promise—including NGAL, IL-18, NHE3, KIM-1, tubular enzymes, and others; urinary NGAL is available as a commercially prepared kit for bedside use. It is unclear when to measure any of the available biomarkers, how frequently to reassess them, or whether intervention will reliably reduce the measured concentration of the assessed biomarker.

Conclusion

AKI is increasingly common and continues to be associated with significant morbidity and mortality. Although the understanding of certain etiologies and mechanisms has improved, the general diagnostic approach remains unchanged. Prevention of initial AKI, as well as prevention of worsening of AKI with supportive therapy, remains the most effective means of managing this insult. Classification of kidney injury with the RIFLE criteria provides a common reference for comparison that can be used for future trials to further elucidate prognosis as well as provide more standardized evidence-based protocols for treatment.

Key references

Bagshaw SM, Carol G, Bellomo R. Early acute kidney injury and sepsis: a multicentre evaluation. *Crit Care.* 2008;12:R47.

Briguori C, Airoldi FD, D'Andrea D, et al. Renal insufficiency following contrast media administration trial (REMEDIAL): a randomized comparison of 3 preventive strategies. *Circulation.* 2007;115(10):1211–1217.

Diskin CJ, Stokes TJ, Dansby LM, et al. Toward the clinical use of the fraction excretion of solutes in oliguric azotemia. *Ren Fail.* 2010;32(10):1245–1254.

Hoste E, Clermont G, Kersten A, et al. RIFLE criteria for acute kidney injury are associated with hospital mortality in critically ill patients: a cohort analysis. *Crit Care.* 2006;10:R73.

Khan FY. Rhabdomyolysis: a review of the literature. *Neth J Med.* 2009;67(9):272–283.

Licurse A, Kim MC, Dziura J, et al. Renal ultrasound in the evaluation of acute kidney injury: developing a risk stratification framework. *Arch Intern Med.* 2010; 170(21):1900–1907.

Lopes JA, Fernandes P, Jorge S, et al. Acute kidney injury in intensive care unit patients: a comparison between the RIFLE and the Acute Kidney Injury Network classifications. *Crit Care.* 2008; 12:R110–117.

Maerz L, Kaplan LJ. Abdominal compartment syndrome. *Crit Care Med.* 2008;36(4):S212–S215.

Mehta RL, Pascual MT, Soroko S, et al. Spectrum of acute renal failure in the intensive care unit: The PICARD experience. *Kidney Int.* 2004;66:1613–1621.

Oliveira JFP, Silva CA, Barbieri CD, et al. Prevalence and risk factors for aminoglycoside nephrotoxicity in intensive care units. *Antimicrob Agents and Chemother.* 2009;53(7):2887–2891.

Palmieri T, Lavrentieva A, Greenhalgh DG. Acute kidney injury in critically ill burn patients. Risk factors, progression and impact on mortality. *Burns.* 2010;36:205–211.

Paul P, Roberts I. Colloids versus crystalloids for fluid resuscitation in critically ill patients. *Cochrane Database Syst Rev.* 2011;3:CD000567.

Podymow T, August P, Akbari A. Management of renal disease in pregnancy. *Obstet Gynecol Clin N Am.* 2010; 37:195–210.

Rabindranath K, Adams J, Macleod AM, et al. Intermittent versus continuous renal replacement therapy for acute renal failure in adults. *Cochrane Database Syst Rev.* 2007;3:CD003773.

Seabra VF, Balk EM, Liangos O, et al. Timing of renal replacement therapy initiation in acute renal failure: a meta-analysis. *Am J Kid Dis.* 2008;52(2):272–284.

Uchino S, Kellum JA, Bellomo R, et al. Acute kidney failure in critically ill patients: a multi-national, multicenter study. *JAMA.* 2005;294(7):813–818.

Chapter 17

Endocrinology in the critically injured patient

Nimitt Patel and Jason Sperry

Although significant advances in the care of the injured patient have occurred over the last decade, those who survive their initial injury continue to be plagued with the development of multiple organ failure, sepsis, and their attributable morbid effects. In these critically injured patients there are many stressors in addition to their injuries, such as infectious complications, various therapeutic interventions, and operative procedures. The injured patient is exposed to these stressors for prolonged periods of time with varying levels of intensity and unpredictability. An injured patient's ability to cope with these factors comprises a complex multi-factorial response in which the endocrine system's involvement, integrity, and flexibility are integral components for survival. The neuroendocrine response is a key factor in maintaining homeostasis and enabling the injured patient to recover.

Hyperglycemia

Hyperglycemia is common in critically injured patients as a result of elevated glucose production in the liver and peripheral insulin resistance, impairing glucose uptake peripherally. Multiple factors contribute to hyperglycemia following injury. The stress response promotes insulin resistance and early glucose mobilization, secondary to the acute effects of endogenous steroids, growth hormone, glucagon, and catecholamine release. This acute stress response following severe injury is different from the response following sepsis or an infectious process. (Figure 17.1). The extent of hyperglycemia in the early postinjury period is proportional to the severity of injury and may be a marker for the physiological derangement that is occurring. The patients in an ICU endure ongoing stressors following injury, which trigger a cascade of events that involve neurohormonal and cytokine pathways, the reaction to which is contingent upon the type and duration of the stressor. During this early period, the liver's ability for autoregulation of glucose is inhibited. Cytokines such as interleukin-1 and tumor necrosis factor-α also contribute to hyperglycemia by further inhibiting insulin release and promoting insulin resistance.

In the last decade, multiple studies have focused on ICU management strategies for hyperglycemia in hopes of improving outcome in critically ill patients.

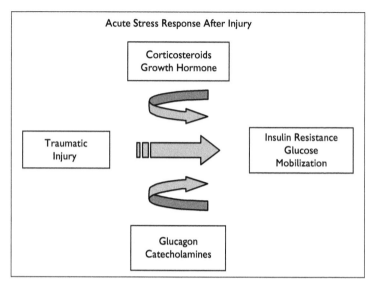

Figure 17.1 Stress response after injury and trauma

In a landmark study, Van den Berghe et al performed a large randomized controlled study on 1548 primarily surgical patients who were assigned to either standard insulin therapy intiated when blood glucose levels were greater than 200 mg/dL or received intensive insulin therapy to maintain blood glucose levels between 80 and 110 mg/dL. Mortality rates at 1 year were reduced from 8% in the conventional insulin therapy to 4.6% in the intensive insulin therapy group. Strict glucose control reduced the average number of blood transfusions by 50%, and resulted in significant decreases in critical illness polyneuropathy, acute renal failure requiring dialysis, and bloodstream infections. A limitation of this study, however, was that the majority of patients were postoperative surgical patients. This group then revisited intensive glucose control in a medical ICU population. They found a mortality benefit in patients who required ICU admission greater than 3 days; but for those who did not require this length of admission a suggestion of higher mortality and three-fold higher incidence of hypoglycemia were found.

These studies were followed by an increasing concern that tight glycemic control may not be generalizable to all critically ill patients, particularly because of the risk for hypoglycemia and its attributable morbidity.

Until recently, the vast majority of prospective hyperglycemia trials contained small proportions, if any, of injured patients. Evidence for the beneficial or detrimental effects of intensive glucose control following injury were limited to retrospective studies. It remained questionable whether tight glycemic control was beneficial following injury, nor was it known if hypoglycemia occurred as commonly as in other patient populations or was associated with poor outcome postinjury. Interestingly, some studies suggest that hyperglycemia may be different following injury as compared to other ICU patients. Multiple large retrospective analyses revealed that early and persistent hyperglycemia following injury was associated with an increased ICU and hospital length of stay, elevated nosocomial infection rates, higher ventilator requirements, and greater mortality; however, little data existed regarding whether aggressive attempts at prevention of hyperglycemia postinjury would result in beneficial effects. Sperry and collegues retrospectively analyzed a large cohort trial of trauma patients for whom a strict glycemic control protocol was utilized. They concluded that early hyperglycemia and persistent hyperglycemia was an independent risk factor for higher mortality and multi-organ failure. Interestingly, this study found that early hyperglycemia was not a significant risk factor for nosocomial infection, as other studies had suggested. The authors hypothesized that the utilization of a strict glycemic control protocol throughout the study may have reduced the risk of nosocomial infection compared to previously studied cohorts.

Most recently, in the largest randomized controlled trial on this topic to date, the Normoglycemia in Intensive Care Evaluation—Survival Using Glucose Algorithm Regulation (NICE-SUGAR) trial attempted to put most of the prior issues regarding the potential benefits of aggressive glycemic control to rest. This study randomly assigned medical and surgical patients to intensive glucose control (81–108 mg/dL) or conventional glucose control (less than 180 mg/dL). The authors reported that severe hypoglycemia was significantly more frequent in the intensive group. Most importantly, there was a significantly higher mortality in the intensive group. They also found no statistically significant difference in the average ICU or hospital length of stay, ventilator days, or need for renal replacement therapy in the two treatment groups. Interestingly, subgroup analyses suggested that intensive glucose control patients who required corticosteroids or were injured had trends towards lower mortality. In contrast, there was no such trend across all medical and surgical patients. This further reinforces the need for further large prospective randomized trials in trauma patients to determine whether intensive glycemic control is indeed beneficial following injury.

In summary, current evidence suggests that intensive glycemic control in the ICU (targeting 80–110 mg/dL) may be harmful and associated with a higher incidence of hypoglycemia and a higher risk of mortality, for most ICU patients. More current guidelines are recommending less aggressive control, targeting glucose level in the 150–180 mg/dL range. Dedicated studies are required to verify any potential benefit of intensive glycemic control following injury.

Adrenal insufficiency

Many disease processes and stressors affect the hypothalamic-pituitary-adrenal (HPA) axis. Normal physiologic response following critical illness or injury results in an increased release of corticotropin-releasing hormone (CRH) from the hypothalamus. This, along with vasopressin, stimulates the release of adreno-corticotropic hormone (ACTH) from the pituitary, which then exerts its effects on the adrenal to release glucocorticoids. The HPA axis has been shown to be vital for the survival of the critically ill patient. Stressors such as severe infection, trauma, burn, or surgery increase cortisol production by as much as 6-fold, proportional to the severity of the stressor. This is the body's physiologic adaptive mechanism to manage any overwhelming inflammatory or stress response.

In critically injured patients a number of factors can cause suboptimal adrenal corticosteroid response following injury. There may be adrenal insufficiency due to physical damage to the HPA axis. The normal secretion of CRH and ACTH in response to stress can be compromised by head injury or pituitary infarction. Adrenal cortical synthesis can directly be affected by multiple mechanisms; one of which is a direct inhibitor effect of inflammatory cytokines. However, the injured patient more commonly will have functional adrenal insufficiency, which is a term used to express the state of adrenal insufficiency without necessarily having any structural damage to the HPA axis.

Severe sepsis and septic shock are leading causes of late death following injury and are associated with reported mortality rates as high as 50%. Overwhelming infection and shock can be associated with a relative or absolute adrenal insufficiency and systemic inflammation-induced steroid receptor resistance.

Many medications can also lead to a functional adrenal insufficiency during illness. Administration of exogenous steroids for any number of medical reasons, the equivalent of at least 30 mg of hydrocortisone or 7.5 mg of prednisone for at least 3 weeks, can suppress the HPA axis and induce adrenal atrophy for months after the cessation of the treatment. These patients often require stress-dose steroid replacement in times of trauma, surgery, or sepsis.

As indicated earlier, cortisol levels vary according to the type and severity of the illness. For this reason it is difficult to ascertain what constitutes a normal physiologic response in these critically ill patients and to what extent the patient needs to be supported with exogenous corticosteroids.

In 1976, a prospective randomized study of surgical patients with septic shock suggested a survival benefit with high-dose steroids. Several subsequent studies refuted any survival benefit with high-dose steroid regimens and showed an increase in super-infection-related mortality. In contrast, more recent studies have shown that low-dose hydrocortisone replacement is beneficial in aiding the reversal of shock and, possibly, decreasing mortality. Annane et al published a randomized double-blind study of low-dose hydrocortisone and fludrocortisone compared to placebo in septic patients. They further classified the patients into the responders and nonresponders to the ACTH stimulation test. There was no difference in survival benefit between patients who responded appropriately to the corticotropin test. However, a lower mortality was found in those patients treated with low-dose steroid replacement who were nonresponders to the ACTH stimulation test. The adverse events were similar in both groups. Subsequent studies of low-dose steroid replacement demonstrated earlier cessation of vasopressor support and a reduction in proinflammatory cytokines. Survival benefit has not been as clear.

More recently, the Corticosteroid Therapy of Septic Shock (CORTICUS) study, a large multi-center, randomized, double-blinded, placebo controlled trial of low-dose steroid replacement versus placebo found that mortality for the two arms was not significantly different overall, even when the groups were stratified by their response to ACTH stimulation. Shock, defined as ongoing vasopressor requirements, was reversed earlier in the hydrocortisone group. However, steroid replacement led to more frequent infectious complications. The authors did not recommend hydrocortisone as a standard therapy in septic patients and deemed the corticotropin stimulation test unreliable to determine which patients might benefit from therapy.

There continues to be controversy regarding utilization of low-dose steroids in adult septic patients who remain poorly responsive or recalcitrant to aggressive fluid and vasopressor therapy. Further studies are required in the trauma population, as it is not clear if the functional adrenal insufficiency in the injured patient and the potential response to hydrocortisone therapy is different relative to that seen in noninjured, septic shock patients in previous trials.

Recently, the use of etomidate in critically ill patients has become a topic of controversy. Etomidate is a short-acting nonbarbiturate sedative with a rapid onset and minimal, if any, cardiovascular side effects. Because of these characteristics, this drug has commonly been used for rapid sequence intubation in patients requiring mechanical ventilatory support. Etomidate causes adrenal insufficiency by reversibly inhibiting the action of an enzyme used in adrenocorticoid steroid synthesis. These deleterious effects can last up to 24 hours after bolus induction. Cuthbertson et al looked at the data from the CORTICUS study to evaluate the effect of etomidate on the adrenal axis and mortality rates at 28 days. They found that the proportion of nonresponders to ACTH stimulation was significantly higher among patients who had been administered etomidate and that etomidate usage was associated with a higher 28-day mortality. Increasing literature in injured patients suggest that the use of etomidate is associated with adrenocortical insufficiency, increased length of stay, and ventilator requirements. It may be an independent risk factor for the adult respiratory distress syndrome. Despite this increasing evidence, etomidate use remains common for rapid sequence intubation due to the minimal effect on the hemodynamics of the critically injured patient. Good prospective studies of etomidate use are still needed.

Endocrinology in the organ donor

Organ transplantation is an evolving field of medicine that has seen enormous technological and medical advancements, which have improved outcomes. Despite these advancements, there is a shortage of organs, which can be further limited secondary to the difficulty associated with post-brain-death management of eligible organ donors. Once a patient becomes brain dead progression to somatic death leads to exclusion of up to 10%–20% of potential donors. Brain death results in many adverse pathophysiologic changes including cardiovascular collapse, severe alterations in organ system homeostasis, upregulation of proinflammatory molecules, and metabolic changes that can ultimately prevent organs from being harvested. Specific changes to endocrine systems result from cessation of pituitary function, acute adrenal insufficiency, and thyroid hormone insufficiency. These adverse changes lead to clinical manifestations including hypotension, severe hyperglycemia, diabetes insipidus, metabolic acidosis, and hypothermia. Management of these endocrine issues is crucial in order to optimize the potential for organ donation in eligible patients.

Adrenal insufficiency and hyperglycemia are common after brain death. Cessation of brain activity leads to anterior pituitary gland dysfunction resulting in HPA axis malfunction and acute adrenal insufficiency. Despite aggressive management, up to 25% of organs are lost as a result of hemodynamic instability. Steroid replacement has been shown to reduce inflammatory cytokine expression and reduce vasopressor requirements by stabilizing and maintaining systemic vascular tone. This reduction in vasopressor requirements is thought to improve organ procurement rates and post-transfusion organ function.

Hyperglycemia is common due to a number of factors, including massive catecholamine release, peripheral insulin resistance, and infusion of dextrose containing solutions. Elevated blood glucose can damage the islet cell of the pancreas in a relatively short time. It is recommended to maintain glucose levels between 80–150 mg/dL to decrease the risk of pancreatic graft dysfunction and minimize associated metabolic abnormalities attributable to ongoing poorly controlled hyperglycemia.

The posterior pituitary is also affected by brain death and leads to undetectable levels of vasopressin in both adult and pediatric organ donors. As a result central diabetes insipidus occurs almost uniformly, leading to polyuria, hypernatremia, and elevated serum osmolality. Diabetes insipidus can directly result in hemodynamic instability if left untreated. The resultant hypernatremia has been shown to increase the risk of graft dysfunction, especially of the liver. The treatment is vasopression replacement either with vasopressin as a continuous infusion or boluses of desmopressin, which acts on V2 receptors. Both minimize excessive urinary fluid loss and correct sodium abnormalities. Effectively treating the diabetes insipidus minimizes the risks to potential donor organs. Many studies have also reported that decreased levels of serum thyroxine (T4) result in hemodynamic instability, necessitating higher levels of vasopressor support. Thyroxine administration in brain-dead patients has been shown to reduce vasopressor requirements and has been associated with an increase in the number of organs harvested. Despite this evidence, treatment with thyroid replacement remains controversial and its use is sporadic in the management of the potential organ donor.

Future endocrine topics following injury

An increasing body of evidence from animal models has revealed that sex-hormones and their derivatives play an intricate role in the pathological response to injury. They have been shown to influence the hemodynamic, immunologic, organ system, and cellular responses to traumatic insult. Studies have demonstrated that both cardiovascular and immunologic function are preserved in female rodents when they are in the proestrus phase (when 17β-estradiol levels are highest). A similar large body of evidence has accumulated concerning the detrimental effects of testosterone and its derivatives following trauma-hemorrhage. These results demonstrate the dichotomous nature of male and female sex-hormones in response to trauma-hemorrhage in animals. Estrogen is protective and immune enhancing, while testosterone is deleterious and immunosuppressant.

Large single and multi-center, retrospective studies that have examined sex-based outcome differences following injury have resulted in conflicting and varied conclusions. Relative to controlled animal experiments, predisposing comorbidities and variable injury characteristics create confounding dilemmas in these types of analyses. Possibly more important is the fact that measurements of the hormonal milieu of the male and female patient at the time of injury are lacking in these prior analyses. Interestingly, a recently published, prospective analysis demonstrated that at 48 hours following injury, estrogen levels were positively associated with a greater risk of mortality, a conclusion which contradicts the majority of the experimental animal literature. This association was found and remained significant in both males and females. This more recent data only adds to any controversy regarding the importance of sex-hormones following injury.

Several groups are currently studying the potential beneficial effects of the administration of estrogen during hemorrhagic shock or traumatic brain injury, as well as progesterone following traumatic brain injury. It is clear that additional studies are needed to decipher the mechanisms responsible for any protective effect of sex-hormone following injury and the potential benefits of hormonal manipulation.

Key references

Annane D, Sebille V, Charpentier C, et al. Effect of treatment with low doses of hydrocortisone and fludrocortisone on mortality in patients with septic shock. *JAMA*. 2002;288(7):862–871.

Cuthbertson B, Sprung C, Annane D, et al. The effects of etomidate on adrenal responsiveness and mortality in patients with septic shock. *Int Care Med*. 2009; 35(11):1868–1876.

NICE-SUGAR Study Investigators. Intensive versus conventional glucose control in the critically ill patients. *N Eng J Med*. 2009;360(13):1283–1297.

Preiser JC, Devos P, Ruiz-Santana S, et al. A prospective randomised multi-centre con-trolled trial on tight glucose control by intensive insulin therapy in adult intensive care units: the Glucontrol study. *Intensive Care Med.* 2009;35(10):1738–1748.

Schumer W. Steroids in the treatment of clinical septic shock. *Ann Surg.* 1976; 184:333–341.

Sperry J, Frankel H, Vanek S, et al. Early hyperglycemia predicts multiple organ failure and mortality but not infection. *J Trauma.* 2007;63(3):487–493.

Sperry J, Frankel H, Avery N, et al. Characterization of persistent hyperglycemia: what does it mean post-injury? *J Trauma.* 2009;66(4):1076–1082.

Sprung C, Annane D, Keh D, et al. Hydrocortisone therapy for patients with septic shock. *New Engl J Med.* 2008;358(2):111–124.

Van den Berghe G, Wouters P, Weekers F, et al. Intensive insulin therapy in the critically ill patients. *N Eng J Med.* 2001;345(19): 1359–1367.

Van den Berghe G, Wilmer A, Hermans G, et al. Intensive insulin therapy in the medical ICU. *N Engl J Med.* 2006;354(5):449–461.

Wood KE, Becker BN, McCartney JG, et al. Current concepts: Care of the potential organ donor. *N Engl J Med.* 2004;351(26):2730–2739.

Chapter 18

Infection and antibiotic management

Jeffrey A. Claridge and Aman Banerjee

Infection in the trauma intensive care unit

Nosocomial infections are a major patient safety issue in the ICU. They cause significant increases in patient morbidity and mortality, as well as increase medical expenses. Trauma patients often sustain multiple injuries—any of which can lead to infection. Critically ill trauma patients have a higher risk of infection compared to other surgical ICU cohorts. Studies estimate infectious complications range from 5.7% to 45%. The etiology is multi-factorial. Trauma patients have higher rates of emergency procedures such as intubation, central venous catheterization, and tube thoracostomy, where the use of sterile technique might not be absolute. Trauma and blood transfusion may also be associated with immunosuppression. Additionally, trauma ICU device utilization rates are among the highest when compared to other ICU types.

Systemic inflammatory response syndrome in trauma

The presence of fever and leukocytosis are often the primary drivers for initiation of an "infection workup." However, the sole use of these clinical parameters is often confounded by the high prevalence of the systemic inflammatory response syndrome (SIRS) within the trauma population on admission and persisting for the first week in 91% of patients. SIRS represents a frequently encountered, but nonspecific finding seen with infection, but it can be caused by many other conditions, most commonly trauma, burn injury, pancreatitis, or major surgery. It is a clinical phenomenon manifested by the interactions of humoral and cellular mediators and cytokines. As a result the intensivist is required to be both watchful for infection and wary of the knee-jerk reaction to initiate a "shotgun" approach to the evaluation of fever and leukocytosis in the trauma population. The practice of "pan-culturing," or obtaining respiratory, blood, and urine cultures in patients suspected of infection has been shown to be inefficient.

Conceptually, it is very helpful to consider the differences among SIRS, sepsis, severe sepsis, and septic shock as outlined in Table 18.1. SIRS is more common in trauma patients than true sepsis.

Table 18.1 Definition of terms for the clinical range of infection

Term	Definition and Criteria
Infection	An identifiable invasion of normally sterile tissue by micro-organism(s)
Systemic Inflammatory Response Syndrome (SIRS)	Two or more of the following: • Temperature ≥ 38°C (100.4°F) or ≤ 36 °C (96.8°F) • Heart Rate > 90 beats/minute • Respiratory rate > 20 breaths/minute, or $PaCO_2$ < 32 mm Hg • White Blood Cell Count > 12,000/mm³, or < 4,000/mm³, or > 10% band forms
Sepsis	The presence of infection with SIRS
Severe Sepsis	Sepsis with end organ dysfunction, hypoperfusion, or hypotension. Can include: • Lactic acidosis • Oliguria • Altered mental status
Septic Shock	Sepsis induced hypotension not responsive to an adequate fluid challenge and/or requiring inotropic/vasoactive agents (e.g., 500 mL fluid infused as a bolus or hypotension persisting > 1 hour)

Infection workup

The decision whether to initiate a focused workup for infection should be assessed daily during rounds by the ICU team. The workup should begin with a review of the patient's injuries and medical history, hospital course, recent procedures and the utilization of devices such as mechanical ventilators, central venous catheters (CVC), urinary catheters, and nasogastric tubes. The physical exam should be used to help determine possible sources of infection and to guide further diagnostic tests. One should pay close attention to the auscultation of the chest, evaluation of IV and CVC sites for local inflammation, a thorough skin exam with attention to drain sites, traumatic and/or surgical wounds, and pressure sores. A review of a chest radiograph should be performed, especially in mechanically ventilated patients. The intensivist should use all available clinical information to determine the need for further diagnostic tests. Table 18.2 outlines the common infections seen in trauma patients, along with diagnostic criteria and preventive strategies.

Diagnostic tests

Blood cultures
Blood cultures are the gold-standard for diagnosing bacteremia. However, their ability to detect bacteremia is low, most likely because of the sporadic nature

Table 18.2 Infectious complications in critically ill trauma patients

Complication	Incidence	Risk Factors	Diagnostic Criteria	Common Organisms	Preventative Measures

Ventilator Associated Pneumonia (VAP)	• 27%–44% cases
	• 1.7–12.3 per 1,000 vent days
		• Duration of mechanical ventilation
		• Head injury
		• Increased injury severity
		• Self-extubation
		• Reintubation
		• Urgent intubation
		• Prolonged bag mask ventilation
		• Chest injury
		• Impaired airway reflexes
		• chronic obstructive pulmonary disease
		• Advanced age
		• Aspiration
		• Supine position
		• Malnutrition
		• Over-sedation
		• Maxillary sinusitis
		• Cardiac disease/arrest
			• Radiographic—
			Two or more serial CXR with new, progressive or persistent infiltrate, cavitation, or consolidation
			• Clinical (one of the following)—
			  – Fever > 38°C with no other recognized cause
			  – WBC < 4,000/mm³ or ≥12,000/mm³
			  – Age ≥ 70 with altered mental status and no recognized cause
			And at least two of the following:
			  – New onset purulent sputum, increased suctioning requirement
			  – Cough, dyspnea, tachypnea
			  – Rales or bronchial breath sounds
			  – Worsening gas exchange, increased O² requirement, increased vent support
			• Microbiology—
			Positive culture result:
			  – blood with no other recognized source
			  – pleural fluid
			  – quantitative culture by BAL or PSB
			  – ≥5% BAL-obtained cells contain intracellular bacteria
				• *Escherichia coli*
				• Enterobacter species
				• Klebsiella species
				• Proteus species
				• *Serratia marcescens*
				• *Haemophilus influenzae*
				• *Staphylococcus aureus* (MSSA and MRSA)
				• *Streptococcus pneumoniae*
				• Anaerobes
				• Legionella species
				• *Pseudomonas aeruginosa*
				• *Acinetobacter baumanii*
					• Standardized ventilator weaning protocol
					• Protocol for administration of sedative medications with daily sedation interruption
					• Elevate head of bed 30°
					• Oral hygiene program (e.g., tooth/gum/tongue brushing, chlorhexadine (0.12%) rinse BID)
					• Use deep suctioning to clear pooled secretions, change suction tip every shift
					• Avoid gastric distention
					• H2-blocker or PPI
					• Hand hygiene program
					• Selective decontamination of the digestive tract

(continued)

Table 18.2 (continued)

Complication	Incidence	Risk Factors	Diagnostic Criteria	Common Organisms	Preventative Measures
Catheter-Related Blood Stream Infections	0.6–4.0 cases per 1,000 central line days	• Duration of intravascular catheterization • Catheter site: femoral > jugular > subclavian • Number of lumens • Parenteral nutrition/ lipid infusion • Urgent placement • Exchange over a wire • Extremes of age • Burns • Use for hemodialysis • Malnutrition	Any of the following in a patient with a CVC: • Fever > 38°C, chills, or hypotension (not attributable to a cardiac event or hypovolemia) Along with one of the following: • Positive semiquantitative or quantitative culture of the catheter • Simultaneous quantitative blood cultures drawn through the CVC and peripheral vein with a ratio of 5:1 or more (CVC vs. peripheral) • Differential time to positivity (CVC culture becomes positive > 2 hours before peripheral culture)	• Staphylococcus aureus (MSSA and MRSA) • Coagulase-negative staphylococci • Gram-negative bacilli • Pseudomonas aeruginosa • Candida albicans	• Early removal • Aseptic technique • Use of maximal barrier precautions • Skin antisepsis with 2% chlorhexidine • Hand-hygiene program
Urinary Tract Infection (UTI)	0.4–7.7 cases per 1,000 urinary catheter days	• Duration of catheterization • Female sex • Catheter insertion outside of operating room • Use of nonclosed system • Age > 50 • Diabetes mellitus	• Clinical (one of the following with a positive urine culture) – Fever > 38°C, urgency, frequency, dysuria, suprapubic tenderness – Positive urine culture: ≥ 10^5 CFUs/mL (no more than 2 species of microorganisms) Or – At least two of the above signs/symptoms	• Escherichia coli • Enterobacter • Enterococci • Klebsiella pneumoniae • Pseudomonas aeruginosa • Candida albicans	• Early removal of catheters with use of nurse-based or electronic protocols • Aseptic technique for insertion • Secure catheter in place with collecting bag with level of bladder

| | | | – Positive urine dipstick for leukocyte esterase or nitrite
– Pyuria with at least 3 WBC per high-power field
– Positive urine Gram stain | | • Maintain unobstructed urine flow
• Maintain closed catheter drainage system
• Hand-hygiene program |
| Surgical Site Infections (SSI) | • 3%–25% | • Extremes of age
• ASA class ≥ 3
• Diabetes
• Obesity
• Degree of wound contamination
• Inadequate antibiotic prophylaxis
• Prolonged operative time
• Hypothermia
• Emergent procedure | **Superficial (both)**
• Within 30 days after an operation
• Involves only skin or subcutaneous tissue of the incision
And one of the following:
• Purulent drainage
• Organisms isolated from aseptically obtained culture of fluid or tissue
• Pain or tenderness, localized swelling, redness, or heat, and superficial incision is opened deliberately by the surgeon
Deep (both)
• Occurs within 30 days of an operation
• Involves deep soft tissue (e.g., fascial and muscle layers) of incision
And one of the following:
• Purulent drainage
• Incision dehisces spontaneously/opened by surgeon along with fever (> 38°C), localized pain, or tenderness
• Presence of abscess by radiographic, reoperation or histopathologic examination | • *Staphylococcus aureus*
• Coagulase-negative staphylococci
• Enterococcus
• E. coli
• *Pseudomonas aeruginosa*
• *Bacteroides fragilis* | • Appropriate administration and redosing of prophylactic antibiotic
• Maintenance of normothermia
• Aseptic technique
• Judicious transfusion of blood products
• Meticulous surgical technique |

(continued)

Table 18.2 (continued)

Complication	Incidence	Risk Factors	Diagnostic Criteria	Common Organisms	Preventative Measures
Intra-abdominal Abscess	• 4.2%–23.5%	• Advanced age • Penetrating abdominal trauma • Colonic and gastric injury	• Occurs within 30 days of an operation • Involves any part of the anatomy (e.g., organs or spaces) other than the incision, which was opened or manipulated during an operation • Presence of abscess by radiographic, reoperation or histopathologic examination – CT with IV contrast showing: rim enhancement, air fluid levels, or nonhomogeneity	• *Escherichia coli* • Streptococci • Enterococcus • *Klesiella pneumoniae* • *Bacteroides fragilis* • *Candida albicans*	• Currently no strong evidence

Sinusitis	• 2%–22.5%	• Duration of nasoenteric tube use
		• Duration of endotrachial intubation
		• Nasotracheal intubation
		• Facial trauma
			• Fever (> 38°C)
			• Purulent rhinorrhea
			• CT sinus showing:
			  – mucosal thickening
			  – opacification
			  – air fluid levels
				• *Staphylococcus aureus*
				• *Pseudomonas aeruginosa*
				• *Klebsiella pneumoniae*
				• *Escherichia coli*
				• Enterobacter
					• Prompt removal of nasal instrumentation

Antibiotic-associated Diarrhea	• 4% • 3.2 cases per 1,000 patient-days	• Antibiotic administration within 30 days • Administration of fluoroquinolones, cephalosporins, clindamycin,	Clinical • > Three watery bowel movements/day containing either blood or mucus • Abdominal pain • Fever (> 38°C) • WBC ≥ 12,000/mm^3	• *Clostridium difficile* • *Staphylococcus aureus* • *Klebsiella oxytoca* • *Clostridium perfringens*	• Barrier infection control policy • Hand hygiene • Restriction of high-risk antibiotics

		Risk factors	Diagnosis	Microbiology	Prevention
		• Use of PPI or H₂-antagonists • Length of stay in hospital/long-term care facility • Age > 65 years • Multiple comorbidities • Kidney disease requiring dialysis	Laboratory diagnosis • Positive cytotoxigenic culture • Positive toxin A/B enzyme immunoassay • Positive toxin B PCR		• Aseptic technique • Early drainage of retained hemothoracis or parapneumonic effusions • Hand hygiene
Empyema	2%–25%	• Duration of tube thoracostomy • Penetrating trauma • Fractures of more than two ribs • Length of ICU stay • Presence of pulmonary contusion • Retained hemothorax • Exploratory laparotomy • Incomplete expansion of lung after placement • Occult diaphragmatic injury	Radiographic • Persistent and loculated pleural fluid collection with or without an air-fluid level despite tube thoracostomy • Residual or reaccumulated loculated pleural fluid collection after removal of the chest tube Associated with: • Fever > 38°C • WBC < 4,000/mm³ or ≥12,000/mm³	• Streptococcus pneumoniae • Staphylococcus aureus • Escherichia coli • Haemophilus influenza • Klebsiella pneumoniae • Pseudomonas aeruginosa • Bacteroides fragilis	

BAL = bronchoalveolar lavage CFU = colony forming units; CT = computed tomography; CVC = central venous catheter; CXR = chest x-ray; MSSA= methicillin sensitive *staphylococcus aureus*; MRSA = methicillin resistant *staphylococcus aureus*; PSB = protected specimen brush; PCR = polymerase chain reaction; PPI = proton pump inhibitor; WBC = white blood cell

CHAPTER 18 **Infection and antibiotic management**

of bacteremia. Cultures should be drawn prior to initiation of antibiotics, if possible. Additionally, up to 50% of positive cultures are the result of contamination rather than true bacteremia. There is no consensus on acceptable clinical predictors of bacteremia. As a result, utilization varies with the physician's experience in estimating the probability of bacteremia in a given population. Based on the available literature, guidelines were proposed to improve the diagnostic yield of blood cultures. The skin site should be disinfected prior to culture. At least two culture sets should be obtained from different sites in a 24-hour period. More blood is better; at least 10–20 mL of blood should be drawn per bottle. Blood drawn from CVC sites should be paired with a peripheral blood culture. Before assuming that a positive culture drawn through a CVC represents true central-line associated bloodstream infection (CLABSI), there must also be a concurrent positive peripheral blood culture. Further evidence of catheter infection would be that the CVC culture becomes positive faster than the peripheral culture.

If the cultures are positive, the clinician is then left to determine whether this result represents true bacteremia or contamination. Findings suggestive of bacteremia are the growth of virulent organisms such as S pneumoniae, Klebsiella species, pseudomonas species, S aureus, Enterobacteriaceae, and Candida species. The presence of predisposing risk factors for bacteremia such as an immunocompromised state, prostheses, or indwelling lines should also be taken into consideration. Finally, the recovery of the same organism from multiple sites is suggestive of true bacteremia.

Findings indicative of a contaminated culture include prolonged incubation period before growth of an organism, the inability to reproduce the microorganism in subsequent cultures, or the presence of multiple organisms in an immunocompetent patient. Also, if the patient's clinical condition is not suggestive of sepsis, contamination should be suspected. The growth of skin flora, such as coagulase-negative staphylococci, diphtheroids, and Bacillus species also suggest contamination. This is especially true if only one culture site is positive. However, up to 15% of coagulase-negative staphylococci represent true pathogens, especially in the presence of a CVC.

Respiratory culture

The use of clinical criteria alone to diagnose ventilator-associated pneumonia (VAP) results in significant misdiagnosis among critically ill patients. Confirmatory laboratory data is essential to establish the diagnosis of VAP, to determine the causative organism, and to determine the organism's antibiotic sensitivity.

Tissue culture and postmortem histology are considered the gold standard for diagnosing VAP. Surrogates for these tests involve performing Gram stains and quantitative cultures on respiratory samples obtained from one of four diagnostic techniques: endotracheal aspiration, bronchoalveolar lavage (BAL), bronchoscope-directed brushing, and blind BAL or protected specimen brushing (PSB). The threshold applied to quantitative cultures for the diagnosis of VAP varies by collection method. For PSB the threshold is 10^3 colony-forming units (CFU) /mL; 10^4 CFU/mL for BAL; and 10^5 CFU/mL or 10^6 CFU /mL for tracheal aspirates.

Endotracheal aspiration is usually performed by the respiratory therapist; it involves the instillation of 5–10 mL of 0.9% saline solution into the airway followed by passage of a suction catheter into the endotracheal (ET) tube to retrieve the sample into a sterile specimen trap. It is the least invasive and most inexpensive technique. However, its utility is hampered by its frequent contamination of the specimen by oropharyngeal flora.

BAL involves the passage of a bronchoscope under visual direction into the area of consolidation. Approximately 100 mL of 0.9% saline is lavaged, and the specimen is suctioned into a Luken's trap. The advantages of BAL are that it samples a larger area than PSB or bronchoscope-directed brushing. It also may provide a therapeutic advantage via aspiration of plugs and mucus to clear the bronchial tree. The reported sensitivity and specificity of BAL to diagnose VAP are as high as 97% and 92%, respectively. The procedure is slightly less expensive than the bronchoscope-directed brushing.

Blind (or "mini") BAL involves the passage of a protected, double catheter, which can be directed to the right or left lung, through the ET tube. The inner cannula is then advanced farther into the airway and lavage is performed as in the bronchoscopic technique. In general, this technique has similar accuracy as the standard BAL.

Bronchoscope-directed brushing involves the visually-directed passage of a bronchoscope down the ET tube into the area of consolidation on chest x-ray. A double-sheathed microbiology brush is then passed along the bronchoscopes instrument port, unsheathed and collects the specimen under direct visualization. It is then resheathed and withdrawn from the bronchoscope. This technique has been shown to have a sensitivity of 100% and specificity of 96% using $\geq 10^3$ CFU/mL. It is the most expensive technique.

Blind PSB refers to the passage of a double-sheathed microbiology brush down the ET tube until it meets resistance. It is then telescoped out to obtain a sample, then resheathed and withdrawn. It is slightly more expensive than the tracheal aspirate due to the cost of the microbiology brush.

Controversy still exists regarding which of these tests represents the gold-standard for diagnosis of VAP. The difference in the threshold for determining VAP according to modality makes it difficult to establish one method as the gold-standard. Comparative studies have not clearly demonstrated better accuracy of one method over the others.

Urine culture

The urine is commonly cultured in the ICU to diagnose a catheter-associated urinary tract infection (CAUTI) or asymptomatic bacteriuria. It is often initiated as part of an "infection" workup associated with fever and leukocytosis. The practice of obtaining a urinalysis prior to sending a urine culture is not uniform in all ICUs, despite the fact that these cultures have a negative predictive value of 90%. Urinalysis is a quick, inexpensive test that requires little expertise to perform correctly. The most useful components for urinary tract infection (UTI) diagnosis are the presence of leukocyte esterase and nitrite. The presence of nitrites has high specificity (96.6%–97.5%) for bacteriuria but low sensitivity (0%–44%). The absence of leukocyte esterase has a negative predicted value of 97%–99%. The presence of both has sensitivity of 98%–99.5%. These results can prove useful in determining whether to begin empiric antibiotic treatment or to order a urine culture. It can also reduce unnecessary urine cultures, resulting in significant cost reductions.

Source control

Source control refers to the use of an intervention to obtain physical control of a focus of infection. The four methods for source control include drainage, debridement, device removal, and performance of a definitive procedure. Drainage describes the removal of an infected fluid collection by an incision or by insertion of a drain. Draining an encapsulated abscess converts it into a controlled sinus or fistula that can then heal by secondary intention. Debridement refers to the removal of devitalized or infected tissue. Removal of necrotic tissue eliminates a nidus of infection. Device removal refers to the removal of a prosthetic device that has become colonized by microorganisms living in a biofilm. Definitive procedures refer to the removal of the focus of infection such as decortication for an empyema or sigmoid colectomy for diverticulitis.

Antibiotic management

Antibiotic stewardship

Life-threatening infection is often the cause for, or consequence of, ICU admission. The prompt administration of appropriate antibiotic therapy can be potentially lifesaving in cases of sepsis or septic shock. In contrast, delay in antibiotic administration, even by a matter of hours, can increase mortality. However, overuse and inappropriate dosing of broad-spectrum antibiotics can contribute to the development of resistant microorganisms or opportunistic infection such as *Clostridium difficile* colitis. The supply of new antimicrobial agents available is also limited. The concept of antibiotic stewardship aims to both optimize antibiotic therapy and minimize the development of bacterial resistance.

Antibiotic stewardship begins with the use of preventative strategies to avoid nosocomial infections. Such stewardship includes adequate hand hygiene, appropriately limited and focused antibiotic prophylaxis, patient decolonization measures, environmental decontamination, and isolation for colonized patients. The use of best practices to avoid VAP, CLABSI and CAUTI must be followed. Care should be taken to select an appropriate antibiotic agent, as well as appropriate dose and duration, in order to minimize resistance and drug toxicity. Finally, antimicrobial de-escalation should be employed. De-escalation refers to the narrowing of the spectrum of antibiotic therapy according to clinical response, culture result, or pathogen susceptibility. In addition, the concept also calls for the cessation of antimicrobial therapy if an infection is not established.

Prophylactic antibiotic use

The benefits of using prophylactic antibiotics in the setting of elective and urgent operations have been well-demonstrated by several studies. The premise behind its use is to establish a tissue-drug concentration of the antibiotic prior to bacterial contamination. This is not feasible in the trauma population. Instead, it has been proposed that the administration of antibiotics after injury assumes the role of a presumptive therapy.

Open fracture

A fracture is considered "open" when the fragments are in communication with the environment through a defect in the skin. Having an open fracture increases the risk of bone and soft tissue infections. The Gustilo classification system is used to categorize the severity of open fractures. Type I consists of a clean open fracture with a skin wound < 1 cm in length. Type II consists of an open fracture with a laceration > 1 cm in length without extensive soft tissue damage, flaps, or avulsions. Type III consists of an open segmental fracture with > 10 cm wound with extensive soft tissue injury or a traumatic amputation. Special categories in Type III include gunshot fractures and open fractures caused by farm injuries. The risk of infectious complications increases with increasing Gustilo stage.

The recent Eastern Association for the Surgery of Trauma (EAST) practice guidelines for antibiotic prophylaxis of open fractures recommends administering systemic antibiotic coverage promptly, directed towards gram-positive organisms after Type I or II injuries and gram-negative coverage should be added for Type III injuries. High-dose penicillin should be administered for open fractures suspected of fecal or clostridial contaminations such as in farm accidents. Single-agent fluoroquinolone therapy is not superior to cephalosporin/aminoglycoside regimens and may be detrimental for fracture healing. This may result in higher wound infections in Type III fractures. For Type III fractures, antibiotics should be continued for no more than 72 hours postinjury. Finally, once-daily aminoglycoside therapy is safe and effective for Type II and III injuries.

Tube thoracostomy

Chest injury is commonly encountered in both blunt and penetrating trauma. The vast majority of these injuries can be managed via a closed-tube thoracostomy. A significant morbidity of this procedure is the complication of empyema. The use of antibiotics to prevent empyema is controversial. The EAST practice guidelines concluded that there is insufficient data to suggest that prophylactic antibiotics reduce the incidence of empyema. Interestingly, the use of a first-generation cephalosporin for up to 24 hours may reduce the incidence of pneumonia, but not empyema.

Basilar skull fracture/cerebrospinal fluid leak

Basilar skull fractures have the potential to place elements of the central nervous system in contact with bacteria from the paranasal sinuses and throat. Traumatic cerebrospinal fluid (CSF) leaks occur most often in young males, occurring in 2% of all patients with head injuries, and 12% to 30% of patients with basilar skull fractures. These patients have the potential to develop meningitis; as a result, some physicians administer antibiotics in an attempt to mitigate this risk. The available evidence from a meta-analysis of several randomized clinical trials does not support the use of prophylactic antibiotics to prevent meningitis in this patient population. Many leaks are self-limiting, but early repair of persistent leaks, within 7 days, may reduce the risk of meningitis.

Empiric antibiotic use

Empiric antibiotic use refers to the practice of administering broad-spectrum systemic antibiotics to patients suspected of infection without diagnostic laboratory evidence. Approximately 26% of patients admitted to a surgical-trauma intensive care unit will receive at least one course of empiric antibiotics. Of those patients, only 20%–25% will actually go on to demonstrate evidence of an infection.

In general, prior to initiation of empiric therapy, cultures should be obtained. Therapy should be initiated promptly when there is a high suspicion of infection, utilizing the hospital's antibiogram to help choose the appropriate agent(s). Dosing should take into consideration penetration of the affected organ (e.g., lung and central nervous system infections frequently need higher doses of some agents) and changes in pharmacokinetics caused by fluid resuscitation, which can significantly increase the volume of distribution of the agent. The duration of therapy should be limited to no more than 3 days without clinical improvement or positive culture result. Therapy can be extended if clinical improvement is observed; however, a stop date should be determined by the intensivist or infectious disease consultant. Finally, antibiotic therapy should be tailored according to culture sensitivities, favoring narrow spectrum agents when possible.

Key resources

Arnold HM, Micek ST, Skrupky LP, Kollef MH. Antibiotic stewardship in the intensive care unit. *Semin Respir Crit Care Med*. 2011;32(2):215–227.

Claridge JA, Golob JF Jr, Leukhardt WH, et al. The "fever workup" and respiratory culture practice in critically ill trauma patients. *J Crit Care*. 2010;25(3):493–500.

Claridge JA, Pang P, Leukhardt WH, Golob JF, Carter JW, Fadlalla AM. Critical analysis of empiric antibiotic utilization: establishing benchmarks. *Surg Infect (Larchmt)*. 2010;11(2):125–131.

Dellinger RP, Levy MM, Carlet JM, et al. Surviving Sepsis Campaign: international guidelines for management of severe sepsis and septic shock: 2008. *Crit Care Med.* 2008;36(1):296–327.

Hoff WS, Bonadies JA, Cachecho R, Dorlac WC. East Practice Management Guidelines Work Group: update to practice management guidelines for prophylactic antibiotic use in open fractures. *J Trauma.* 2011;70(3):751–754.

Hoover L, Bochicchio GV, Napolitano LM, et al. Systemic inflammatory response syndrome and nosocomial infection in trauma. *J Trauma.* 2006;61(2):310–316.

Kumar A, Roberts D, Wood KE, et al. Duration of hypotension before initiation of effective antimicrobial therapy is the critical determinant of survival in human septic shock. *Crit Care Med.* 2006;34(6):1589–1596.

Luchette FA, Barie PS, Oswanski MF, et al. Practice Management Guidelines for Prophylactic Antibiotic Use in Tube Thoracostomy for Traumatic Hemopneumothorax: the EAST Practice Management Guidelines Work Group. Eastern Association for Trauma. *J Trauma.* 2000;48(4):753–757.

Marshall JC, al Naqbi A. Principles of source control in the management of sepsis. *Crit Care Clin.* 2009;25(4):753–768, viii–ix.

Porzecanski I, Bowton DL. Diagnosis and treatment of ventilator-associated pneumonia. *Chest.* 2006;130(2):597–604.

Chapter 19

Hypothermia and trauma

Samuel A. Tisherman

Introduction

Spontaneous, uncontrolled hypothermia occurs in up to half of the victims of major trauma. Trauma patients are unable to maintain normal temperature homeostasis because of the effects of shock, alcohol and drug intoxication, sedation, and anesthesia. Anesthesia alone may decrease heat production by 20%. In addition, the administration of room-temperature fluids and exposure for evaluation and operative interventions can increase heat loss. The more severe the injury, the greater the risk of hypothermia.

Hypothermia and outcome from trauma

Multiple studies have demonstrated a strong association between this uncontrolled hypothermia and mortality in trauma patients, even controlling for confounding variables, such as injury severity, presence of shock, and transfusion requirements. Wang et al (2005), using a large, statewide trauma database and applying advanced, multiple regression analysis, demonstrated an independent association between hypothermia and mortality. Age, sex; injury severity score; head, abdominal, and skin abbreviated injury scale; systolic blood pressure; mechanism of injury; intravenous fluids; route of temperature measurement; and history of asthma or alcoholism were independent predictors of hypothermia. Yet the adjusted odds ratio for death in patients who became hypothermic was 3.03 (95% CI: 2.62–3.51). A similar association was shown for patients with isolated traumatic brain injury. The odds ratio for death in patients with isolated traumatic brain injury who became hypothermic was 2.30 (CI: 1.68–3.13).

Physiologic effects of hypothermia

Exposure hypothermia has been variably defined by certain temperature levels. Mild hypothermia is typically 32–35°C, moderate 28–32°C, and severe below 28°C. It is critical in these patients to measure core temperature; typically, rectal, bladder, or esophageal temperature is used. Rectal temperature is often preferred because of ease of use.

In healthy individuals, normal temperature is maintained within a narrow range by multiple centrally and peripherally mediated responses, decreasing heat loss and increasing metabolism. These responses are typically blunted in trauma patients. Shivering, however, may be counterproductive because it causes an increase in oxygen consumption for which the patient may not be able to physiologically compensate, vasodilatation that may cause more heat loss, and metabolic acidosis. When and how to stop shivering is controversial. No single agent is ideal, although opioids or neuromuscular blockers are frequently used.

Hypothermia affects multiple organs in both positive and negative ways. Overall, cellular metabolism decreases proportionally with temperature, which may be beneficial when perfusion is limited. The clinical effects of hypothermia are subtle at mild levels, but become more severe and predictable with lower temperatures.

From a respiratory standpoint, mild tachypnea may occur with mild hypothermia. Apnea occurs with deeper levels of hypothermia. Although arterial oxygenation is typically well-maintained, tissue oxygenation may be impaired by vasoconstriction. In addition, there is a leftward shift of the hemoglobin dissociation curve, which may further decrease tissue oxygenation. Hypothermia alters the measured arterial pH, PCO_2, and PO_2, tempting some to suggest "correcting" blood gas values for the patient's temperature ("pH stat" approach) before treating the values, given that blood gas analyzers typically warm the sample to 37°C. This is unnecessary as there is no proven benefit in using the corrected values. In fact, the "alpha-stat" approach utilizing noncorrected values may even be better in some circumstances.

From a cardiac standpoint, mild hypothermia may cause tachycardia, with bradycardia more common at deeper levels of hypothermia. On the electrocardiogram, J (Osborn) waves may be seen, as well as widening of the PR, QRS, and QT intervals. Atrial arrhythmias are common. With severe hypothermia, ventricular tachycardia, ventricular fibrillation, or asystole can occur. With mild-to-moderate hypothermia, blood pressure is typically adequate for the level of tissue metabolism. Vasodilatation can occur at mild hypothermia levels if shivering is present. Vasoconstriction occurs at lower temperatures, sometimes making pulses difficult to feel. If hypothermia is the only disturbance, blood pressure is usually adequate for tissue oxygenation at that body temperature.

From a neurologic standpoint, mild-to-moderate hypothermia typically causes confusion, agitation or apathy, and loss of coordination. It is important to keep in mind that hemorrhagic shock, intoxication, or traumatic brain injury may cause similar findings. These causes should be ruled out before assuming that hypothermia alone explains an altered mental status. With severe hypothermia, coma, and possibly electroencephalogram silence, may be seen. If these findings are purely the result of the hypothermia, they are typically reversible.

From a renal standpoint, hypothermia decreases the absorption of fluid by the kidneys, which may lead to an inappropriate "cold" diuresis, further complicating hemodynamics. Urine output, therefore, has limited utility as a marker of adequate organ perfusion.

Coagulation abnormalities are frequently thought of as the major complications of hypothermia in trauma patients. Decreased enzyme function, proportional to temperature decrease, leads to dysfunction of the clotting cascade. Platelets are decreased in number because of sequestration. They may also be dysfunctional. Increased fibrinolysis may be present. Tissue trauma itself, however, may cause a consumptive coagulopathy. Metabolic acidosis, which is common because of shock and/or hypothermia, independently impairs clotting. Studying coagulation in hypothermic patients is confounded by the fact that standard laboratory instruments warm blood to 37°C.

Severely injured trauma patients often develop the potentially lethal triad of hypothermia, coagulopathy, and acidosis. The exact contribution of each factor to mortality is difficult to determine definitively. To break the cycle of bleeding, transfusion, worsening coagulopathy, worsening hypothermia, and more bleeding, the "damage control," abbreviated laparotomy (rapid control of active bleeding and contamination, packing the abdomen, with rewarming and restoration of homeostasis in the ICU) has been life-saving.

Prevention

Heat loss occurs via radiation, conduction, convection, and evaporation. Consideration of these factors can help plan techniques to minimize additional heat loss. Otherwise healthy hypothermic patients can minimize heat loss by behavioral responses (moving to a warmer environment and wearing warm clothing) and cutaneous vasoconstriction. Trauma patients lack these responses, so more active measures are needed to prevent hypothermia.

Ideally, hypothermia should be actively prevented as soon as possible in the field and emergency department. This should be continued into the operating room and ICU. The environment should be kept as warm as possible. Warm, humidified oxygen can be administered. All fluids should be warmed prior to infusion. They can be stored in warm storage units. They can also be warmed during infusion with countercurrent heating devices. More active warming devices can also be used, including heating blankets, servo-controlled surface warming devices (e.g., the Artic Sun®, Medivance Corp, Louisville, CO), and convection air warmer (e.g., Bair Hugger®, Arizant, Eden Prairie, MN). Intravascular temperature management systems involving the circulation of water through a sheath surrounding a central venous catheter (e.g., Thermogard XP®, Zoll, Chelmsford, MA) are being used more frequently. An even more aggressive warming technique involves arterial and venous cannulation and extracorporeal rewarming using a Level I countercurrent warming device, but this has only been utilized in a few centers.

Treatment of the hypothermic patient

Treatment of the hypothermic patient, like all trauma patients, should begin with a primary survey. The adequacy of the airway and spontaneous breathing should be assessed. If the patient only has exposure hypothermia, without concern for trauma, endotracheal intubation may not be necessary unless apnea or profound obtundation is present. In a severely hypothermic patient, spontaneous breathing suggests acceptable cerebral perfusion, even if pulses are difficult to palpate. On the other hand, presence of ventricular arrhythmias or asystole should prompt initiation of external chest compressions.

Management of cardiac arrest from hypothermia is complicated by the fact that arrhythmias tend to be refractory to defibrillation and anti-arrhythmics. It is reasonable to attempt up to three shocks and administer small doses of anti-arrhythmics, but aggressive rewarming with ongoing cardiopulmonary resuscitation is the best approach. Closed-chest, cardiopulmonary bypass, if available, is also a good option.

It is worth keeping in mind that unnecessary manipulations, such as placement of a central venous catheter or placement of an endotracheal tube, can cause ventricular arrhythmias and cardiac arrest. Moreover, administration of most medications should be limited because they are typically ineffective, but nonetheless accumulate, leading to toxic levels with rewarming.

The choice of rewarming technique is dependent upon the patient's body temperature, the clinical effects of hypothermia, and available resources. For patients with mild hypothermia, passive warming devices, such as insulating blankets, typically are sufficient. Active, external rewarming using heating blankets or convective air warmers may also be useful. For patients with moderate hypothermia, more active rewarming is usually needed. Simple, external rewarming can theoretically lead to "after drop," a decrease in core temperature during active warming because of the resultant vasodilatation of the extremities leading to sudden return of cold blood to the core. Convective air warmers remain very effective. Body cavity lavage (e.g., stomach, bladder, pleural space, peritoneum) with warm fluids has been used extensively in the past, but if the body cavity is not already accessible, the risks involved in placing pleural or peritoneal catheters make this approach unnecessary considering the efficacy of other techniques. Intravascular warming catheters are also very helpful. For the severely hypothermic patient without arrhythmias, the techniques noted above may be effective. On the other hand, if rewarming remains difficult or if arrhythmias develop, the use of cardiopulmonary bypass should be considered.

Drowning

Drowning is a common cause of accidental death, particularly in children and adolescents. Diving accidents, alcohol and drug intoxication, and exhaustion are common precipitating factors. The great majority of submersion victims have inhaled a significant amount of water. Whether this is fresh or salt water, acute lung injury often ensues. Supportive care is needed.

The bigger, long-term issue in these patients is the degree of hypoxemia and resultant neurologic deficit. Early on, this is difficult to predict. If the drowning was in cold water, it is possible for the brain to have cooled to a protective level prior to cardiac arrest, lending some increased potential for recovery.

Frostbite

Frostbite is a local complication of hypothermia involving exposed surfaces of the body. This results in tissue freezing and microvascular occlusion, leading to tissue ischemia and death. Management involves local warming, ideally by immersion in warm water (38–41°C). Elevation can help decrease tissue edema. Administration of tetanus toxoid is indicated. Because the true extent of irreversible injury is difficult to determine initially, it is best to defer debridement or amputation until clear demarcation has occurred.

Therapeutic hypothermia

Mild therapeutic hypothermia has become the standard of care for comatose patients after cardiac arrest. The mechanisms of benefit from therapeutic hypothermia clearly go beyond simply decreasing metabolism. Decreased oxidant injury and inflammation have been demonstrated. Recommendations from the American Heart Association suggest that patients who remain comatose after resuscitation from an out-of-hospital cardiac arrest caused by ventricular tachycardia/fibrillation should be cooled to 32–34°C for 12–24 hours. They further suggest that therapeutic hypothermia may also offer benefits after in-hospital cardiac arrest and after cardiac arrest from other causes. For comatose trauma patients, without traumatic brain injury, who have suffered a cardiac arrest, therapeutic hypothermia may be considered if there is no clear contraindication, such as coagulopathy.

There has been ongoing interest in whether or not mild hypothermia could be of benefit during or after other ischemic insults, including hemorrhagic shock. Consequently, therapeutic, controlled hypothermia has been studied in laboratory experiments using traumatic hemorrhagic shock models. Beneficial effects have been demonstrated on the heart, liver, and skeletal muscle. More importantly, hypothermia consistently improves survival. The studies have included models of pure hemorrhage shock and combinations of hemorrhagic shock and tissue trauma.

Why is there such a dichotomy between the beneficial effects of hypothermia demonstrated in the laboratory and the strong clinical association between hypothermia and worse outcomes in patients? Coagulopathy certainly could be part of the explanation, though coagulation studies at 34°C, and experience with therapeutic hypothermia after cardiac arrest or traumatic brain injury, do not suggest clinically relevant coagulation abnormalities at this temperature. It is possible that the amount of tissue trauma commonly seen in trauma patients may not be well-replicated in the laboratory. Another important factor that has not been adequately studied in this situation is the effect of transfusions of banked blood on outcome, another variable not included in the laboratory studies. At this time, active rewarming of hypothermic trauma patients remains the standard of care.

For the trauma patient who has suffered a cardiac arrest, the survival rate overall is < 10%. Survival is significantly lower with blunt trauma, compared to penetrating, or with non-chest-trauma. If the patient has suffered exsanguinating hemorrhage, there is not enough time to control bleeding and restore circulation before significant ischemic damage has occurred in the most vital organs, the brain and heart. A novel approach under investigation to manage this situation, called Emergency Preservation and Resuscitation, includes rapid cooling of the entire body via an intra-arterial flush of ice-cold fluids to use deep levels of hypothermia to preserve organ viability until hemostasis can be achieved. This approach will be tested in a safety and feasibility trial soon.

Laboratory studies have demonstrated that mild-to-moderate hypothermia can improve many physiologic parameters and outcome after traumatic brain injury (TBI). Clinically, one single-center randomized, controlled trial of early, post-TBI hypothermia demonstrated benefit in a subset of patients with initial Glasgow Coma Scale (GCS) of 5 to 7 at 6 months, but not 12 months. Subsequent multi-center studies have failed to demonstrate benefit. A separate area of interest is the use of therapeutic hypothermia later in the patient's course, once intracranial hypertension has been demonstrated. Definitive studies of this approach are lacking. It is clear, however, that fever is detrimental in patients with TBI. Aggressive prevention of fever seems worthwhile.

Given that therapeutic hypothermia has benefit in patients with neurologic impairment from cardiac arrest and there are laboratory suggestions of benefit following stroke and TBI, there has been interest in treating spinal cord injury with therapeutic hypothermia. Benefit has been demonstrated in laboratory studies, but clinical studies have not been completed yet.

Key references

Fukudome EY, Alam HB. Hypothermia in multisystem trauma. *Crit Care Med.* 2009; 37(suppl):S265–S272.

Gentilello LM, Jurkovich GJ, Stark MS, et al. Is hypothermia in the victim of major trauma protective or harmful? *Ann Surg.* 1997;226:439–447.

Laniewicz M, Lyn-Kew K, Silbergleit R. Rapid endovascular warming for profound hypothermia. *Ann Emerg Med.* 2008;51:160.

Morita S, Seiji M, Inokuchi S, et al. The efficacy of rewarming with a portable and percutaneous cardiopulmonary bypass system in accidental deep hypothermia patients with hemodynamic instability. *J Trauma.* 2008;65:1391.

Peberdy MA, Callaway CW, Neumar RW, et al. Part 9: post-cardiac arrest care: 2010 American Heart Association Guidelines for Cardiopulmonary Resuscitation and Emergency Cardiovascular Care. *Circulation.* 2010;122(suppl 3):S768–S786.

Taylor EE, Carroll JP, Lovitt MA, et al. Active intravascular rewarming for hypothermia associated with traumatic injury: early experience with a new technique. *Proc. (Bayl Univ Med Cent).* 2008;21(2):120–126.

Tisherman SA. Hypothermia and injury. *Curr Opinion in Critical Care.* 2004;10:512–519.

Wang HE, Callaway CW, Peitzman AB, Tisherman SA. Admission hypothermia and outcome after major trauma. *Crit Care Med.* 2005;33:1296–1301.

Chapter 20

Nutrition

Juan B. Ochoa and Jodie Bryk

Introduction

Critical illness profoundly disrupts the ability to maintain volitional oral intake, which without intervention can lead to prolonged starvation, the progression towards malnutrition, and the development of malnutrition-related organ dysfunction and complications. In addition, lack of oral intake in another human being elicits emotional responses by both well-intentioned family and healthcare providers prompting the unnecessary provision of inappropriate nutrition intervention during illness. Far from being supportive, however, prescription of inappropriately indicated forms of nutrition intervention in the critically ill patient can result in significant side effects and may worsen outcomes. Nutrition intervention has evolved into a medical discipline with goals that are more complex than simply providing calories and nitrogen. Nutrition intervention is not intuitive and requires a careful understanding of metabolism during health and disease, as well as knowledge of the different forms of nutrition intervention. This chapter aims to provide a basic understanding of nutrition intervention in the critically ill while providing guidelines that can help physicians in their day-to-day practices.

The necessity of nutrition intervention

It is appropriate that care of nutritional needs is secondary to the care of primary concerns including cardiopulmonary stabilization. Consequently, patients frequent are kept "nil per os [NPO]." In addition, on the days that follow, patients frequently are fed below their caloric and nutritional needs. What are the consequences of starving a patient for several days? Is this well-tolerated, inconsequential, or does this negatively affect outcome?

The starvation response is a physiologic process that enables an otherwise normal individual to more efficiently utilize nutrient stores in the event of inadequate intake. Metabolic changes observed during starvation include a significant decrease in energy expenditure with ensuing hypothermia, listlessness, and bradycardia along with decreased protein turnover. These metabolic changes protect the patient and lengthen the amount of time that normal organ function is preserved. Starvation, however, like other compensatory mechanisms, cannot be prolonged indefinitely and it eventually fails, leading to malnutrition.

Understanding malnutrition

Malnutrition ensues as a result of prolonged starvation; different from starvation, malnutrition is a pathologic condition characterized by organ dysfunction associated with inadequate supply of one or more nutrients. Malnutrition invariably leads to poor outcomes in all illnesses. Malnutrition is a highly significant independent predictor of increased morbidity and mortality in postoperative or critically ill, hospitalized patients. Malnutrition increases length of stay in the hospital, augments the utilization of resources, and increases cost. Malnutrition occurs surprisingly often in our institutions and may be present in up to 30% or more of patients, perhaps even more commonly in critically ill patients.

Intuitively, most clinicians believe that treatment and/or prevention of malnutrition should improve outcomes and decrease cost. Two main approaches have been used to solve this:

(1) Quality-practice improvement aimed at preventing prolonged starvation while in the hospital
(2) Basic and clinical research aimed at understanding how critical illness affects metabolic responses, facilitating the design of treatments aimed at preventing the progression to malnutrition.

The lessons learned from these two approaches have shaped clinical practices and led to the development of guidelines. Significant enough progress has been made so that effective nutrition intervention can be applied to most patients.

Attempts at relieving or preventing malnutrition have made it evident that our current understanding of malnutrition is limited, and that under certain circumstances, treatment is frustratingly ineffective. Three types of malnutrition have been identified, based on their etiology:

(1) Starvation-related malnutrition. Malnutrition secondary to lack of intake is the classic form of malnutrition that can be observed under circumstances of environmental and/or social factors (e.g., natural disasters or war). Starvation-related malnutrition is effectively treated with dietary replacement. This form of malnutrition is surprisingly prevalent in certain populations such as the elderly and institutionalized.
(2) Malnutrition due to immune activation leads to significant changes in metabolism including increased energy utilization, resistance to the use of glucose as an energy source, and increased destruction of protein. These changes are the result of classic "inflammatory" signaling.

Progression to malnutrition is accelerated during illness due to increased utilization of nutrient stores. The degree of progression towards malnutrition is determined in part by the acuity of illness. Jensen and colleagues have therefore defined illness-related malnutrition into two further categories:

(a) Malnutrition related to acute illnesses (e.g., sepsis and severe trauma).
(b) Malnutrition secondary to chronic inflammation (such as that observed in cancer and obesity).

Outcomes during both acute and chronic inflammatory processes are negatively affected by the presence of malnutrition. This has led to the development of nutrition interventions aimed at curtailing the progression to malnutrition during illness. In contrast to the treatment of starvation-related malnutrition, however, the nutritional management of illness-related malnutrition is far more challenging. For example, approaches aimed at providing supraphysiologic amounts of nutrients (hyperalimentation) in these patients have uniformly failed and ultimately been largely abandoned. Nonetheless, nutrition intervention is essential and causes a significant difference in outcome.

Avoiding Starvation in the Hospital. On average in the United States, patients are kept NPO over 56 hours (> 2 days) after arrival to the intensive care unit (ICU). Not surprisingly, most nutrition intervention plans fail to achieve desired nutritional goals (often measured as caloric/energy goals). There is a wide variation in practices in ICUs around the world. Worldwide, patients fed through enteral nutrition (EN) tend to achieve 70% of their caloric goals, although in the United States patients received on average approximately only 48% of their caloric goals.

Stress produced through injury or after infection is associated with a metabolic response that is diametrically different from that observed during starvation. Neuroendocrine responses and immune activation during critical illness lead to insulin resistance and the destruction of muscle protein as a source of substrate for gluconeogenesis. The catabolic stress of critical illness predominates over that of anabolic responses leading to a negative nitrogen balance and an accelerated progression towards malnutrition. In addition, energy expenditure is normal or increased in a critically ill patient. As a result of this metabolic response, progression towards exhaustion of available nutrients and the appearance of malnutrition is faster than that observed in a classic starvation response. The critically ill patient is thus poorly equipped to tolerate even modest periods of starvation.

Nutrition intervention in the form of early EN or oral intake in those patients who can has been systematically evaluated in critically ill and surgical patients. The goal of early EN is to minimize the amount of time that the patient is kept NPO. Multiple studies in different patient populations, including critically ill medical patients, trauma victims, and patients with elective surgery demonstrate that early EN is associated with significant benefits including improved gastrointestinal function, improved EN tolerance, decreased infection rates, and a possible decrease in length of stay. Meta-analyses in critically ill and elective-surgery patients suggest that early EN may be associated with decreased mortality. Other markers of improved outcomes associated with early EN may include decreased ventilator days and need for dialysis.

Quality of the studies of early EN has been variable. Regardless, the preponderance of evidence does suggest that EN should be started as soon as possible in critically ill patients, preferably within 24 hours.

Caloric intake

Malnutrition that results from starvation in an otherwise normal individual is indeed responsive to nutrition intervention. Early clinical observations suggested that the catabolic response to critical illness could be curtailed with the provision of energy (caloric intake) above that of resting energy expenditure (REE) in what became known as "hyperalimentation." Delivery of large amounts of nutrients became possible with the advent of Total Parenteral Nutrition (TPN). Contrary to expectations, hyperalimentation not only failed to prevent progression towards malnutrition in critical illness, but it was also associated with a significant increase in side effects including hyperglycemia, liver dysfunction, and when compared to EN, a trend towards increased mortality.

Virtually all studies that compare EN with TPN demonstrate that achieving caloric goals is far easier with the latter. These studies repeatedly demonstrate that patients on EN routinely achieve 50%–70% of caloric goals while patients on TPN achieve near 100% of proposed caloric intake. And yet, most studies demonstrate that outcomes using EN are better than when TPN is used. These observations beg the question of what is the ideal caloric intake for a critically ill patient.

The determination of energy requirements in a critically ill patient can be done using different techniques. The simplest is the calculation that overall critically ill patients require approximately 25 Kcal/kg/day (ideal body weight [IBW]) to meet caloric needs. There is however, a significant margin of error attributable to this calculation. Other more sophisticated calculations include the Harris-Benedict formula and the Ireton-Jones formula. Indirect calorimetry, which calculates energy expenditure based on the consumption of oxygen and generation of CO_2 provides the most accurate method of calculating actual energy expenditures. To date, however, indirect calorimetry remains a relatively difficult and expensive technology. Furthermore, despite its accuracy it has been difficult to prove that the use of indirect calorimetry as a tool is associated with improved clinical outcomes.

The laws of thermodynamics dictate that failing to meet the provision of caloric goals in a given patient results in a negative energy balance; also called a *caloric deficit*. In 2007, Villet et al demonstrated that in critically ill patients the caloric deficit accumulated was associated with worsened outcomes, including increased mortality. Though this study was only observational and thus did not determine causality, it prompted the concern that providing addition supplement parenteral nutrition with EN was necessary to correct the caloric deficit. So far, studies have only demonstrated the benefit of supplementing EN with TPN after 7 days of failing to achieve caloric goals with EN.

Current recommendations suggest that clinicians should attempt to meet at least 50%–65% of caloric goals through EN in the first week of hospitalization in the ICU. In the previously healthy patient, TPN should be started after 7 days in the ICU if unable to achieve adequate EN intake.

Protein intake

Provision of adequate amounts of protein during critical illness is essential. Protein balance is achieved through anabolism and catabolism, two closely regulated processes that are altered during illness. Balance between anabolism and catabolism is achieved when the same amount of protein is deposited as that which is catabolized. Proteins are the sole source of nitrogen and thus measures of nitrogen intake and loss are used to estimate protein balance.

Increased catabolism of protein beyond that which can be achieved through anabolic responses is observed in critically ill patients. Neurohormonal changes and immune activation observed in critical illness forces breakdown of protein to be used as an energy source, for tissue repair, as well as for the synthesis of new proteins and peptides. The muscle provides a significant amount of protein and, as a result, loss of muscle mass may be prominent during acute illness. Catabolic protein responses can only partially be curtailed with dietary provision of nutrients.

Average protein intake to achieve adequate nitrogen balance in a healthy adult is approximately 0.75 g/kg/day. In the critically ill adult, current recommendations suggest that protein intake should be increased to 1.2–2 g/kg/day. Further increase in protein intake, based on IBW, is recommended for the morbidly obese patient.

Digestibility of protein may be impaired in a number of illnesses, thus leading to malabsorption of protein. Some illnesses associated with decreased capacity to digest protein include malnutrition, acute/chronic pancreatitis, cystic fibrosis, intestinal ischemia, enteritis, autoimmune disease, and inflammatory bowel disease. The incidence of inappropriate protein digestion and malabsorption in the ICU is unknown. Specialized diets may contain predigested protein and are known as peptide-based diets. Peptide-based diets may be better tolerated and may decrease the incidence of diarrhea.

Benefits of enteral nutrition

It is apparent from the studies reported above that EN benefits outcome in critically ill patients through mechanisms that are independent of the amount of caloric intake. It has also become clear that nutrition intervention alone fails to curtail a negative nitrogen balance and the continued loss of muscle mass in critically ill patients, particularly those with severe inflammatory states. Malnutrition induced by inflammatory states is best treated by correcting the underlying acute illness, thus controlling the inflammatory response.

The benefits of EN go beyond creating a positive nitrogen balance. The possible benefits include maintaining gut trophism and function, modulation of the immune response, and delivery of essential nutrients, including those that become specifically necessary during illness.

The gastrointestinal tract is benefited by the presence of luminal nutrients. Luminal nutrients maintain gut trophism and may protect against the negative effects of shock by preventing increased intestinal permeability. Luminal nutrients may help regulate the gastrointestinal microbiome, which is easily disrupted during illness. In addition, gastrointestinal motility is stimulated with EN, serving both to prevent and/or to manage ileus. Finally, nutrients in the intestinal lumen appear to be essential in maintaining a healthy gut associated lymphoid tissue, including secretion of immunoglobulin A.

All these beneficial effects are independent of reaching caloric goals. In fact, only small amounts of nutrients are necessary to maintain adequate gastrointestinal function. Recently, one study compared the use of "trophic" feeding, delivering only 10 mL/hr enterally, with full caloric feeding during the first week in the ICU, in an open-label prospective randomized trial in patients with respiratory failure. Mortality, number of ventilator days, and number of infections were similar in both groups. On the other hand, patients on trophic feeds exhibited fewer episodes of elevated gastric residual volumes.

Modification of immune responses with nutrients (Table 20.1). Nutrients, in addition to their physiologic roles as food, can modify and benefit physiological functions. Attention has been drawn to nutrients that help modify immune responses to illness. This is particularly important as underlying paradigms of illness in the ICU suggest that an uncontrolled immune response is responsible for tissue damage (described as the systemic inflammatory response syndrome [SIRS]). Conversely, paralysis of immune responses, particularly those of adaptive immunity, may be responsible for increased susceptibility to infection and is thought to be part of a compensatory anti-inflammatory response syndrome (CARS). The modulation of SIRS and the prevention of CARS have been at the center of multiple pharmacologic and intervention trials. Although specific

Table 20.1 Nutrients that may modify immune function, decrease oxidative stress, or act as signaling molecules
Amino Acids
Arginine—Precursor of the formation of nitric oxide, essential for T lymphocyte function.
Glutamine—Fuel for enterocytes and lymphocytes. Signaling molecule inducing HSP 70.
Citrulline—Precursor of arginine. May serve as an antioxidant.
Cysteine—Tested as an antioxidant
Vitamins
Vitamin A—Multiple functions
Vitamin C—Used as an antioxidant in burn patients
Micronutrients
Zinc—Micronutrient acting in multiple enzymatic pathways.
Selenium—Used as an antioxidant.

nutrients may have had benefit in small trials most of these trials produced disappointing results.

Arginine remains the best studied amino acid in critical illness and in other patient populations. Arginine is a precursor of nitric oxide and is necessary to maintain normal T lymphocyte function. Arginine metabolism in the absence of illness is governed by a balance between intake and endogenous generation in the kidneys versus protein turnover.

Arginine exerts little influence on immune function in the absence of immune activation, but its metabolism changes dramatically during illness. Arginine deficiency states are observed under a growing number of conditions including certain cancers (renal cell carcinoma), chronic infections, and after trauma (physical injury). High-dose arginine administration can decrease postoperative infections (by approximately 40%) in patients undergoing major elective surgery.

Glutamine is the most abundant circulating amino acid. Like arginine, glutamine levels decrease during critical illness. Glutamine is extensively metabolized by the intestinal mucosa to citrulline, which is metabolized to arginine in the kidneys. As a result of this metabolism, supplementation of glutamine in enteral diets increases plasma circulating citrulline and arginine, but fails to increase circulating glutamine levels. Glutamine delivered intravenously increases circulating glutamine but fails to generate citrulline or arginine. Intravenous glutamine supplementation is associated with a significant decrease in mortality (approximately 30%) from sepsis. Enteral glutamine supplementation does not provide the same benefit.

Lipids are seen mainly as a source of energy. Two polyunsaturated fatty acids (PUFAs),linoleic acid and alpha linolenic acid, are essential lipids that need to be provided in the diet. Deficiencies of essential fatty acids can cause severe skin changes, immune dysfunction, visual disturbances, and neurological manifestations. PUFAs are classified according to where the first double bond is present in the carbon chain starting to count from the last (ω) carbon. Alpha linoleic acid (LA—18:2) is a ω-6 fatty acid. Alpha linolenic acid (ALA—18:2) is an ω-3 fatty acid. The products of ALA and LA, however, exhibit significantly different biological properties.

Dietary intake of LA, ALA and their derivatives is frequently reported as a ratio (LA:ALA). Dietary changes in the last 50 years favor a high intake of ω-6 fatty acids over ω-3 fatty acids, which favors chronic immune activation and may be associated with atherosclerosis, certain forms of cancer, and some autoimmune diseases. Omega-3 fatty acids (ω-3 FA) are concentrated in certain fish, particularly in the liver. Docohexanoic acid (DHA) and eicosapentanoic acid (EPA) form the main ω-3 fatty acids in fish oil. In critical illness, there are now several available diets that promote a more physiologic ratio of ω-6:ω-3 fatty acid intake with concentrations of fish oil that approach those recommended by the American Heart Association (AHA) for a heart-healthy diet.

Different types of oils have been used in supraphysiologic concentrations as "pharmaconutrients" in an attempt to modify inflammatory responses. Trials of fish and borage oils in patients with respiratory failure suggest that this combination of fish oil, gamma linolenic acid (GLA) (a ω-6 FA from borage oil), and several antioxidants improve pulmonary function and decrease mortality in patients with acute respiratory distress syndrome (ARDS). The benefits reported have generated a Grade A recommendation for use in ARDS by the American Society of Parenteral and Enteral Nutrition (ASPEN) and the Society of Critical Care Medicine (SCCM). A more recent trial, however, did not show benefit.

Exact micronutrient requirements during critical illness are mostly unknown. It appears clear, however, that traditional micronutrient requirements in normal individuals are inadequate and that further research in this area is badly needed. Although the list of micronutrients that hold promise is long, some micronutrients do deserve mention.

Nucleotides form the backbones of RNA and DNA, are necessary in multiple metabolic processes, and are particularly important during cellular proliferation and tissue repair. As such, nucleotides may need to be supplemented during critical illness and may support mucosal trophism in the intestinal lumen, as well as play key roles in proliferation of lymphocytes. Nucleotide supplementation has been incorporated into commercial diets for the critically ill, and is generally added to arginine and/or omega-3 fatty acids. Studies of the effects of nucleotide supplementation alone are lacking.

Nutrients such as vitamin C, selenium, and zinc are cataloged as antioxidants, although all of them play multiple other roles. Antioxidants have been studied for multiple diseases, including cancer; for aging; and for critical illness.

Techniques for delivery of enteral nutrients

Oral intake is the most logical route of nutrient delivery and should be encouraged in most patients capable of engaging in it. However, oral intake is significantly impaired in acutely critically ill patients and thus has to be replaced in a large number of patients in the ICU.

Oral nutritional supplements (ONS) allow dietary complementation in patients whose intake appears to be inadequate. These supplements may provide additional protein and energy. Specialized ONS may offer significant specialized benefits, such as providing improved consistency of liquids in patients with dysphagia or providing supraphysiologic quantities of arginine and supplemental ω-3 fatty acids prior to surgery. Studies of ONS with an increased proportion of protein suggest decreased morbidity and mortality in certain patient populations, such as elderly patients undergoing hip replacement.

Feeding tubes bypass the patient's inability to eat and/or swallow. Various types of feeding tubes, and techniques to place them, are available. Nasogastric tubes provide a temporary route of delivery of nutrients into the stomach. Nasoenteral feeding tubes deliver nutrients beyond the pylorus. Gastrostomies and jejunostomies (and their combinations) achieve a more stable form of enteral access when compared to nasogastric or nasoenteral feeding tubes, though their placement requires more sophisticated surgical or endoscopic techniques and may have additional associated complications.

The selection of one type of enteral access over others in a given patient is dictated by the patient's clinical condition, the availability of the different options in a given institution, and technical expertise in placement and management. Decisions regarding the need to place a feeding tube and the type of feeding tube to place should be done as early as possible in the course of patient care. This is particularly important in surgical patients where the option to place a gastrostomy or a jejunostomy should be considered if a laparotomy is performed. Lack of planning may lead to inappropriate use of feeding tubes.

Available enteral diets. Literally hundreds of enteral formulas and enteral supplements are available, though evidence for clinical effectiveness varies widely. Availability of the different formulas is dictated in great part by contracts with specific companies.

Enteral nutrition formulas can be classified in various ways. Based on their capacity to deliver recommended dietary allowances (RDAs), enteral formulas can be classified as complete (when they could be considered as the sole source of nutrition) or supplemental (when they are considered additive to complete formulas). The type and quantity of macronutrient delivered provides distinctive differences.

Complete formulas frequently contain 1 cal/cc of formula. Calorically dense formulas exist that deliver 1.5 or 2.0 cal/cc are also available. The source of calories can vary significantly. Carbohydrate sources can be defined by their complexity and/or glycemic index and content. The amount of lipid and carbohydrates are often altered in an attempt to better control glycemia in diabetic and critically ill patients with glucose intolerance. The source of lipids can also vary significantly. Different types of vegetable oils may be used. The amount, type, and quantity of protein can also vary significantly. Patients with malabsorption may benefit from elemental diets that include simple carbohydrates, medium chain triglycerides, and protein hydrolysates, which are readily absorbed.

Monitoring nutrition and side effects. Delivery of nutrition intervention requires careful monitoring to determine tolerance, the effectiveness of therapy, and side effects. Evidence demonstrates that the use of quality practice improvement processes, with careful adherence to checklists, achieves the best nutrition goals and clinical outcomes. Appropriate protocols improve the time to initiation of therapy, avoiding significant delays and inappropriate discontinuation.

Contrary to common belief, initiation of EN does not require evidence of bowel motility. Waiting for bowel sounds or passage of flatus may actually delay initiation of nutrition intervention. Cessation of feeding occurs frequently and significantly decreases the delivery of EN. It is estimated that more than 65% of the reasons given to stop delivery of EN are avoidable or unnecessary. Adequate education and team efforts can avoid inappropriate delays.

Gastric residuals are often used as a measure of monitoring for tolerance of EN. Gastric residuals of < 500 cc should not prompt cessation of nutrition intervention as they do not predict tolerance. Monitoring of tolerance requires significant clinical experience.

Side effects are observed with all forms of nutrition intervention. Total parenteral nutrition is more frequently associated with fluid and electrolyte disturbances, hyperglycemia, and immune dysfunction. Gastrointestinal side effects are observed with EN. Side effects may increase morbidity, mortality, and cost. Preventive measures and careful monitoring of all forms of nutrition intervention will decrease the incidence of side effects.

Overfeeding is a particularly troublesome problem and is more frequently observed with the use of TPN. Overfeeding leads to significant metabolic and immune abnormalities including hyperglycemia, dyslipidemia, cholestasis, azotemia, and fluid overload. Overfeeding is avoided by carefully monitoring and adhering to the established nutrition requirements necessary for a given individual.

Morbidity and mortality are observed with complications arising from feeding tubes. Nasogastric feeding tubes may increase incidence of aspiration. Inadvertent placement of feeding tubes into the airway may lead to pneumothorax and death. Erosion of the feeding tube into adjacent tissues may result in significant local injury. Contamination of feeding tubes may lead to infection, though the incidence of this problem is unknown. Colonization of feeding tubes may lead to creation of biofilms that may enhance protein precipitation and clogging of feeding tubes. Feeding tubes can be dislodged by inadvertent traction. To avoid these complications, careful protocols in feeding tube placement and maintenance should be instituted.

Diarrhea is a particular problem in critically ill patients using EN. Diarrhea increases cost of care and may diminish the effectiveness of medical nutrition intervention. Diarrhea can result from many different causes including the use of medications that will promote diarrhea. Equally, inadequate digestion and absorption of proteins, lipids, or carbohydrates may result in diarrhea. Elemental formulas may be beneficial in this situation.

Intestinal ischemia may be observed infrequently with EN, particularly in patients with hemodynamic instability.

Nutrition in the morbidly obese. Obesity is the most significant underlying nutrition-related illness in ICUs across the United States and is becoming a significant issue in many other countries including third-world countries. A recent evaluation suggests that over 25% of patients in the ICU are obese, 8% are morbidly obese, and 25% are overweight. Obesity creates significant challenges towards providing adequate nutrition intervention. Major challenges include

(1) Malnutrition among the morbidly obese is poorly recognized by physicians.

(2) Obesity significantly alters the immune responses and is associated with chronic inflammatory responses.
(3) Obesity is associated with significant insulin resistance and hyperglycemia.
(4) Obesity is frequently comorbid with coronary artery disease, hypertension, diabetes, and certain forms of cancer.
(5) Most clinicians appear to assume that patients may have the "reserves" to tolerate starvation. An evaluation by Alberda and colleagues (2009) demonstrated that the amount of calories received in the ICU was inversely proportional to patients' body mass index, so that morbidly obese patients received a mere 5 Cal/kg/day. It is thus wrong to assume that morbidly obese patients are well-nourished.

Nutrition intervention in the morbidly obese patient is particularly challenging. Placement of feeding tubes can be anatomically difficult. Surgical and endoscopic procedures may result in a higher incidence of complications in these patients. Transport of the patients to the operating room or endoscopy/fluoroscopy suites may be difficult. Calculation of caloric/protein needs may be extremely difficult and require the use of metabolic carts. Insulin resistance may be a significant problem that limits the amounts of carbohydrates that can be delivered. The use of protocols and specialized nutrition intervention teams may be of particular importance in these patients.

Conclusions

Nutrition evaluation and intervention in the acutely and critically ill patient is an essential aspect of care. Adequate nutrition intervention is not intuitive and requires careful understanding of basic biological principles. Early nutrition evaluation and intervention improves prognosis. Delivery of nutrition intervention can be better achieved through quality practice improvement that involves the use of protocols and checklists. Nutrition intervention should be considered a team activity in the ICU. Specialized nutrition intervention teams may assist in the care of particularly challenging patients. Progress in nutrition intervention has allowed for the development of recommendations and guidelines. New knowledge in controversial areas of critical care nutrition is being constantly developed and will help clinicians achieve better goals. Nutrition intervention, when adequately done, is associated with decreased morbidity, mortality, and cost.

Key references

Alberda C, Gramlich L, Jones N, et al. The relationship between nutritional intake and clinical outcomes in critically ill patients: results of an international multicenter observational study. *Intensive Care Med.* 2009; 35:1728–1737.

Caba D, Ochoa JB. How many calories are necessary during critical illness? *Gastrointest Endosc Clin N Am.* 2007;17:703–710.

Casaer MP, Mesotten D, Hermans G, et al. Early versus late parenteral nutrition in criti-cally ill adults. *N Engl J Med.* 2011;365:506–517.

Drover JW, Dhaliwal R, Weitzel L, et al. Perioperative use of arginine-supplemented diets: a systematic review of the evidence. *J Am Coll Surg.* 2011;212:385–399.

Jensen GL, Mirtallo J, Compher C, et al. Adult starvation and disease-related malnutri-tion: a proposal for etiology-based diagnosis in the clinical practice setting from the International Consensus Guideline Committee. *JPEN: J Parenter Enteral Nutr.* 2010;34:156–159.

Lewis SJ, Andersen HK, Thomas S. Early enteral nutrition within 24 h of intestinal sur-gery versus later commencement of feeding: a systematic review and meta-analysis. *J Gastrointest Surg.* 2009;13:569–575.

McClave SA, Kushner R, Van Way CW, et al. Nutrition therapy of the severely obese, critically ill patient: summation of conclusions and recommendations. *JPEN: J Parenter Enteral Nutr.* 2011;35:88S–96S.

McClave SA, Martindale RG, Vanek VW, et al. Guidelines for the Provision and Assessment of Nutrition Support Therapy in the Adult Critically Ill Patient: Society of Critical Care Medicine (SCCM) and American Society for Parenteral and Enteral Nutrition (A.S.P.E.N.). *JPEN: J Parenter Enteral Nutr.* 2009;33:277–316.

Rice TW, Mogan S, Hays MA, et al. Randomized trial of initial trophic versus full-energy enteral nutrition in mechanically ventilated patients with acute respiratory failure. *Crit Care Med.* 2011;39:967–974.

Rice TW, Wheeler AP, Thompson BT, et al. Enteral omega-3 fatty acid, gamma-linolenic acid, and antioxidant supplementation in acute lung injury. *JAMA.* 2011;306:1574–1581.

Villet S, Chiolero RL, Bollmann MD, et al. Negative impact of hypocaloric feeding and energy balance on clinical outcome in ICU patients. *Clin Nutr.* 2005;24:502–509.

Zhu X, Herrera G, Ochoa JB. Immunosupression and infection after major surgery: a nutri-tional deficiency. *Crit Care Clin.* 2010;26:491–500, ix.

Chapter 21

Venous thromboembolism prophylaxis

Louis H. Alarcon

Introduction

Venous thromboembolism (VTE) is a common problem in trauma patients and can potentially lead to significant morbidity, mortality, and resource expenditure. Hospitalized patients recovering from traumatic injury experience the highest rates of VTE among all subgroups of patients. Complications from VTE are the third leading cause of death in hospitalized trauma patients who survive beyond the first 24 hours after injury. Depending on the patient cohort and diagnostic modality, rates of deep venous thrombosis (DVT) and pulmonary embolism (PE) may be as high as 40% and 20% or higher, respectively, in trauma patients without VTE prophylaxis. Although the most serious consequence of VTE is the development of massive PE and death, DVT and PE can also lead to significant morbidity and long-term sequelae.

Although numerous prophylactic interventions have been studied for preventing VTE in trauma patients, the optimal method of prophylaxis, one that will balance risk of VTE with risk of complications, remains elusive. Several evidence-based guidelines have been proposed with varying degrees of adherence and effectiveness, primarily due to concerns of increased bleeding in the multi-trauma patient. What is clear is that delay in the initiation of prophylaxis is associated with a 3-fold increase in the incidence of VTE (Knudson et al, 2004). This increased incidence in VTE occurring with delayed initiation is likely secondary to an earlier than expected development of VTE. In fact, VTE has been diagnosed in a significant number of patients within the first 24 hours after injury. Approximately one-third of all cases of VTE are diagnosed within 1 week of injury. Unfortunately, the lack of level 1 evidence in this regard hampers the development of consensus guidelines for prophylaxis in trauma patients, and highlights the need for adequately designed prospective evaluations to define optimal practice in this area.

Risk of VTE in the injured patient

The risk of VTE after major trauma is well-established and understood by most clinicians. In a prospective observational study of injured patients not receiving

VTE prophylaxis, Geerts et al (1996) reported an incidence of lower extremity DVT documented by venography of 58%, with 18% of individuals having proximal thrombus extension. In subsequent studies, several patient and injury-specific risk factors have been identified that place the injured patient at increased risk for VTE. These include injury severity score (ISS) > 15, massive blood transfusion, requirement for surgery, lower-extremity long-bone fracture, pelvic fracture, spinal cord injury, closed head injury, surgical repair of venous injury, insertion of a femoral venous central line, prolonged immobilization, and delayed initiation of pharmacologic VTE prophylaxis. The two most powerful risk factors for VTE in meta-analysis of available studies were vertebral fractures and spinal cord injury.

Given the recognized relatively high risk of VTE among trauma patients, strategies directed toward prevention are essential. As a result, VTE prophylaxis in some form is considered standard-of-care for hospitalized trauma patients. Hospitals caring for injured patients must have protocols guiding VTE prophylaxis in conjunction with quality assurance measures to document compliance and effectiveness. Unfortunately, prophylactic measures only reduce the incidence but do not eliminate the occurrence of VTE. Even with the use of routine thromboprophylaxis, the incidence of DVT and PE in trauma patients is still estimated to be as high as 31% and 6%, respectively. Clinicians caring for acutely injured patients should maintain a high index of suspicion for VTE development, despite strict adherence to protocols. In fact, only 1% of patients with VTE manifest any clinical evidence before diagnosis, thus emphasizing the role of screening of patients at increased risk.

Prophylaxis against venous thromboembolism in trauma

The ideal prophylactic strategy would be very safe (zero risk of bleeding) and highly effective in preventing VTE. This ideal modality does not yet exist. To reduce the risk of VTE, both mechanical and pharmacologic methods have been advocated. Mechanical prophylaxis includes intermittent pneumatic compression devices (PCD), and vena cava filters (VCF). Pharmacologic prophylaxis presently includes unfractionated heparin (UFH) and low molecular weight heparin (LMWH), with the potential use of Factor Xa inhibitors in the future.

Mechanical prophylaxis: intermittent pneumatic compression devices

Mechanical methods of VTE prophylaxis include a variety of foot pumps and sequential compression devices (SCD). The devices are thought to mediate their effect through an increase in venous flow and a reduction in venous stasis. In addition, PCDs have been shown to have a direct effect on the fibrinolytic pathway via shortening of the euglobulin lysis time, increasing the activity of anticoagulant proteins, and increasing plasminogen activation.

Despite these theoretical benefits, the literature supporting the use of these devices has methodological limitations and shows limited benefit in trauma patients. Although PCDs have demonstrated a reduction in the risk of DVT in a number of patient subgroups compared with no prophylaxis, they do not reach the protection offered by pharmacologic prophylaxis. Furthermore, a meta-analysis of trials evaluating PCDs found no reduction in the incidence of DVT in trauma patients compared to those who received no prophylaxis. Similarly, mechanical prophylaxis interventions have not been shown to reduce the risk of PE or death. Despite these limitations, the combination of both mechanical and pharmacologic prophylaxis may result in increased efficacy over each individually. Overall, the primary advantage of these mechanical devices over pharmacologic prophylaxis is the low risk of bleeding complications. Many centers routinely order them for injured patients. However, these devices have been associated with skin and soft tissue injury, wound complications, and relatively poor compliance with utilization even when routinely ordered. As a result, proper application must be ensured when applied.

Mechanical prophylaxis: vena cava filter

Although use of vena cava filters is well-established for the treatment of patients with established VTE who fail medical therapy or have a contraindication to anticoagulation, the prophylactic use of VCFs is controversial. Some retrospective studies suggest that the prophylactic placement of VCFs may result in a reduction in the incidence of PE in trauma patients unable to be anticoagulated for a number of reasons, while other studies found no difference. A meta-analysis of the available prospective studies found no difference in the rates of PE among trauma patients with and without prophylactic VCFs. In addition, it should be remembered that without other forms of VTE prophylaxis, VCFs do nothing to prevent or treat DVT and its sequelae. Furthermore, there is some evidence that trauma patients who receive a prophylactic VCF may be at increased risk for the development of DVT.

VCF insertion and retrieval are associated with a number of complications, including insertion site DVT, caval DVT, and filter migration. Despite these limitations, a growing interest in prophylactic VCF use in the trauma setting has resulted from the emergence of retrievable VCFs with an acceptable safety profile. However, there is insufficient long-term data on the prophylactic use of retrievable VCFs to make solid recommendations at this time. Another challenge is defining the patient population at the appropriate high risk for the development of VTE despite pharmacologic VTE prophylaxis. At present, this high-risk patient population is thought to consist of patients with severe traumatic brain injury defined as a Glasgow Coma Scale less than 8, spinal cord injury with paraplegia or tetraplegia, complex pelvic fracture with associated long-bone fractures, multiple long-bone fractures, and massive transfusion. However, there is insufficient evidence showing that the prophylactic use of retrievable VCFs is effective at preventing PE, either when implemented in all high-risk trauma patients or when coupled with use of noninvasive screening modalities. Additionally, the rate of removal of these retrievable VCFs remains relatively low, although our institution has demonstrated that an institutional protocol can significantly increase the retrieval rate of prophylactic VCFs. Given that the efficacy and safety of prophylactic VCF insertion in the setting of trauma remains debated, there is significant practice variability among trauma centers in this regard. Important questions remain unanswered regarding the use of prophylactic VCFs: Do VCFs reduce the incidence of clinically significant PE in patients who are able to receive LMWH? If so, is there is group of high-risk patients who will develop VTE despite "optimal" prophylaxis? Is VCF insertion cost-effective? Do retrievable VCFs have a role in the patient whose risk of VTE or contraindication to LMWH is temporary? Until better data are available on the utilization of prophylactic VCF to reduce the incidence of PE in high-risk injured patients, the one universally accepted indication for VCF insertion will remain those patients who have a documented VTE and contraindications for anticoagulation.

Pharmacological prophylaxis: aspirin and other antiplatelet agents

Aspirin and other antiplatelet agents have been evaluated in a number of studies to assess their effectiveness in preventing VTE. Some studies have suggested a modest benefit of these agents in reducing the incidence of VTE in surgical and medical patients, while other studies show that aspirin has no benefit in reducing the incidence of VTE in hospitalized patients. Therefore, aspirin cannot be recommended as a prophylactic agent for any group of hospitalized patients, including trauma patients.

Pharmacological prophylaxis: unfractionated heparin

Heparin is a naturally occurring polysaccharide with a molecular weight varying between 3 and 30 kDa. The main anticoagulant activity of UFH is mediated by augmenting the activity of anti-thrombin III, which is an inhibitor of activated factor X and thrombin. UFH is the traditional pharmacologic VTE prophylaxis in medical and surgical patients. Although UFH has been used extensively in hospitalized patients, prospective data demonstrating efficacy in trauma patients remains lacking.

Although many of the studies examining the effect of UFH in trauma have methodological shortcomings, available evidence suggests that UFH is ineffective in preventing VTE in severely injured patients, especially at a dose of only 5,000 units administered subcutaneously twice per day. The potential benefit of dosing three times per day is unclear but has been shown to have increased benefit in some trials. Based on the current literature, UFH cannot be recommended as being effective for VTE prophylaxis in trauma patients. Many clinicians use UFH in trauma patients with a relative contraindication to LMWH, such as renal insufficiency, although data supporting this practice is lacking.

Pharmacological prophylaxis: low molecular weight heparin

LMWHs vary in molecular mass between 2 and 9 kDa. The molecules contain a unique pentasaccharide that imparts specific binding to antithrombin III, but in a lower proportion than UFH. LMWH has proportionally more anti-Xa activity compared to anti-factor II activity. The use of LMWH after trauma, in the form of enoxaparin or daltaparin, for the prevention of VTE has been demonstrated to be superior to PCDs or UFH in multiple studies. In a landmark prospective study, Geerts et al (1996) randomized 344 patients after major trauma to either LMWH or UFH for VTE prophylaxis. Administration of these agents was initiated within 36 hours of injury, and all patients underwent a screening venogram within 14 days of randomization. Exclusion criteria included intracranial hemorrhage, ISS < 9, or evidence of ongoing bleeding or coagulopathy. In comparison to patients who received UFH, LMWH was associated with a 30% reduction in all DVT (44% with UFH vs. 31% with LMWH, $p = 0.014$) and a 58% reduction in proximal DVT (15% with UFH vs. 6% with LMWH, $p = 0.012$). Major bleeding complications were infrequent (1.7%) although there was a slight increased risk of bleeding complications in patients receiving LMWH, which did not reach statistical significance (0.8% with UFH vs. 3.9% with LMWH). This study is the basis for the recommendation that LMWH is the preferred prophylactic agent for injured patients, and has become the standard of care for VTE prophylaxis in the trauma-patient population. For trauma patients, daily dosing is probably inadequate, and twice daily dosing is preferable. Formal economic analysis suggests that the use of LMWH in the trauma setting is cost-effective.

The safe administration of LMWH is complicated by variations in patient demographics and comorbid conditions. As a result, several investigators have suggested altering the dose of LMWH based on these specific characteristics. Included among the patient characteristics are obesity, renal failure, and edema. Although effectiveness of LMWH can be followed using anti-Xa levels, the practicality of this strategy remains problematic. Also, pharmacokinetic studies demonstrate that the standard dose of enoxaparin recommended for the prevention of VTE following multiple trauma (30 mg SQ Q12 hr) may provide inadequate anti-Xa activity, and is affected by the presence of peripheral edema. In addition, since renal clearance is the primary mode of elimination of LMWH, these drugs will accumulate and may be associated with increased risk of bleeding complications in patients with renal insufficiency. Patients with renal insufficiency should either receive UFH or have appropriate reduction of the dose of LMWH if the CrCl < 30 mL/min. With these modifications, no substantial risk of increased risk for VTE or bleeding has been reported.

Trauma patients often have injuries that place them at risk for complications associated with pharmacologic VTE prophylaxis. Various injuries are associated with either an increased risk of bleeding or excessive morbidity should a bleeding event occur, and constitute a relative contraindication to the administration of LMWH. These situations include traumatic brain injury with intracranial hemorrhage, ongoing hemorrhage, coagulopathy, intra-abdominal solid organ injury managed nonoperatively, and vertebral fractures associated with epidural hematoma. To complicate matters further, prophylaxis with LMWH may not reduce the incidence of VTE in some subsets of patients, including patients with traumatic brain injury during rehabilitation post-acute-care.

The prophylactic use of LMWH, started once hemostasis has been achieved, is the most efficacious and simplest option for the majority of medium- and high-risk trauma patients. The bleeding concerns associated with the use of LMWH in trauma patients with multiple injuries may delay the administration of VTE prophylaxis. Despite these concerns, studies demonstrate that LMWH has an acceptable safety profile when administered to patients with traumatic brain injury and/or solid organ trauma. Nonetheless, the decision as to whether and when LMWH can be safely prescribed after major trauma is left to clinician discretion. However, this discretion leads to variations in practice patterns that may delay initiation of prophylaxis, thereby increasing the risk for VTE. The risk of delayed initiation of prophylaxis appears to increase significantly by 4 days after injury, with a 3-fold increased risk of VTE. As a result, a number of investigators have suggested early initiation of prophylaxis within 24–48 hours for solid organ injury and 72 hours for head injury. Furthermore, despite common practice, LMWH need not be discontinued or held for most surgical procedures performed on the trauma patients.

Although bleeding remains the most common complication of both UFH and LMWH administration, patients should be carefully monitored for the development of heparin-induced thrombocytopenia (HIT). This prothrombotic syndrome is a result of the development of antibodies against platelet factor 4-heparin complexes. Binding of the platelet factor 4-heparin-antibody complex to the platelet surface Fcγlla receptor causes platelet activation, thromboembolic complications, and the paradoxical thrombocytopenia. The larger more sulfated heparins, such as UFH, are more commonly associated with HIT than the LMWH, although some studies show no difference in incidence of HIT between UFH and LMWH. Although thought to occur only in approximately 1% of patients receiving heparin, injured patients and those with previous exposure to heparin are at increased risk. As a result, therapy for patients suspected of having HIT should begin with immediate discontinuation of heparin in any form followed by pharmacologic inhibition of thrombin (e.g., recombinant hirudin, argatroban, danaparoid sodium).

The duration of LMWH prophylaxis after injury is an area that merits additional study; the current literature does not provide enough evidence to support consensus recommendations in this regard. It is clear that some trauma patients remain at increased risk for VTE after discharge from the acute-care setting; identifying and prophylaxing these patients may be beneficial. Data in patients undergoing surgery for elective hip replacement or hip fracture support a duration of VTE prophylaxis of 4–6 weeks postoperatively. Although it is difficult to extrapolate these conclusions to the general trauma patient population, it stands to reason that injured patients with hip or pelvic fractures and other injures would be at similar or higher risks of VTE during the recovery phase. Most experts agree that VTE prophylaxis should continue throughout hospitalization for trauma patients, and should continue through the period of rehabilitation for patients with impaired mobility, pelvic fractures, and long-bone fractures, spinal cord injury, etc.

Venous thromboembolism prophylaxis in patients with neuraxial analgesia

Several studies have demonstrated the benefits of neuraxial blockade (epidural and paravertebral regional blocks) in trauma patients. However, the risk of a rare but potentially devastating complication, spinal or epidural hematoma, is increased with the concomitant use of anticoagulant drugs. Although the true incidence is not well-established, the seriousness of this complication mandates extreme caution when using anticoagulation in patients with epidural or spinal catheters. In 1997, the Food and Drug Administration issued a public health advisory reporting that a series of patients developed perispinal hematoma after receiving LMWH in conjunction with spinal or epidural anesthesia. Although many patients had other factors that may have predisposed them to bleeding complications (e.g., underlying hemostatic abnormalities, anatomic or vascular vertebral column abnormalities, or traumatic needle insertion), some patients who suffered a perispinal hematoma after epidural anesthesia while on LMWH experienced sustained neurologic impairment despite surgical decompression. Therefore, LMWH should be used with caution or avoided entirely in patients receiving spinal or epidural analgesia. In addition, patients should be monitored closely for the development of any new signs of spinal cord compression.

Screening for venous thromboembolism in injured patients

Early identification of DVT and PE in trauma patients would allow treatment to be initiated and reduce the potential for complications. Venous Doppler and duplex ultrasonography are currently the most widely used methods for the diagnosis of lower extremity DVT because they can be performed at the bedside, are fairly accurate, widely available, and noninvasive. Doppler ultrasound has a sensitivity of 85% and specificity of 88% to detect proximal DVT in *symptomatic* patients. Duplex ultrasound employs real-time B-mode scanning with Doppler ultrasound. Duplex ultrasound has a 96% sensitivity and specificity to diagnose proximal lower extremity DVT in *symptomatic* patients. Both modalities are operator dependent, and are less sensitive for the detection of DVT in asymptomatic patients or for DVT below the knee. Furthermore, the presence of splints and dressings may limit adequate visualization of extremity veins by Doppler ultrasonography. Deep pelvic veins, which are often the source of emboli after pelvic fracture, are rarely visualized. In retrospective studies, screening duplex examinations detect a significant number of subclinical DVTs, although these studies have not shown an impact on patient outcomes. In addition, most of the studies on ultrasonographic screening for DVT in trauma patients have methodology flaws and did not employ confirmatory venography, the gold standard to diagnose DVT. Significant variability in screening practice has led to variability in the published risk of DVT. The costs of routine screening even among high-risk trauma patients are also prohibitive. There is no evidence that screening provides incremental gain in patient protection over the early, appropriate use of VTE prophylaxis. Selective screening might be beneficial in the subgroup of high-risk patients in whom early thromboprophylaxis has not been initiated due to the presence of bleeding risk.

Other less frequently used screening tools consist of imaging with magnetic resonance venography and laboratory evidence of clot formation with D-dimer. Although infrequently used, magnetic resonance venography can demonstrate asymptomatic deep pelvic vein thrombosis in patients with pelvic fractures undergoing operative fixation. Identification of these deep pelvic vein thromboses is usually not possible with venous Doppler ultrasonography. However, the majority of these patients had other sites of DVT that would have been detected by venous Doppler ultrasonography.

D-dimer, on the other hand, is a simple and inexpensive laboratory study that has been used to rule out VTE in medical patients. Although D-dimer has been associated with a negative predictive value for VTE as high as 100% in some studies, other studies have demonstrated no predictive value in trauma patients to the use of D-dimer due to injury-induced elevations that can persist for prolonged periods in the most seriously injured. Thus, until further large prospective studies are performed, the routine use of D-dimer as a screening tool cannot be advocated in the trauma population.

Strategy for venous thromboembolism prevention

Despite the extensive evidence supporting the use of VTE prophylaxis in hospitalized patients, adherence with this key patient safety practice remains suboptimal. Hospitals should have an active strategy that addresses the prevention of VTE in hospitalized patients in the form of a written, institution-wide VTE prophylaxis policy. Strategies that have been shown to increase adherence to VTE prophylaxis guidelines include the use of computerized decision support systems and automatic alerts, preprinted order sets, and periodic audit and feedback. Passive methods, such as the simple distribution of educational materials, are not as effective in ensuring long-term compliance.

Key references

Carlile M, Nicewander D, Yablon SA, et al. Prophylaxis for venous thromboembolism during rehabilitation for traumatic brain injury: a multicenter observational study. *J Trauma.* 2010;68:916–923.

Davidson BL, Buller HR, Decousus H, et al. Effect of obesity on outcomes after fondaparinux, enoxaparin, or heparin treatment for acute venous thromboembolism in the Matisse trials. *J Thromb Haemost.* 2007;5:1191–1194.

Ekeh AP, Dominguez KM, Markert RJ, et al. Incidence and risk factors for deep venous thrombosis after moderate and severe brain injury. *J Trauma.* 2010;68:912–915.

Geerts WH, Jay RM, Code KI, et al. A comparison of low-dose heparin with low-molecular-weight heparin as prophylaxis against venous thromboembolism after major trauma. *N Engl J Med.* 1996;335:701–707.

Geerts WH, Bergqvist D, Pineo GF, et al. Prevention of venous thromboembolism: American College of Chest Physicians Evidence-Based Clinical Practice Guidelines (8th edition). *Chest.* 2008;133:381S–453S.

Gorman PH, Qadri SF, Rao-Patel A. Prophylactic inferior vena cava (IVC) filter placement may increase the relative risk of deep venous thrombosis after acute spinal cord injury. *J Trauma.* 2009;66:707–712.

Haas CE, Nelsen JL, Raghavendran K, et al. Pharmacokinetics and pharmacodynamics of enoxaparin in multiple trauma patients. *J Trauma.* 2005;59:1336–1343; discussion 1343–1334.

Karmy-Jones R, Jurkovich GJ, Velmahos GC, et al. Practice patterns and outcomes of retrievable vena cava filters in trauma patients: an AAST multicenter study. *J Trauma.* 2007;62:17–24; discussion 24–15.

Knudson MM, Ikossi DG, Khaw L, et al. Thromboembolism after trauma: an analysis of 1602 episodes from the American College of Surgeons National Trauma Data Bank. *Ann Surg.* 2004;240:490–496; discussion 496–498.

Lim W, Dentali F, Eikelboom JW, et al. Meta-analysis: low-molecular-weight heparin and bleeding in patients with severe renal insufficiency. *Ann Intern Med.* 2006;144:673–684.

Malinoski D, Jafari F, Ewing T, et al. Standard prophylactic enoxaparin dosing leads to inadequate anti-Xa levels and increased deep venous thrombosis rates in critically ill trauma and surgical patients. *J Trauma.* 2010;68:874–880.

McMullin J, Cook D, Griffith L, et al. Minimizing errors of omission: behavioural reenforcement of heparin to avert venous emboli: the BEHAVE study. *Crit Care Med.* 2006;34:694–699.

Mohta M, Verma P, Saxena AK, et al. Prospective, randomized comparison of continuous thoracic epidural and thoracic paravertebral infusion in patients with unilateral multiple fractured ribs—a pilot study. *J Trauma.* 2009;66:1096–1101.

Morris TA, Castrejon S, Devendra G, et al. No difference in risk for thrombocytopenia during treatment of pulmonary embolism and deep venous thrombosis with either low-molecular-weight heparin or unfractionated heparin: a meta-analysis. *Chest.* 2007;132:1131–1139.

Napolitano LM, Garlapati VS, Heard SO, et al. Asymptomatic deep venous thrombosis in the trauma patient: is an aggressive screening protocol justified? *J Trauma.* 1995;39:651–657; discussion 657–659.

Norwood SH, Berne JD, Rowe SA, et al. Early venous thromboembolism prophylaxis with enoxaparin in patients with blunt traumatic brain injury. *J Trauma.* 2008;65:1021–1026; discussion 1026–1027.

Pierce CA, Haut ER, Kardooni S, et al. Surveillance bias and deep vein thrombosis in the national trauma data bank: the more we look, the more we find. *J Trauma.* 2008;64:932–936; discussion 936–937.

Rogers FB, Cipolle MD, Velmahos G, et al. Practice management guidelines for the prevention of venous thromboembolism in trauma patients: the EAST practice management guidelines work group. *J Trauma.* 2002;53:142–164.

Stannard JP, Lopez-Ben RR, Volgas DA, et al. Prophylaxis against deep-vein thrombosis following trauma: a prospective, randomized comparison of mechanical and pharmacologic prophylaxis. *J Bone Joint Surg Am.* 2006;88:261–266.

Chapter 22

Sedation and analgesia in the intensive care unit

A. Murat Kaynar

Sedation

Most patients admitted to intensive care unit (ICUs) require sedation and analgesia to minimize discomfort, anxiety, dyspnea, pain, and risks associated with agitation, such as inadvertent removal of tubes or catheters. The level of sedation required should be defined as early as possible in the course of a patient's stay in the ICU. As stated in the Society of Critical Care Medicine (SCCM) Guidelines for sedation and analgesia, *The desired level of sedation should be defined at the start of therapy and reevaluated on a regular basis as the clinical condition of the patient changes. Regimens should be written with the appropriate flexibility to allow titration to the desired endpoint, anticipating fluctuations in sedation requirements throughout the day.* The clinical practice of sedation and analgesia in the ICU has been hampered by the lack of patient-focused treatments, by the illusion that a "well" sedated patient is adequately cared-for, and by our inertia in limiting the use of these medications. Thus, patient-focused sedation should incorporate the concept that the need for sedation and analgesia differs among patients and within patients over time during the course of their illnesses. There is no "one size fits all" regimen of sedatives and analgesics in the ICU. These medications should be titrated to effect. For example, converting orotracheal intubation to tracheostomy has been shown to reduce the use of sedatives and analgesics and also shorten the duration of deeper sedation. On the other hand, a history of alcohol abuse leads to greater medication requirements. Importantly, the requirements for sedatives are dynamic and, in general, decrease as the patient improves.

As much as the therapies need to be individualized, the approach to sedation and analgesia is better accomplished in a multi-disciplinary fashion, including the perspectives of nurses, pharmacists, and physicians and amalgamating them into a functional and patient-oriented medical plan. One has to remember that medications help to achieve sedation, but inadequate analgesia can lead to agitation and discomfort, which cannot be relieved with sedatives alone. On the other hand, sedatives could lead to adverse outcomes including unnecessarily prolonged mechanical ventilation, ICU length of stay, and increased morbidity and mortality. The intensivist must be vigilant to use just the right amount of medications for the proper amount of time.

The care of agitated and distressed patients begins by considering predisposing and precipitating factors, such as pain, metabolic syndromes, acute neurologic disorders, underlying dementia, medications (including benzodiazepines and opioids), withdrawal states, poisons, infections, postoperative states, underlying mental illnesses, ICU procedures, and sleep deprivation. Once other treatable causes are ruled out, the clinician has to be able to assess the clinical severity of agitation using reproducible metrics. Several such scales and assessment tools have been developed to assist clinicians in determining a patient's possible need for sedation therapy and response to interventions. Most of the sedation scales are descriptive assessments of a patient's level of anxiety or agitation. (Tables 22.1–4). Unless a patient is in extremis and requiring more than usual doses of sedatives, an ICU clinician could define the optimal level of sedation as a patient being calm, comfortable, and easily arousable. This would correspond to a *Ramsay Scale* score of 2, a *Sedation-Agitation Scale* score of 4, a *Richmond Agitation-Sedation Scale* score of 0, or a *Motor Activity Assessment Scale* score of 3. Although these sedation goals are ideal, they are far from realistic. Estimates are that more than 70% of ICU patients respond to the ICU experience with some level of anxiety. Minimizing stimuli that could provoke anxiety, such as unnecessary lights, noises, sleep interruption, and procedures, can decrease the need for medications. This should be part of a patient-focused and functional sedation plan.

Sedative medications are often administered by continuous infusion for a smooth clinical course, but this has been linked to prolonged sedation and longer ICU stay. Daily interruption of sedatives, with restarting at a decreased dose, can decrease use of sedatives, days on mechanical ventilation, and ICU length of stay.

Table 22.1 Riker sedation-agitation scale

Score	Description	Explanation
7	Dangerously agitated	Thrashing side-to-side, trying to remove catheters or tubes, trying to get out of bed, physically attacking staff
6	Very agitated	Requires restraints, must be frequently reminded of correct behavior
5	Agitated	Physically anxious/agitated, calms with verbal directions
4	Calm and cooperative	Easily arousable, follows verbal commands
3	Sedated	Hard to arouse, will awaken with verbal or gentle physical stimuli, can follow simple commands but will drift off if unstimulated
2	Very sedated	Arouses only to physical stimuli, does not respond or follow commands, does/can have spontaneous movement
1	Unarousable	No or minimal response to noxious stimuli, does not follow commands or respond

Table 22.2 Richmond agitation-sedation scale

Score	Description	Explanation
+4	Combative	Violent, danger to staff or self
+3	Very agitated	Aggressive, tries to removes catheters and tubes
+2	Agitated	Numerous nonpurposeful movements, fights the ventilator
+1	Restless	Displays anxiety, nonaggressive movements
0	Calm and alert	
−1	Drowsy	Not fully alert but will respond to voice with > 10 s eye opening
−2	Light sedation	Awakens with eye contact, < 10 s
−3	Moderate sedation	Eye opening or movement to voice; no eye contact
−4	Deep sedation	No response to verbal stimuli; eye opening or movement to physical stimuli
−5	Unarousable	No response to verbal or physical stimuli

Sedatives in the intensive care unit

There are many agents appropriate for sedation in the ICU. And it is important to remember that the sedative agents listed (Table 22.5) do not have any analgesic properties except for dexmedetomidine. Previously, the most common sedatives employed in the ICU were either benzodiazepines or opioids.

Among the benzodiazepine sedatives, midazolam and lorazepam are still widely used. Their lack of hemodynamic effects, low cost, and significant

Table 22.3 Motor activity assessment scale

Score	Explanation
6	Dangerously agitated; no external stimulus is required to elicit movement and patient is uncooperative, pulling at tubes or catheters, or thrashing side-to-side or striking at staff or trying to climb out of bed and does not calm down when asked
5	Agitated; no external stimulus is required to elicit movement; attempts to sit up or moves limbs out of bed and does not consistently follow commands (e.g., will lie down when asked but soon reverts back to attempts to sit up or move limbs out of bed)
4	Restless and cooperative; no external stimulus is required to elicit movement and patient is picking at sheets or tubes or uncovering self; follows commands
3	Calm and cooperative; no external stimulus is required to elicit movement and patient is purposefully adjusting sheets or clothes; follows commands
2	Responsive to touch or name; opens eyes or raises eye brows or turns head toward stimulusor, moves limbs when touched or name is spoken loudly
1	Responsive only to noxious stimulus; opens eyes or raises eyebrows or turns head toward stimulus or moves limbs with noxious stimulus
0	Unresponsive; does not move with noxious stimulus

Table 22.4 Ramsay scale

Score	Explanation
1	Awake; patient anxious and agitated or restless or both
2	Patient cooperative, oriented, and tranquil
3	Patient responds to commands only
4	Asleep; a brisk response to a light glabellar tap or loud auditory stimulus
5	A sluggish response to a light glabellar tap or loud auditory stimulus
6	No response to a light glabellar tap or loud auditory stimulus

amnestic effect make them good choices. For long-term sedation, they are still the drugs of choice. These medications are commonly administered by continuous infusion or intermittent boluses. The 2002 SCCM practice guidelines suggested lorazepam as the preferred sedative for prolonged use, whereas midazolam was recommended for short-term use due to the unpredictable nature of awakening after its prolonged use. Midazolam may accumulate in the setting

Table 22.5 Sedatives

Diazepam

Agent/Dose	Metabolism	Metabolites	Side effects
Bolus—0.03 to 0.1 mg/kg, may repeat every 0.5 to 6 hours	Desmethylation and hydroxylation	Active, can lead to prolonged sedation	Phlebitis

Midazolam

| *Bolus*—0.02 to 0.08 mg/kg, may repeat every 0.5 to 2 hours
Infusion—0.04 to 0.2 mg/kg per hour | Oxidation | Active, can lead to prolonged sedation especially with renal failure | None |

Lorazepam

| *Bolus*—0.02 to 0.06 mg/kg, may repeat every 2 to 6 hours
Infusion—0.01 to 0.1 mg/kg per hour | Glucuronidation | None | Solvent related acidosis/renal failure in high doses |

Propofol

| *Bolus*—1.5 to 2.5 mg/kg (induction of general anesthesia)
Infusion—0.3 to 4.0 mg/kg per hour | Oxidation | None | Pain on injection, elevated triglycerides, hypotension with bolus dosing, and propofol infusion syndrome |

Dexmedetomidine

| *Bolus*—0.5 µg/kg over at least 10 minutes
Infusion—0.2 to 0.7 µg/kg hour | Glucuronidation and conjugation | None | Possible hypotension and bradycardia |

of liver dysfunction; or its active metabolite, α-hydroxymidazolam, may accumulate in renal dysfunction. On the other hand, prolonged use of lorazepam could lead to the accumulation of the vehicle, propylene glycol, with resultant renal dysfunction, metabolic acidosis, and altered mental status. Toxicity is usually observed after prolonged use (~1 week) or high doses (> 14 mg/hr), and could be detected by increased osmolal gap.

Propofol, a phenol derivative commonly used as an induction agent in the operating room, is very popular for infusions in the ICU. While bolus dosing can result in hypotension, a titrated infusion can provide sedation and stable hemodynamics. Propofol is officially approved for < 48 hours of use, but it is frequently used beyond these limits. Propofol has been shown to decrease ventilator weaning time compared to midazolam infusion. Despite its beneficial properties, one has to be cognizant of the side effects of propofol infusion, including hypertriglyceridemia, hemodynamic compromise, and the propofol infusion syndrome with metabolic acidosis, rhabdomyolysis, renal failure, and cardiac depression.

The most recent entry into the sedation field is dexmedetomidine, an α2-adrenergic agonist with a short half-life. Dexmedetomidine combines a sedative effect with an opioid-sparing analgesic effect. It has been shown to result in decreased days of mechanical ventilation and length of stay following cardiac surgery. Dexmedetomidine has no significant depressive effects on respiratory drive. It has been shown that the use of dexmedetomidine could decrease the opioid use and facilitate extubation in "difficult-to-wean" patients. It has also been used in the management of alcohol withdrawal successfully. However, it can cause bradycardia and dystonia due to acetylcholine release.

Analgesia

Analgesia is defined as the "the blunting or absence of sensation of pain or noxious stimuli." Just as sedation scales are used to provide better care for patients, analgesia should also be measured and assessed to determine appropriate dosing of analgesic agents. Pain is relatively easy to assess in coherent, awake patients. To facilitate this assessment in intubated or aphasic patients, a Visual Analog Scale (VAS) has been developed, with 0 being no pain to 10 being the worst pain imaginable. Patients can state or point to the appropriate value, and clinicians would adjust the therapy accordingly. The VAS has been modified to ease a patient's understanding (particularly with pediatric patients) to a "smiley face scale" of all smiles to frown to grimaces corresponding to the level of a patient's discomfort. Bedside caregivers should also note the physiologic responses to activities or procedures that could produce discomfort and then treat as indicated. A Behavioral Pain Scale has since been introduced that attempts to correlate the level of discomfort with patient behavior. Behavioral Pain Scale and other similar tools are based on the recognition of typical behaviors, such as grimacing due to pain, restless movements, and rigid limbs. The Behavioral Pain Scale (Table 22.6) may help identify patients who cannot otherwise voice their level of discomfort. This scale may be useful, especially when a

Table 22.6 Behavioral pain scale

Behavior	Description	Score
Facial expression	Relaxed	1
	Partially tightened	2
	Fully tightened	3
	Grimacing	4
Upper limb movements	None	1
	Partially bent	2
	Fully bent, fingers flexed	3
	Permanently retracted	4
Compliance with mechanical ventilation (MV)	Tolerating movement	1
	Coughing but tolerating MV	2
	Fighting MV	3
	Unable to control ventilation	4

patient's hemodynamic responses maybe limited by medication or the patient's underlying condition. Although the pain scales have been validated in various ICU cohorts, surveys suggest that the clinical penetration of these tools is still limited to half of clinicians.

Analgesics in the intensive care unit

Opioids are the main analgesics used in the ICU. Table 22.7 lists some of the more common agents. They vary in potency and duration of action. The synthetic opioids, fentanyl and remifentanil, are more potent than morphine and are suitable for infusions in the ICU. Their short duration of action also make them appropriate for small bolus dosing when patients must undergo short painful procedures. All of the opioids also have some sedative properties, which can be beneficial.

Opioids function via the μ1 and μ2 receptors. All cause dose-dependent respiratory depression, which can limit their usefulness in spontaneously breathing patients. Other side effects are muscle rigidity, hypotension, gastroparesis, nausea and vomiting, urinary retention, and pruritus. As noted in Table 22.7, the clinician needs to be aware of the metabolism of opioids, such as morphine, which will accumulate in the setting of renal dysfunction due to its active metabolite, morphine-6-glucuronide, leading to prolonged opioid effects. The commonly used agents in the United States include fentanyl, hydromorphone, and morphine sulfate, although sufentanil is commonly used in Europe.

Ketamine (ketamine hydrochloride) is a centrally acting dissociative anesthetic, providing pain relief with preservation of pharyngeal and laryngeal reflexes. This property makes ketamine a very good agent for analgesia for the nonintubated patient during very painful procedures. However, while the airway is maintained, secretions are significantly increased and patients may have difficulty in clearing these secretions. It has hypnotic, analgesic, and amnesic effects. Ketamine can cause mild stimulation of the cardiovascular system. Benzodiazepines are often administered prior to ketamine to minimize the dissociative hallucinations or nightmares some patients may experience. "Flashbacks" may be a concern as ketamine is closely related to phencyclidine. Given in combination with other agents, either a benzodiazepine or mixed with propofol, this is not a real problem.

Ketorolac, a nonsteroidal anti-inflammatory drug, may be useful for patients requiring occasional dosing for mild-to-moderate pain. It has no sedative properties or effect on respiration; however, it may lead to gastrointestinal and coagulation problems. Use of ketorolac or other nonsteroidal anti-inflammatory agents may decrease the need for opioids.

Acetaminophen, or paracetamol, has also been added to our list of nonopioid medications in the management of pain in our ICUs, but the clinical data available is still sporadic and needs to be evaluated further.

In Table 22.7, the dosages for the commonly used analgesics are given as a range. Thus it is imperative that clinicians carefully titrate these agents. All of

Table 22.7 Analgesics

Morphine

Agent/Dose	Metabolism	Metabolites	Side Effects	Equivalent Dose Half-life
Bolus—0.01 to 0.15 mg/kg every 1 to 2 hours	Glucuronidation	Renal failure leads to accumulation	Histamine release	10 mg 3–7 h
Infusion—0.07 to 0.5 mg/kg per hour				

Hydromorphone

Bolus—10 to 30 μg/kg every 1 to 2 hours	Glucuronidation	None	None	1.5 mg 2–3 h
Infusion—7 to 15 μg/kg per hour				

Fentanyl

Bolus—0.35 to 1.5 μg/kg every 0.5 to 1.0 hour	Oxidation	None	Large doses will cause muscle rigidity	200 μg 1–6 h
Infusion—0.7 to 10 μg/kg per hour				

Remifentanil

Bolus—Not usual	Plasma esterase	None	Rigidity with large bolus	3–10 min
Infusion—0.6 to 0.15 μg/kg per hour				

Ketorolac

Bolus—15 to 30 mg every 6 hours, decrease with renal insufficiency or older patients	Renal	None	Risk of bleeding	2–8h
Infusion—None				

the agents (except ketamine) have some potential for lowering blood pressure and cardiac output; some directly, but mostly by attenuation of the patient's sympathetic response to pain. Almost all of the agents will produce some level of sedation as well. Therefore, administration of adequate analgesics may allow reduction in the doses of the sedatives to maintain the same level of sedation for an individual patient. Using a sedation scale along with a VAS for pain can result in an optimized, patient-focused regimen.

Consideration must also be given for pain relief for temporary intense discomfort associated with procedures in the ICU. Utilization of an agent with a short half-life would be most appropriate in this situation. A clinician should also consider adding a short-acting sedative/amnestic.

Regional anesthetics are certainly underutilized in the ICU. A thoracic epidural or paravertebral anesthesia may be the treatment of choice for a patient with rib fractures or an abdominal surgical wound. Often employing a combination of a low-dose local anesthetic and a lipophilic narcotic, such as fentanyl or sufentanil, an epidural can provide remarkable pain relief without the side effects of respiratory depression or significant sedation. However, epidural analgesia requires expertise in insertion, limiting its use. Caution is also required as low-dose anticoagulation for deep venous thrombosis prophylaxis is often a contraindication for epidural insertion.

Delirium

Delirium is an acute disorder of attention and global cognitive function, characterized by acute onset and fluctuating symptoms. It is common among critically ill patients and possibly worsens outcomes, including increased long-term mortality. Delirium is a syndrome caused by physiologic consequences of a medical disturbance. Symptoms include changes in awareness and consciousness, memory deficits, hallucinations, and disturbances in sleep. It is important to establish a patient's baseline, that is, his or her mental status prior to ICU admission. Delirium, comes on quickly (hours to a few days), and should be distinguished from dementia, which comes on gradually (months to years). Dementia is almost always a progressive, permanent condition; delirium often clears in several days to weeks. Metabolic disturbances are the most common causes for delirium. Pharmacologic agents are another significant cause. Other causes include central nervous system disorders, withdrawal states, poisons, infections, diabetes, electrolyte abnormalities, hypoxia, hypercarbia, organ dysfunction, postoperative state, mental illness, pain, surgical/ICU procedures, and sleep deprivation/altered sleep patterns. Factors that are more common in patients who suffer from delirium include serious illness, older age, and a history of a previous mental disease.

Although most delirium cases present in the hyperactive form, a hypoactive delirious state is also common among ICU patients. Of the various causes of delirium, there is emerging evidence that the hypoactive delirium in the ICU is related to the use of sedatives, especially lorazepam.

Evaluation of a patient for diagnosis of delirium

Two commonly accepted methodologies exist to assess whether or not a patient is suffering from delirium. The Confusion Assessment Method (CAM) requires a patient to be able to verbalize. Because this may not be possible in many ICU patients, the CAM-ICU was developed to assess nonverbal patients. The CAM identifies delirium based on four features:

(1) Acute onset of fluctuations or variability in the course of mental status
(2) Inattention
(3) Disorganized thinking
(4) Altered level of consciousness.

Delirium is diagnosed if the patient has both of the first two symptoms and also has either the third or fourth symptom. Treatment of delirium is based on finding the underlying cause, if possible, and correcting or minimizing its effect. Among the reversible causes of delirium, administration of pharmacologic agents has the best prognosis for improvement. In addition, methods to reduce anxiety in ICU patients can reduce the incidence of delirium. Pain may be one of many factors contributing to a patient's delirium and should always be addressed. Following the preventive measures, the pharmacologic treatment of delirium is most often accomplished with antipsychotics.

Haloperidol is often the drug of choice, as it has few anticholinergic side effects and is not likely to cause hypotension or sedation. Haloperidol may be given intravenously (IV), intramuscularly, or by mouth. The IV route is reported to result in fewer extrapyramidal symptoms. It may be useful in doses as low as 0.25 to 0.50 mg every 4 hours but is usually started at 1 to 2 mg every 4 hours and titrated to higher doses as required. For severe cases, an infusion of 5 to 10 mg/h may be started after a bolus dose of 10 mg. Some newer antipsychotic medications (risperidone, olanzapine, and quetiapine) have been used in the treatment of patients with delirium. Patients receiving antipsychotic medications should have a baseline electrocardiogram and have their electrocardiograms monitored during therapy. A rate-corrected QT interval greater than 450 ms or more than 25% over baseline may warrant a reduction or discontinuation of the antipsychotic medication. Other significant side effects of haloperidol are tardive dyskinesia and muscle rigidity, which are due to extrapyramidal effects of the agent. Recent work suggests that these side effects are less commonly observed in patients receiving olanzepine. Benzodiazepines are the treatment choice for extrapyramidal effects.

A benzodiazepine would be the agent of choice for delirium related to withdrawal states. A benzodiazepine may also be added to a lower dose of an antipsychotic in patients who may not tolerate a higher dosage of the antipsychotic. A cholinergic agent, physostigmine, may be used if the state of delirium has been caused by an anticholinergic agent. Patients who are truly "psychotic" may require restraints, sedation, and even the use of a neuromuscular-blocking agent to protect themselves.

Neuromuscular blockade in the intensive care unit

Clinicians should consider many issues when initiating therapy including neuromuscular blockers (NMB) in the ICU and should have a logical reason for using them (Table 22.8). The patient's condition may dictate which agent or class of agents should be used. The pharmacology of NMB agents (metabolism, active metabolites, and clearance) is especially important in the ICU because NMBs are often given by infusion rather than a single bolus as in the operating room, and patients frequently have renal or hepatic dysfunction. Side effects of some of the agents range from trivial to unacceptable depending on a patient's condition.

Clinically useful neuromuscular blocking agents are of two types, benzylisoquinolinium or aminosteroidal compounds. The benzylisoquinolinium compounds are related to curare. Fortunately, the clinically used agents atracurium and cisatracurium lack the ganglionic blockade effect of curare. Both atracurium and cisatracurium are eliminated by Hoffman elimination (nonenzymatic degradation), making them especially important for use in patients with renal or hepatic insufficiency. The aminosteroidal compounds pancuronium, vecuronium, and rocuronium are metabolized by the liver and excreted by the kidneys. Renal or hepatic insufficiency can prolong the action of pancuronium and vecuronium. Rocuronium may have prolonged action with hepatic disease, though fewer data exist on the prolonged duration of rocuronium infusions compared with pancuronium or vecuronium.

Although the side effects of individual agents must be considered in critically ill patients, especially those with organ dysfunction, it is prolonged neuromuscular blockade or weakness that is the most worrisome problem. In the 1990s, numerous case reports of prolonged weakness or blockade were published coining the term critical illness polyneuro-myopathy. The aminosteroidal compounds were at first the most frequent culprits. Then, even the benzylisoquinolinium compounds were associated with polyneuro-myopathy in a number of cases. Patient conditions associated with the potential for prolonged blockade include organ dysfunction, sepsis, concomitant magnesium therapy, hypothermia, acidosis, prolonged NMB infusion, and systemic steroid therapy.

When using NMB, train-of-4 monitoring with a peripheral nerve stimulator should be used along with clinical observation of the patient. Whether the NMB is used to decrease oxygen consumption, facilitate mechanical ventilation, reduce intracranial pressure, or to protect the patient, the need for NMB must be defined and continually reassessed (Figure 22.1). If muscular relaxation fails to achieve the stated goal, it probably should not be maintained. A once-daily interruption of NMBs and sedatives has been proposed to allow better observation of those drugs' effects and whether they are still required.

Table 22.8 Neuromuscular blocking agents

Agent/Dose	Active Metabolite	Metabolism	Elimination	Side Effects
Pancuronium				
Bolus/intermittent dosing—0.1 to 0.2 mg/kg; redose 0.1 mg/kg every 1 to 3 hours as clinically needed or when train-of-4 monitoring indicates need. *Infusion*—rarely used	Yes	Liver	Renally excreted	Vagolytic
Vecuronium				
Bolus/intermittent dosing—0.08 to 0.10 mg/kg; redose with 0.01 to 0.15 mg/kg every 20 to 45 minutes. May give higher dose to facilitate faster onset, 0.3 mg/kg (clinical examination and train-of-4 monitoring to determine when subsequent doses are required) *Infusion*—Bolus of 0.08 to 0.10 mg/kg, then after 20 to 30 minutes start 1 (xg/kg per minute (range 0.8 to 1.2 µg/kg per hour)	Yes	Liver	Renally excreted	None
Rocuronium				
Bolus/intermittent dosing—0.6 mg/kg; redose with 0.1 to 0.2 mg/kg as clinically needed or when train-of-4 monitoring indicates need. May give larger dose to facilitate faster onset, 1.2 mg/kg per minute, useful for rapid-sequence intubation *Infusion*—Bolus of 0.6 mg/kg per minute, then infusion of 0.01 to 0.012 mg/kg per minute	No	Liver	Renally excreted	None
Cisatracurium				
Bolus/intermittent dosing—0.15 to 0.2 mg/kg; redose with 0.03 mg/kg every 40 to 60 minutes (clinical examination and train-of-4 monitoring to determine when subsequent doses are required) *Infusion*—Bolus of 0.15 to 0.2 mg/kg, then 1 to 3 µg/kg per minute (range 0.5 to 10 µg/kg per minute)	No	None	Hoffman elimination	None

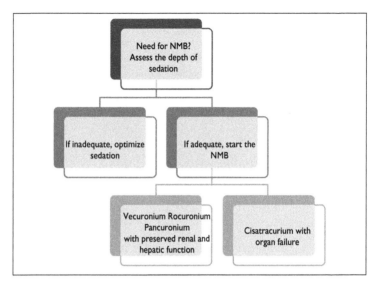

Figure 22.1 Algorithm for initiation of neuromuscular blockade

Protocolized care

Protocolized care for use of sedatives can improve the quality of care and outcomes for ICU patients. The two landmark research protocols involved (1) nurse-driven algorithms to decrease the use of sedatives and (2) daily interruption of sedation. Both studies showed significant reduction in the duration of mechanical ventilation, ICU stay, and hospital length-of-stay.

Key references

Devlin JW, Roberts RJ, Fong JJ, et al. Efficacy and safety of quetiapine in critically ill patients with delirium: a prospective, multicenter, randomized, double-blind, placebo-controlled pilot study. *Crit Care Med.* 2010;38(2):419–427.

Ely EW, Inouye SK, Bernard GR, et al. Delirium in mechanically ventilated patients: validity and reliability of the confusion assessment method for the intensive care unit (CAM-ICU). *JAMA.* 2001;286(21):2703–2710.

Girard TD, Kress JP, Fuchs BD, et al. Efficacy and safety of a paired sedation and ventilator weaning protocol for mechanically ventilated patients in intensive care (Awakening and Breathing Controlled trial): a randomised controlled trial. *Lancet.* 2008;371(9607):126–134.

Ho AM, Karmakar MK, Critchley LA. Acute pain management of patients with multiple fractured ribs: a focus on regional techniques. *Curr Opin Crit Care.* 2011;17(4):323–327.

Jacobi J, Fraser GL, Coursin DB, et al. Clinical practice guidelines for the sustained use of sedatives and analgesics in the critically ill adult. *Crit Care Med*. 2002;30(1):119–141.

Kress JP, Pohlman AS, O'Connor MF, et al. Daily interruption of sedative infusions in critically ill patients undergoing mechanical ventilation. *N Engl J Med*. 2000;342(20):1471–1477.

Murray MJ, Cowen J, DeBlock H, et al. Clinical practice guidelines for sustained neuromuscular blockade in the adult critically ill patient. *Crit Care Med*. 2002;30(1):142–156.

Sessler CN, Gosnell MS, Grap MJ, et al. The Richmond Agitation-Sedation Scale: validity and reliability in adult intensive care unit patients. *Am J Respir Crit Care Med*. 2002;166(10):1338–1344.

Chapter 23

Pediatric trauma

Daniel Rutigliano and Barbara A. Gaines

Epidemiology

Childhood injury is the leading cause of morbidity and mortality among children (ages 0–19 years) in the United States. These injuries represent an enormous burden both financially and emotionally to families and society alike. According to the Centers for Disease Control (CDC), from 2000–2006, on average, 12,175 children in the United States died each year from unintentional injuries. Risk for injury and death vary by race. In the United States, injury death rates are highest for Native Americans and Alaska Natives and are lowest for Asian or Pacific Islanders. Overall death rates for whites and African-Americans are approximately the same. The World Health Organization (WHO) reported in 2008 that unintentional injury resulted in the deaths of over 800,000 children worldwide in 2004.[3] After 10 years of age, childhood injury was the number one cause of death amoung children worldwide.

The 2010 National Trauma Database (NTDB) Pediatric Report on childhood injuries highlights the typical pattern of injuries seen in this population. A bimodal distribution of incidents by age is seen, with the first peak at 0–2 years of age and the second peak occuring after 15 years of age. Fatalities by age also follow a similar distibution. Males are more likely than females to be injuired in all age groups, with males having a 2-fold higher death rate.

Injury characteristics differ by age. Falls, motor vehicle trauma (MVT), and pedestrian-motor vehicle collisions are the leading causes of injury in the United States. Falls are the most common cause of injury until 15 years of age, with the vast majority of injuries occuring within the 0-–10-year-old age range. After 15 years of age, MVT becomes the leading cause of injury. (Figure 23.1) For children under 1 year of age, suffocation is the leading cause of mortality, while from ages 1–64 years MVT is the leading cause of death. Firearms deserve special mention here because they result in the highest percentage of fatality per incidence in the pediatric population even if the overall incidence is relatively low.

The head, upper extermity, and face are the most common regions of the body injured. In children with multiple injuries, head, thorax, and lower extremity injuries are prevalent. Fatal injuries typically involve injuries to the head, thorax, and abdomen, with most of these being associated with MVT and tramatic brain injuries (TBI). Trauma to the neck is a rare occurrence, but it results in a 25% fatality rate.

Rank	Less Than 1 (n=5,883)	1 to 4 (n=10,203)	Age Group in Years 5 to 9 (n=7,144)	10 to 14 (n=9,088)	15 to 19 (n=40,734)
1	Suffocation 66%	Drowning 27%	MVT - Occupant 22%	MVT - Occupant 26%	MVT - Occupant 41%
2	MVT - Occupant 8%	Pedestrian 15%	MVT - Unspecified 15%	MVT - Unspecified 15%	MVT - Unspecified 28%
3	Drowning 7%	Fires/Burns 14%	Pedestrian 14%	Pedestrian 12%	Poisoning 7%
4	MVT - Unspecified 5%	MVT - Occupant 13%	Fires/Burns 13%	Drowning 10%	MVT-Other 6%
5	Other Injuries 5%	MVT - Unspecified 9%	Drowning 13%	MVT - Other 9%	Pedestrian 5%
6	Fires/Burns 6%	Suffocation 8%	Other Injuries 7%	Other Injuries 8%	Drowning 5%
7	Poisoning 2%	Other Injuries 8%	MVT - Other 6%	Fires/Burns 6%	Other Injuries 5%
8	Falls 2%	Falls 2%	Pedal Cyclist 4%	Pedal Cyclist 6%	Falls 1%
9	Pedestrian 1%	Poisoning 2%	Suffocation 4%	Suffocation 4%	Fires/Burns 1%
10	MVT - Other 0.5%	MVT - Other 2%	Falls 1%	Poisoning 2%	Suffocation 1%
11	Pedal Cyclist 0.02%	Pedal Cyclist 0.3%	Poisoning 1%	Falls 2%	PedalCyclist 1%

Figure 23.1 Leading causes of unintentional injury death among children 0–19 years of age. Adapted with permission from the Center for Disease Control Childhood Injury Report: Patterns of Unintentional Injuries among 0–19 Year Olds in the United States, 2000–2006.

The practicing physician should be aware of some unique injury presentations in the pediatric population. Drowning and suffocation, as well as accidental poisoning, are more likely in children. Infants can drown in as little as one inch of water. Animal bites, especially to the face and hands, are also more common in the pediatric population because children tend to have less awareness of the dangers an animal might present.

Unfortunately, child abuse is also something that physicians must consider. Chronic patterns of abuse can be difficult to identify, but once recognized, require immediate action and involvement of child protective services.

Emergency department management

Resuscitation of a pediatric trauma patient follows the basic principles defined by the Advance Trauma Life Support (ATLS) program, namely the ABCs of airway, breathing, and circulation. However, because of the wide range in patients' size and patterns of injury, as well as various physiologic presentations, physicians who treat children must recognize and understand important distinctions from adult trauma management.

The smaller body mass of children, thus the energy force per unit body area, is much higher in pediatrics than in adults, resulting in a greater risk for severe injuries. Significant injury can result even from relatively low-impact/velocity mechanisms. The incomplete ossification of the skeleton and growth plates also makes children more susceptible to injury. Because of the pliable skeleton, internal organ damage can occur without obvious overlying external fractures (e.g., severe pulmonary contusions without rib fractures). Children have a large surface-area-to-body volume, thus hypothermia is more of a concern. Increased physiological reserve allows near-normal maintenance of vital signs even in the presence of severe shock; hypotension is a *late* sign of shock and pediatric patients tend to become unstable later in the assessment period as compared to adults.

Airway management in children differs from the adult due to unique anatomic variations. (Figure 23.2) Children have an anterior larynx, which makes it harder to visualize; in addition, the anterior larynx position makes the angle between the base of the tongue and the glottic opening more acute; the epiglottis is large, floppy, and does not lift up as easily. The large tongue can easily obstruct the airway and make laryngoscopy more difficult. As a result of these differences, use of a straight blade with the laryngoscope is recommended to create a more direct visual plane from the mouth to the glottis. Care must be taken in the presence of loose teeth as these can easily be dislodged and cause airway obstruction. The cricoid ring is the narrowest part of the airway in children (as opposed to the vocal cords in adults) and it tends to form a natural seal with the endotracheal tube (ETT)—low pressure cuffed tubes are important to use to minimize the risk of pressure necrosis. The trachea is also shorter in pediatric patients than in adults; as a result it can be very easy to intubate the right main-

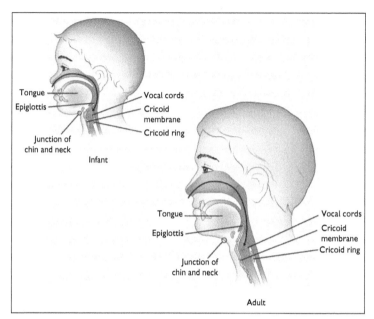

Figure 23.2 Anatomic airway differences between children and adults. The anatomic differences particular to children include: (1) Higher, more anterior position for the glottic opening (Note the relationship of the vocal cords to the chin-neck junction.); (2) relatively larger tongue in the infant, lying between the mouth and the glottic opening; (3) relatively larger and more floppy epiglottis in the child; (4) cricoid ring is the narrowest portion of the pediatric airway (In adults, the narrowest portion is the vocal cords.); (5) position and size of the cricothyroid membrane in the infant; (6) sharper, more difficult angle for blind nasotracheal intubation; (7) larger relative size of the occiput in the infant. *From Auerbach: Winderness Medicine, 5th ed. Mosby 2007, chapter 19- redrawn from figure 19.1 Walls RM, Murphy MF, Luten RC, Schneider RE, eds. Manual of Emergency Airway Management, 2nd ed. Philadelphia: Lippincott Williams & Wilkins, 2004*

stem bronchus; even minimal movement of the patient can cause dislodgement of the ETT.

Orotracheal intubation is the preferred route of definitive airway management. Nasotracheal intubation is not recommended because of an increased risk of pharyngeal/adenoid bleeding and the relatively acute angle of the posterior nasopharynx. Depending on the urgency of the airway, preoxygenation with mask ventilation is recommended followed by rapid sequence induction with inline cervical spine immobilization. In patients with a difficult airway, the ability to ventilate via the bag-valve-mask technique is critical and may be just as effective when compared with endotracheal intubation for transport. A recent study looking at the effect of endotracheal intubation in the out-of-hospital setting versus bag-valve-mask ventilation did not demonstrate any survival improvement in those patients who underwent intubation for short transports. If establishment of an orotracheal airway is not possible, then a surgical airway is necessary. For children 10 years and older, a cricothyrotomy is the preferred approach because of its superficial location and the ease with which it may be converted to a formal tracheostomy once the patient has stabilized. In younger children, the cricoid cartilage provides a large amount of support for the trachea and damage to it can result in long-term tracheomalacia. For this reason children younger than 10 years should undergo a needle cricothyrotomy with jet ventilation, usually with a 12- to 14-gauge needle. This is only useful as an emergent temporizing measure until an orotracheal airway can be established or a formal tracheotomy can be created.

Selection of the ETT size varies with the age of the patient. Approximating the diameter of the patient's little finger can provide a guide for size selection but may be unreliable. Use of the Broselow pediatric emergency tape can provide a rapid assessment of patient size and weight based on their length, from 3 to 35 kg. Based on the tape measurement, patients are then placed into a color category, with the documentation on the tape providing recommendations on ETT size as well as medication dosing for intubation if needed. Several formulas also exist to calculate proper ETT size based on age, such as cuffed ETT size = (age in years/4) + 3. The insertion depth of the ETT (cm) can also be calculated—for children under 1 year of age = weight/2 + 8; for children over 1 year = age/2 + 12. Once the ETT is in place, it is important to confirm proper position and secure the tube with the neck in a neutral position. Due to the short length of the pediatric trachea, any movement of the neck can result in tube dislodgement. Neck flexion can push the tube farther in, possibly resulting in a right mainstem intubation, and neck extension can result in the tube being pulled out of the airway.

During ventilation, if any change in the patient's respiratory status occurs, it is helpful to remember the acronym DOPE—Displacement, Obstruction, Pneumothorax, Equipment. It is important to remember that smaller ETTs have narrow lumens that can get easily blocked with secretions, blood, etc., resulting in rapid desaturation. The high compliance of the pediatric airway also makes it very susceptible to dynamic collapse in the presence of airway obstruction or pneumothorax. Finally, physicians need to be aware that aggressive ventilation, especially in neonates/infants, can easily cause iatrogenic pneumothoraces. Judicious use of positive end-expiratory pressure with weight-appropriate tidal volumes is a must.

The management of circulation and obtaining vascular access also differs among children. As always, attempts should be made to obtain two large-bore IVs during the primary survey. After two unsuccessful attempts, the next approach is usually an intraosseous (IO), which is a simple, safe, and effective means of obtaining access. (Figure 23.3) With the development of new IO insertion devices, individuals with little training can place these lines within a minute. The preferred site is approximately 2–3 cm below the tibial plateau, through the flat anteromedial portion of the bone. The distal femur can also be used if the tibia has been injured. If both bilateral lower extremity long bones have been injured, then the humerus

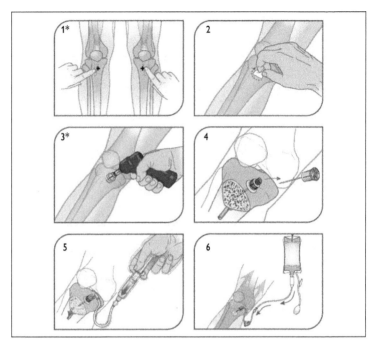

Figure 23.3 Illustration of the Steps for Intraosseous (IO) Insertion *(adapted from EZ-IO Intraosseous Infusion System)*

or iliac crest may be appropriate. IO access is temporary and should be removed within 24 hours of insertion or once definitive IV access has been obtained.

If neither peripheral nor IO access is successful, central venous access can be attempted. In general, central venous percutaneous catherization is avoided during emergency resuscitation, especially in younger children, because of risk of injury to adjacent arteries and/or lacerations of the vessel. If attempted in older pediatric patients the femoral approach is preferred. In addition, for older children a greater saphenous vein cutdown at the ankle can be used. In younger patients, saphenous vein access can be obtained via a groin cutdown secondary to the small size of the vessel at the level of the ankle.

Once IV access has been obtained, fluid resuscitation of the pediatric trauma patient is begun, usually with a 20 cc/kg bolus of fluid, typically an isotonic solution such as lactated Ringer's or normal saline. The 20 cc/kg bolus can be repeated 1–2 times in an attempt to correct hypovolemia and improve perfusion. If shock persists despite a total of 40–60 cc/kg of fluid, the administration of packed red blood cells is warranted. This is usually given as a bolus of 10 cc/kg while a maintenance rate of crystalloid fluid is infused. Massive transfusion protocols should be activated in trauma cases where greater than 400 cc/kg of blood are expected to be transfused or greater than one total blood volume for an infant (80 cc/kg). Current recommendations are based on U.S. Army protocols in adults recommending 1:1:1 transfusion of packed red blood cells, fresh frozen plasma, and platelets. This protocol is useful for older children as well and can be modified to a weight-based protocol for younger children as 30 cc/kg:20 cc/kg:20 cc/kg.

After the primary survey is completed, the secondary survey of the pediatric trauma patient continues in much the same way as in adults. All patients should have an appropriate size cervical collar in place for c-spine stabilization. Treatment of life-threatening injuries, such as tension pneumothorax (via needle decompression and chest tube insertion); cardiac tamponade (via pericardiocentesis); and open-book pelvis fractures (via application of a sheet tied tightly around the pelvis to reduce volume) should all be managed in the trauma bay as appropriate. Gastric decompression with a oral gastric tube may be necessary in patients who underwent extensive bag-mask ventilation prior to intubation because severe gastric dilation can result in vagally mediated bradycardia and vomiting/aspiration risks. Finally, although exposure of the trauma patient is critical, the pediatric patient is much more likely to become hypothermic during this evaluation. Use of warm blankets and warmed IV fluids, as well as increasing the trauma room temperature, can be helpful for maintaining the patient's temperature.

Initial imaging of the c-spine, chest, and pelvis with x-rays is generally obtained prior to transporting the patient to a different area of the emergency department (ED) or for additional tests. Concern over the long-term effects of medical radiation, particularly computed tomography (CT) scanning, has lead to a re-evaluation of the need for routine imaging studies. (Table 23.1) For example, perhaps pelvic radiographs in a stable blunt-trauma patient should be avoided, given that this may avoid excess radiation exposure to the reproductive organs of children. There are advocates for the ALARA principle (As Low As Reasonably Achievable) when it comes to the use of radiation and the need for CT scan in the pediatric trauma patient. This includes a reduction in repeat scans and the number of phases used while undergoing a scan. Although CT scan remains an important diagnostic modality for the pediatric trauma surgeon its use must be

Table 23.1 Radiation doses from various types of medical imaging procedures		
Type of Procedure	**Average Adult Effective Dose (mSv)**	**Estimated Dose Equivalent (No. of Chest X-rays)**
Dental X-ray	0.005–0.01	0.25–0.5
Chest X-ray	0.02	1
Mammography	0.4	20
CT	2–16	100–800
Nuclear Medicine	0.2–41	10–2050
Interventional Fluoroscopy	5–70	250–3500

tempered against its potential risk. This is in stark contrast to the adult trauma environment in which a "pan-scan" approach has become standard.

Alternate means of imaging are being increasingly evaluated as substitutes for a CT scan. Focused Assessment by Sonography in Trauma (FAST) is routinely used in the adult trauma population as a quick means to evaluate an unstable trauma patient for evidence of cardiac or intra-abdominal injury. The thinner abdominal wall found in pediatric patients has the potential to allow for greater visualization of the abdominal cavity, though studies have not yet determined usefulness of ultrasound in evaluating pediatric trauma. Currently, abdominal ultrasound may be a useful screening test to determine who may need further imaging via CT scanning rather than as a specific diagnostic tool. As improvements in ultrasound technology occur and training with its use increases, it may become a more valuable tool in the evaluation of the pediatric trauma patient and may aid in the avoidance of excessive radiation.

Brain and spinal injuries

TBI is one of the leading causes of mortality and long-term morbidity in children in the United States. Brain injury and neurologic failure are a common cause of death in children admitted to a pediatric intensive care unit. Approximately 35% of all unintentional pediatric injuries involve the head, with another 10% involving the spine. These injuries result in approximately 500,000 ED visits annually and cost upwards of $1 billion in care per year.

TBI is usually subdivided into two groups based upon the patient's initial Glasgow Coma Scale (GCS) at the time of presentation. Severe TBI is defined as a GCS < 8. Mild-moderate TBI is defined as GCS 9–14. The GCS has been found to correlate well with outcomes. The verbal portion of this score should be adapted for nonverbal infants and children as their response to comfort and soothing. (Table 23.2) With the increased availability of CT scanners, a subgrouping of patients based on type of injury has also developed: focal injury versus diffuse injury. Most current practice guidelines recommend an immediate head CT upon evaluation of a trauma patient with suspected severe brain injury. (Figure 23.4) This initial head CT is often critical in identifying those patients who require urgent neurosurgical intervention.

The basic principles underlying treatment of TBI in the pediatric population are not that different from those for adults. The fully developed skull provides a solid and rigid protective case for the brain. The primary driving force behind maintaining adequate nutrition and oxygen to the brain is the cerebral perfusion pressure (CPP). The CPP itself is determined by the difference between the mean arterial blood pressure (MAP) and the intracranial pressure (ICP); $CPP = MAP - ICP$. A bare minimum CPP of 40 mm Hg is needed to maintain adequate delivery of oxygen and nutrients to the brain. A CPP of 40–65 mm Hg represents a generally accepted age-related continuum for optimal treatment

Table 23.2 Modification of Glasgow Coma Scale for use in infants and children

Glasgow Coma Scale Score			Modified Coma Scale for Infants		
Activity	Best Response	Score	Activity	Best Response	Score
Eye opening	Spontaneous	4	Eye opening	Spontaneous	4
	To Verbal Stimuli	3		To speech	3
	To Pain	2		To pain	2
	None	1		None	1
Verbal	Oriented	5	Verbal	Coos, babbles	5
	Confused	4		Irritable, cries	4
	Inappropriate words	3		Cries to pain	3
	Nonspecific sounds	2		Moan to pain	2
	None	1		None	1
Motor	Normal spontaneous movements	6	Motor	Normal spontaneous movements	6
	Localizes pain	5		Withdraws to touch	5
	Withdraws to pain	4		Withdraws to pain	4
	Abnormal flexion (decorticate rigidity)	3		Abnormal flexion (decorticate rigidity)	3
	Abnormal extension (decerebrate rigidity)	2		Abnormal extension (decerebrate rigidity)	2
	None	1		None	1

thresholds; however, no study has demonstrated that active maintenance of CPP at a specific value improves morbidity or mortality.

Primary brain injury refers to the immediate damage caused by the traumatic event, such as hematoma, contusion, and diffuse axonal injury. Secondary injury refers to ongoing cerebral damage caused by inadequate delivery of oxygen and nutrients to both the injured brain tissue as well as the surrounding healthy tissue. The primary goal of ICU treatment is to correct underlying hypoxemia and hypotension to minimize secondary injury.

CPP can be altered by a number of factors; for example, hemorrhage and shock can decrease MAP while extra-axial blood collections or diffuse cerebral edema can increase ICP. The rigid skull does not allow passive expansion of the swelling and injured brain, ultimately resulting in herniation and/or compression of the brainstem if the process is not ameliorated. In contrast, infants may have an advantage because the skull bones have not fused, thereby allowing some expansion of the brain and maintenance of a lower ICP.

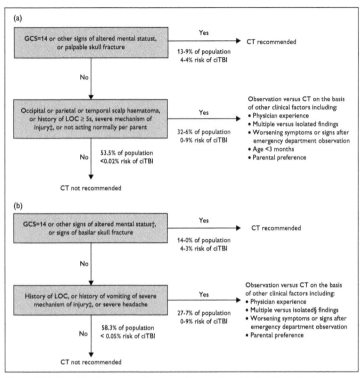

Figure 23.4 Algorithm for computed tomographic scanning of the head in pediatric trauma patients. Reprinted with kind permission from Kuppermann N, Holmes JF, Dayan PS, et al. Identification of children at very low risk of clinically-important brain injuries after head trauma: a prospective cohort study. *Lancet* 2011;374:1160–1170

Secondary measures for treatment of TBI include surgical drainage of extra-axial collections, placement of ICP monitors and extra-ventricular drains, correction of coagulopathy, and, when needed, induction of a barbiturate coma. The goals of therapy, particularly in patients with persistent GCS < 8, are to maintain adequate CPP, minimize ICP elevation, and correct underlying acidosis and hypoxia. Treatment for elevated ICP should begin at > 20mm Hg. Although control of ICP elevation improves survival and long-term neurologic sequelae, the modality of therapy appears to be less important.

Two novel means to treat TBI in children have recently been studied: decompressive craniectomy and induction of hypothermia. Use of decompressive craniectomy, previously only used as a last resort, has demonstrated some benefit and improvement in outcome. Studies have suggested improvements in ICP reduction, higher CPP, and improved return to function. A 2006 Cochrane review noted a reduced risk of death and poor outcome. Additional studies are needed before this technique can become standard-of-care.

Despite a significant amount of laboratory data, induced hypothermia to 32–34°C, typically within the first 8 hours after the event with gradual re-warming after a 24-hour period has not clearly improved outcomes.

Second-impact syndrome is a very rare condition in which a second concussion occurs before a first concussion has properly healed, causing rapid and severe brain swelling and often catastrophic results. Second-impact syndrome can result from even a very mild concussion that occurs days or weeks after the initial injury. Because the brain is more vulnerable and susceptible to injury after an initial brain injury, it only takes a minimal force to cause irreversible damage. The brain's inability to self-regulate following injury can result in increased cerebral blood flow and edema, which can occur rapidly and result in brain death in as little as 3–5 minutes. Because brain death is so rapid, second-impact syndrome has a high fatality rate in young athletes.

Spinal injuries in children are less common than in adults, secondary to the greater mobility and flexibility of the pediatric spine. Normal variations in pediatric cervical spine can make interpretation of x-rays difficult, as up to 40% of children may have pseudo-subluxation of C2 on C3. The larger head size in proportion to body size, however, does predispose younger children to upper cervical injuries, from the occiput to the C3. All patients initially should be immobilized in an age/size appropriate c-collar. Of those patients with spine injury, pediatric patients are more likely to have multiple levels of injury. Assessment should include imaging of at least three levels above and three levels below a known injury to evaluate for additional trauma.

Clearance of the pediatric c-spine is evolving as the desire to avoid unnecessary radiation increases. CT scans of the neck are rarely warranted given that adequate 3-view c-spine x-rays can typically be obtained in children due to their small body size and muscle mass. Teenagers can usually be managed as adults. For patients < 3 years of age, a recent multi-center study found the incidence of cervical spine injuries following blunt trauma to be < 1%. Risk factors included GCS < 14, involvement in a motor vehicle crash, GCS-eye = 1, and age > 2 years.

Another abnormality seen more commonly in children than adults is spinal cord injury without radiographic abnormality (SCIWORA). This typically results from a hyperflexion or hyperextension injury and may be related to the high elasticity of pediatric spinal ligaments. These patients can have various signs of neurologic injury, though these may be delayed. Patients suspected for this injury should undergo magnetic resonance imaging (MRI) to establish the diagnosis. Treatment usually consists of neck immobilization with a cervical collar for 8–12 weeks and follow-up with a pediatric spine specialist.

Thoracic injury

The chest wall of the pediatric age group is much more pliable than that seen in adults. As a consequence, rib fractures are less common, while pulmonary contusions and pneumothoraces present as the more common intra-thoracic injuries. Aortic and great vessel injuries are uncommon in the pediatric population due to greater vessel elasticity and mobility within the chest cavity and lower velocity injury mechanisms. A chest x-ray is the standard diagnostic imaging needed to obtain a diagnosis in most cases; CT scan of the chest is rarely warranted following a normal chest x-ray. Treatment of these injuries should follow ATLS guidelines.

Pulmonary contusion is a common finding after blunt chest trauma and can vary widely in severity. Clinical suspicion is important in the diagnosis, because chest x-ray findings may not be evident for up to 48 hours postinjury. The presence of rib fractures with underlying contusions in children is concerning due to the high amount of force needed to fracture the pliable ribs of a child. This finding should prompt a workup for additional injuries that may be related to a high force or impact. Management ranges from supplemental oxygen delivery and pain control to intubation with mechanical ventilatory support. Development of pneumonia or acute respiratory distress syndrome (ARDS) are possible, although ARDS is considerably less frequent in children than in adults.

The finding of pneumomediastinum after blunt thoracic injury may prompt evaluation of the aerodigestive tract. Significant injury is rare with isolated pneumomediastinum in otherwise asymptomatic children.

Abdominal and pelvic trauma

Ten to fifteen percent of pediatric trauma patients suffer an injury to the abdomen/pelvis; and 10% of deaths related to trauma involve injuries to the abdomen and pelvis. Initial management should include fluid resuscitation, gastric decompression, and stabilization of the pelvis. The most commonly injured organ is the spleen followed closely by the liver, in contrast to the adult where the liver is the most commonly injured. Children have a more densely packed abdominal cavity with less intra- and extra-abdominal fatty layers, thus allowing for greater direct transmission of force as compared to adults. In addition, the lack of a fully ossified pelvis and chest wall further increases the vulnerability of intra-abdominal structures. As a result, relatively low-energy mechanisms can result in significant intra-abdominal injury.

The diagnosis of abdominal trauma begins with a thorough physical examination that can present clues to suspected underlying injuries. Examples of important findings include the "seat belt" sign from the lap belt compressing against the abdomen in an MVC or the "handle bar" sign seen in bicycle accidents.

Chest and pelvic x-rays, along with pertinent laboratory work, such as hepatic and/or pancreatic enzymes, may help diagnostically. The most useful imaging study is an abdominal CT scan with the administration of IV contrast, which is excellent in identifying solid organ and vascular injuries, including grading of these injuries for treatment protocols. (Figure 23.5) CT is limited, however, when it comes to the diagnosis of intestinal injury, especially within the tightly packed abdominal cavity of children. The benefit of using PO contrast is controversial.

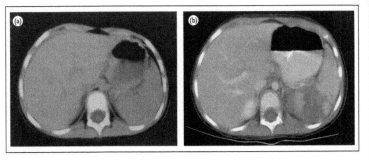

Figure 23.5 Computed tomography of the abdomen demonstrating splenic injuries

In younger children with a paucity of intra-abdominal fat, oral contrast may help with visualization of the c-loop of the duodenum and pancreatic head.

Although children who present in extremis and shock from a high-grade injury require operative intervention, hepatic, splenic, and renal injuries are now managed primarily in a nonoperative fashion with success rates of 90%–95%. ICU care is warranted in those patients with higher-grade injury by CT, hemodynamic abnormality, and/or multiple injuries. ICU stay is usually limited to the first 24–36-hour period if stable. Transfusion for bleeding is usually unnecessary as children can tolerate hemoglobin levels of 6–7 without sequelae. Failure of nonoperative management is determined by evidence of ongoing bleeding, persistent hemodynamic compromise, and uncorrectable acidosis. Attempted splenic preservation may be difficult in a multi-trauma patient in shock but may be attempted in isolated injuries once bleeding has been controlled and the patient is adequately resuscitated. Hepatic and renal injuries are treated in similar fashion to adults, with every attempt made to preserve organ function and repair damaged tissue.

It is important to note that children who have their spleen removed are at risk for development of overwhelming postsplenectomy infection (OPSI), a fulminate bacterial infection that can rapidly lead to coma and death within a 24-hour period. Children under age 5 appear to be particularly at risk, with a reported incidence of 10% compared to that seen in adults of only 1%–2%. It also appears to be more likely in children who have had their spleens removed secondary to hematologic causes in comparison to traumatic causes. Infections caused by encapsulated organisms appear to be responsible for the majority of OPSI cases. Current recommendations are for vaccinations against *Streptococcus pneumoniae*, *Haemophilus influenzae* type B, and *Neisseria meningitides*, preferably at the time of discharge. Antibiotic prophylaxis with daily penicillin is also recommended until age 18 years.

Pancreatic and small-bowel injuries, though rare in pediatric blunt trauma, commonly result from direct blows to the epigastrium, such in as handlebar or seatbelt injury. In addition, young children under 4 years old who present with signs of abdominal trauma and are found to have an unexpected duodenal injury should be suspected victims of abuse. These injuries can be difficult to diagnose because they may present without any tenderness at first, only to later develop extreme abdominal pain, nausea, bilious vomiting, and fevers. Duodenal and small-bowel perforations require exploration. Lacerations should be repaired primarily if possible. Pancreatic contusions and duodenal contusions/hematomas should be managed nonoperatively with NPO orders and nasogastric decompression. Resolution of a duodenal hematoma can take as long as 2–3 weeks and patients may require parenteral nutrition during this period. Distal pancreatic injuries are managed nonoperatively unless ductal disruption is identified, in which case a distal pancreatectomy may be needed.

Laparoscopic evaluation of stable trauma patients is becoming more common, as it may spare the patient an unnecessary laparotomy. Laparoscopy may identify occult injury and can be used for control of bleeding and repair of simple bowel injuries or a distal pancreatectomy.

Child abuse

Child abuse is defined as the physical, emotional, and/or sexual abuse of a child as well as neglect of their well-being. It crosses all socioeconomic classes and all ethnic and cultural boundaries. Child abuse is reported every 10 seconds in the United States, with five children dying each day as a result of it, most of them younger than 4 years of age. Physicians treating pediatric trauma must be ever vigilant to recognize the signs of abuse and by law are obligated to report those findings to child protective services.

Identification of the abused child can be difficult. Abused children are often withdrawn and may not respond to questions for fear of further injury by the abuser. Any child that frequently returns to the ED with signs of injury should raise suspicion. Signs of abuse can include malnutrition and/or failure to thrive; torn frenulum of upper lip; retinal hemorrhages; burns in unusual areas; bite marks; injury to genital, periauricular, or perianal regions; rib fractures; multiple old fractures; and bruising in various stages of healing. Some type of fracture is seen in approximately 80% of abuse victims. Spiral fractures are the result of torsional force applied to an extremity, while transverse fractures occur as a result of a direct force against the bone. Any child who has difficulty walking or who demonstrates decreased movement of one extremity should be evaluated for occult fractures. Multiple rib fractures in a young child are virtually pathognomonic of abuse.

Abusive head injury, the "shaken baby syndrome," is the result of violent acceleration and deceleration forces within the cranium. This can result in extra-axial hematomas as well as diffuse axonal shearing, often with devastating results to the child. Outcomes in abusive-head-injury children are significantly worse than in those whose injuries were accidental. Patients with suspected abusive head trauma need a head CT and an examination by ophthalmology to look for the presence of retinal hemorrhages that are associated with abusive head trauma.

A complete workup of an abused patient includes a thorough physical examination from head to toe with documentation of all suspected bruising or markers of abuse. In addition, a complete skeletal survey is also required to look for and to document occult fractures or old, healing fractures that can identify a repetitive pattern of abuse.

Treatment of the abused child lies in supportive care and correction of underlying injuries. Suspected victims of abuse must be admitted to the hospital for a full medical evaluation and protective services evaluation. Child protective services and social work should be contacted to make arrangements for the care of the child, if needed, as well as to coordinate any ongoing investigation. In addition, child protective services are responsible for assessing the risk to other children in the home. The role of the treating physician should be to focus on the care of the child.

Burns

Burns can be a common finding of child abuse. Concerning patterns of burns include punctate burns in one or more locations, possibly from cigarettes; burns to the buttocks or perineum or burns with clear lines of demarcations suggesting immersion burns. It takes approximately 1.5 seconds to cause a second-degree burn in 150°F water.

Regardless of the method of injury, all burns in children should be treated with standard burn care. Children differ from adults because they have greater body surface area in relation to weight—particularly the child's head. This has important implications for determining the total body surface area burned and thereby the initial resuscitation strategy. The "rule of nines" needs to be modified. (Figure 23.6) Resuscitation based on the Parkland formula (fluid requirement = total body surface area x weight x 4 cc) is most commonly used, but practitioners should be aware that this formula might under-resuscitate the pediatric patient.

Unique critical care issues in pediatric surgery

Ventilatory management

For infants and younger children without existing lung disease, a tidal volume of 4–8 mL/kg to be delivered at a rate of 30–35 breaths per minute is adequate. For older children traditionally 10 mL/kg was used but this has been shown to cause barotrauma; 6 to 8 mL/kg is now common practice. In infants and children, it is unclear what level of peak airway pressure may cause damage. In general, keeping peak pressures below 30 cm H_2O is desirable.

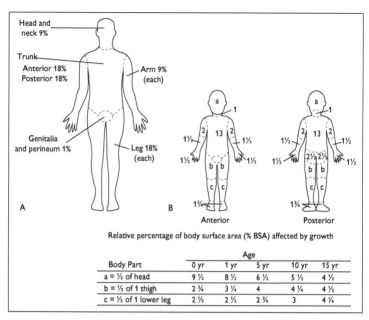

Relative percentage of body surface area (% BSA) affected by growth

Body Part	Age				
	0 yr	1 yr	5 yr	10 yr	15 yr
a = ½ of head	9 ½	8 ½	6 ½	5 ½	4 ½
b = ½ of 1 thigh	2 ¾	3 ¼	4	4 ¼	4 ½
c = ½ of 1 lower leg	2 ½	2 ½	2 ¾	3	4 ¼

Figure 23.6 Diagram Illustrating the "Rule Of Nine" in an Adult (A) and in a Child (B). The younger the child the larger the percentage of body surface area that is represented by the head and the smaller the percentage for the legs. Reprinted with kind permission from Springer Science + Business Media: Sciemionow MZ, Eisenmann-Klein M, eds. *Plastic and Reconstructive Surgery. 2010*

Although ARDS can occur in children, particularly those suffering from an underlying lung infection such as respiratory syncytial virus (RSV), ARDS does not appear to occur as frequently after traumatic resuscitation or surgery as is seen in the adult population. Treatment follows established ARDS guidelines in adults, including low-tidal-volume ventilation and permissive hypercapnia. If conventional ventilation fails, use of high frequency oscillatory ventilation (HFOV) may be helpful. (Figure 23.7) Use of supplemental therapies, such as surfactant administration and inhaled nitric oxide, useful in neonatal populations, do not appear to improve outcomes in pediatric ARDS. As a last resort, extracorporeal membrane oxygenation (ECMO) may be indicated.

Shock

Management of hemodynamic compromise in pediatrics differs slightly compared to that in adults. Pediatric shock is usually related to severe hypovolemia. With septic shock, in contrast to adults, low cardiac output instead of low systemic vascular resistance, appears to be more prevalent and associated with

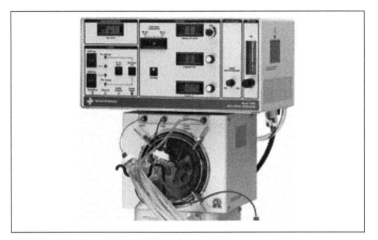

Figure 23.7 High frequency oscillatory ventilator

subsequent mortality. Recommendations for the management of fluid refractory shock are to begin blood pressure support with dopamine followed by epinephrine if needed. A vasodilating agent, such as nitroprusside or milrinone, may be needed if the patient demonstrates evidence of high systemic vascular resistance ("cold shock") to further improve cardiac output. (Figure 23.8) ECMO is very rarely indicated and may be contraindicated because of the need for anticoagulation.

Treatment of shock in the pediatric population, as in adults, should be goal-directed. Patients should have continuous monitoring present, central venous access placed, arterial pressure monitoring, and strict measurement of urine output. Early goal directed end-points include a capillary refill of < 2 sec, urine output of > 1 cc/kg, and warm extremities. Further end-points beyond the initial resuscitation period should include normal perfusion pressure for age/weight, improvement in cardiac output, correction of acidosis and base deficit, clearance of serum lactate, and normalization of mixed-venous oxygen saturation (SvO_2). Admission base deficit and lactate levels may also be useful as markers for long-term prognosis after a severe trauma.

Nutritional support

In comparison to adults, children have higher energy expenditure per kg of body weight, require better intestinal perfusion to absorb calories and prevent mucosal ischemia, shunt energy expenditure from growth in response to injury, have a higher protein turnover rate, and have more complications from profound malnutrition and protein loss. Brain neurons will die nearly as quickly from lack of glucose as they will from hypoxia. The strategy for nutritional support should be goal-directed and based on reassessment after initiation.

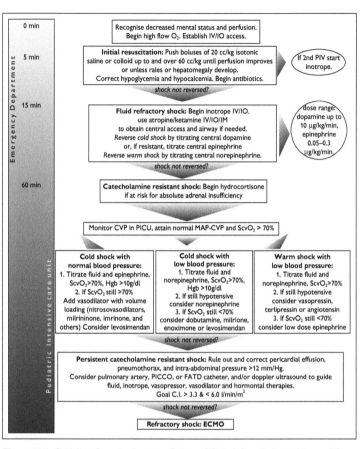

Figure 23.8 Guidelines from the American College of Critical Care-Pediatric Advance Life Support Algorithm for the Management of Pediatric Septic Shock. *With kind permission from publisher Wolters Kluwer Health, Crit Care Med. 2009; 37(2): 680 Figure 2*

The catabolic response to injury in children, as in adults, includes glucagon, cortisol, and catecholamines. Children, especially infants, have much lower stores of glucose, fat, and protein compared to adults. Although these catabolic effects on carbohydrate and fat metabolism threaten children, the real danger lies in protein loss as the lean body mass of children magnifies this effect. Without adequate protein, loss of muscle protein from diaphragmatic and intercostals can result in respiratory failure.

Nutritional requirements for children vary with age. An infant will need, on average, 100 kcal/kg of body weight to maintain baseline energy expenditures while a teenager will use 30–60 kcal/kg. (Table 23.3) Equations to

Table 23.3 Estimated protein and energy requirements if different age groups

Age	Protein (g/kg/day)	Energy (kcal/kg/day)
Neonates	2.2	120
Children (age 10 yr)	1.0	70
Adults	0.8	35

(adapted from Holcomb and Murphy: Ashcraft's Pediatric Surgery). With kind permission from Elsevier who granted permission for reuse and adaptation. Figure was published in Ashcroft's Pediatric Surgery 2010 table 2–2

measure a patient's resting energy expenditure can be used, including the Harris-Benedict, World Health Organization, and Schofield equations. These equations unfortunately do not account for the changes that occur in homeostasis after a traumatic injury (e.g., increased energy requirements following burns or decreased requirements during sedation and paralysis following severe TBI). The equations serve to provide a good first approximation. Caloric intake can then be adjusted based on the patient's clinical picture and various nutritional markers such as albumin, pre-albumin, BUN, and pCO_2 levels.

Early nutritional support can ameliorate the effects of protein catabolism, speed the rate of recovery, and lessen the risk of late complications (i.e., infection, dehiscence, death). Although total parenteral nutrition (TPN) has traditionally been used to provide adequate nutrition to children, especially in the very young or early in the course of illness, enteral feeding, if feasible, has become the preferred method of feeding. Gastric feeding, as well as postpyloric feeding, are acceptable means of enteral access. The need for vasoactive agents in hypotensive patients has been thought to be a relative contraindication to enteral feeding. However, patients who are on low-dose medication can tolerate trickle feeding (10%–20% of goal rate), which may be enough to provide the added benefits shown for enteral feeding.

Summary

Management of pediatric trauma and the care of critically ill children are complex and evolving fields. Traumatic injury is the number one cause of pediatric morbidity and mortality in the United States, as well as globally. Practitioners caring for these children should take note of the differences in injury patterns as well as the response to injury and critical illness of children in comparison to adults; children should not be managed as "little adults." Whenever possible exposure to radiation should be kept to a minimum, nonoperative management of solid organ injuries is standard-of-care, and early nutritional support is paramount to recovery. Children with severe traumatic brain injury and/or complex chest and abdominal injuries would best be served by transfer to the nearest high-level pediatric facility.

Key references

Adelson PD, Bratton SL, Carney NA, et al. Guidelines for the acute medical management of severe traumatic brain injury in infants, children, and adolescents. Chapter 8. Cerebral perfusion pressure. *Pediatr Crit Care Med*. 2003;4(suppl 3):S31–S33.

Adelson PD, Bratton SL, Carney NA, et al. Guidelines for the acute medical management of severe traumatic brain injury in infants, children, and adolescents. Chapter 4. Resuscitation of blood pressure and oxygenation and prehospital brain-specific therapies for the severe pediatric traumatic brain injury patient. *Pediatr Crit Care Med*. 2003;4(suppl 3):S12–S18.

Adelson PD, Bratton SL, Carney NA, et al. Guidelines for the acute medical management of severe traumatic brain injury in infants, children, and adolescents. Chapter 17. Critical pathway for the treatment of established intracranial hypertension in pediatric traumatic brain injury. *Pediatr Crit Care Med*. 2003;4(suppl 3):S65–S67.

Adelson PD, Bratton SL, Carney NA, et al. Guidelines for the acute medical management of severe traumatic brain injury in infants, children, and adolescents. Chapter 14. The role of temperature control following severe pediatric traumatic brain injury. *Pediatr Crit Care Med*. 2003;4(suppl 3):S53–S55.

Carcillo JA, Fields AI, American College of Critical Care Medicine Task Force Committee Members. Clinical practice parameters for hemodynamic support of pediatric and neonatal patients in septic shock. *Crit Care Med*. 2002;30(6):1365–1378.

Cigdem MK, Onen A, Siga M, Otcu S. Selective Nonoperative Management of Penetrating Abdominal Injuries in Children. *J Trauma*. 2009;67(6):1284–1287.

Dehmer JJ, Adamson WT. Massive transfusion and blood product use in the pediatric trauma patient. *Semin Pediatr Surg*. 2010;19(4):286–291.

Gaines BA. Intra-abdominal solid organ injury in children: diagnosis and treatment. *J Trauma*. 2009;67(suppl):S135–S139.

Gaines BA, Ford HR. Abdominal and pelvic trauma in children. *Crit Care Med*. 2002;30(suppl 11):S416–S423.

Gaines BA, Shultz BS, Morrison K, Ford HR. Duodenal injuries in children: beware of child abuse. *J Pediatr Surg*. 2004;39(4):600–602.

Gaines BA, Rutkoski JD. The role of laparoscopy in pediatric trauma.*Semin Pediatr Surg*. 2010;19(4):300–303.

Gausche M, Lewis RJ, Stratton SJ, et al. Effect of out-of-hospital pediatric endotracheal intubation on survival and neurological outcome: a controlled clinical trial. *JAMA*. 2000;283(6):783–790.

Hindy-François C, Meyer P, Blanot S, et al. Admission base deficit as a long-term prognostic factor in severe pediatric trauma patients. *J Trauma*. 2009;67(6):1272–1277.

Hutchison JS, Ward RE, Lacroix J, et al. Hypothermia therapy after traumatic brain injury in children. *N Engl J Med*. 2008;358(23):2447–2456.

Jagannathan J, Okonkwo DO, Dumont AS, et al. Outcome following decompressive craniectomy in children with severe traumatic brain injury: a 10-year single-center experience with long-term follow up. *J Neurosurg*. 2007;106(suppl 4):268–275.

Joffe A, Anton N, Lequier L, et al. Nutritional support for critically ill children. Cochrane database of systematic reviews (Online). 2009;(2):CD005144.

Kreykes NS, Letton RW. Current issues in the diagnosis of pediatric cervical spine injury.*Semin Pediatr Surg*. 2010;19(4):257–264.

Soundappan S, Smith NF, Lam LT, et al. A trauma series in the injured child: do we really need it? *Pediatr Emerg Care*. 2006;22(10):710–716.

Stuhlfaut JW, Soto JA, Lucey BC, et al. Blunt abdominal trauma: performance of CT without oral contrast material. *Radiology*. 2004;233(3):689–694.

Chapter 24

Critical care and trauma in pregnancy

Joshua Brown and Gary T. Marshall

Intensive care unit (ICU) admission is required in < 1% of pregnant women; however, maternal and fetal mortality can increase several-fold in critically-ill pregnant patients. Trauma is one of the frequent causes of maternal/fetal mortality, along with venous thromboembolism, hemorrhage, and hypertensive disorders. Diligent management of maternal conditions and risk factors carries the greatest benefit to the fetus. Early involvement of obstetric expertise is strongly advised in all cases.

Critical care considerations

Normal changes to anatomy and physiology (Table 24.1), as well as unique risk factors, require a tailored approach to the pregnant patient in the ICU.

Cardiovascular system and hemorrhage

Pregnant patients have an elevated heart rate and lower blood pressure compared with nonpregnant patients. These changes may mimic vital sign changes in hemorrhage. Because increased plasma volume is present, significant alterations in maternal vital signs are not present until up to one-third of maternal blood volume is lost. In addition, compression of the uterus on the inferior vena cava can decrease venous return, exacerbating hypotension. Pregnant patients should be positioned with a roll under the right flank to alleviate this compression. A high index of suspicion is essential for early recognition of hemorrhage and appropriate resuscitation.

Hemorrhage in the third trimester is commonly due to placental abruption. Abruption occurs with disruption of maternal vessels in the deciduas basalis, commonly in the setting of trauma, hypertension, or cocaine use. Pain and vaginal bleeding are common, although up to 20% will not have evident bleeding. Ultrasound may be useful for diagnosis of a retroplacental hematoma. Fluid and blood resuscitation should be promptly instituted. Continuous fetal heart rate (CFHR) monitoring is essential. Cesarean delivery should be performed if maternal hypotension or non-reassuring fetal heart tones are observed in an otherwise viable fetus.

Table 24.1 Physiologic and anatomic changes with pregnancy	
Cardiovascular	Cardiac output increases up to 40%
	Heart rate increases up to 15 beats/minute
	Systemic vascular resistance decreases, diastolic blood pressure falls 5–10 mmHg
	Decreased central venous pressure
	Heart displacement leads to left axis deviation and t-wave flattening on electrocardiogram.
Respiratory	Increased minute ventilation, due to increased tidal volume
	Respiratory rate is relatively unchanged
	Functional Residual Capacity decreases due to diaphragmatic elevation
Hematologic	Blood volume increases by 50%
	Plasma expansion greater than red cell mass expansion resulting in lower hematocrit
	Increased clotting factor levels
Renal	Increases in renal blood flow resulting in increased glomerular filtration rate (GFR)
	Decreased glucose reabsorption
Gastrointestinal	Delayed gastric emptying
	Increased gastric acid production
	Impaired gallbladder contraction
Anatomic Changes	Uterus becomes intra-abdominal by week 12 and can compress the inferior vena cava in the supine position
	Heart is displaced superiorly
	Diaphragm elevated up to 4 cm, with increased excursion
	Gastroesophageal junction anatomy is distorted
	Small bowel is displaced from the abdomen
Lab Value Alterations	Sodium decreases by up to 5 mEq/L
	Bicarbonate decreases (20–25 mEq/L) to compensate for increased minute ventilation
	Blood urea nitrogen decreases (4–7 mg/dL) as well as creatinine (0.4–0.7 mg/dL) with increased glomerular filtration rate (GFR)
	Hematocrit decreases (32–36%)
	White blood cell count increases (18–25 WBC/mm^3)
	Albumin is decreased (< 2.9 gm/dL) due to volume expansion

Several pharmacologic agents are useful in the setting of postpartum hemorrhage:

- Oxytocin 10–40 units IV
- Methylegonovine 0.2 mg IM (maximum 5 doses)
- Prostaglandin F2 Alpha 250 mcg IM
- Misoprostol 1000 mcg PR

When vasopressor use is required for maternal hypotension, limited evidence suggests that ephedrine is the preferred agent due to its ability to increase maternal and uterine blood flow with few side effects. Phenylepherine is an acceptable alternative; however, maternal bradycardia can occur. Norepinephrine and epinephrine should be avoided when possible due to deleterious effects on uterine blood flow.

Venous thromboembolism

Venous thromboembolism (VTE) is a common problem, particularly in trauma patients, and pregnancy increases the risk 4- to 7-fold. Early recognition is often impaired because many signs of deep vein thrombosis (DVT) and pulmonary embolism (PE) overlap with normal changes in pregnancy, including lower extremity swelling, mild dyspnea, and tachycardia. Further, the A-a gradient is normal in up to 58% of pregnant patients with PE. If suspected, lower extremity duplex or computed tomography (CT) angiography should be performed. CT angiography involves less radiation than a V/Q scan. If radiation is a concern, an echocardiogram may be a good initial test to evaluate for right-heart strain. Initial therapy is a heparin infusion that can later be transitioned to low molecular weight heparin, both of which are safe in pregnancy. Warfarin is contraindicated due to teratogenic effects.

Respiratory support

Pregnant patients have a chronic respiratory alkalosis due to increased minute ventilation. Consequently, normal arterial blood gases will reveal a slightly higher pH, up to 7.47, and pCO_2 near 30 mmHg. For patients requiring mechanical ventilation, minute ventilation should be adjusted to a pCO_2 of 30–32 mmHg. A pCO_2 less than 30 mmHg should be avoided as this reduces uterine blood flow. In cases for which permissive hypercapnea is indicated, exposure to a pCO_2 of up to 60 mmHg has not adversely affected long-term fetal outcomes. Pregnant patients have reduced reserve and are prone to rapid oxygen desaturation.

In patients requiring a chest tube, placement must be anatomically higher than the standard site of insertion due to elevation in the diaphragm (4 cm) to avoid intra-abdominal placement.

Neurologic system

Analgesic and sedative medications are routine in the ICU, but these may enter the fetal circulation. Opioids are preferred. Nonsteroidal anti-inflammatory drugs are avoided as they can cause early closure of the ductus arteriosus. Limited evidence suggests teratogenic effects of lorazepam, thus midazolam is the sedative of choice. For neuromuscular blockade, cisatracurium is the preferred agent because its metabolism is independent of renal and hepatic function. Vecuronium is an acceptable alternative. Duration of this therapy should be limited when possible.

Patients requiring anticonvulsant therapy should be given benzodiazepines or barbiturates in moderate doses. Phenytoin is contraindicated due to teratogenic effects.

Both local and general anesthetics are considered safe. Local anesthetics cross the placenta, thus large doses should be avoided.

Gastrointestinal prophylaxis

Alteration in the gastroesophageal junction places patients at particular risk for aspiration. Head of bed elevation is necessary. Antiemetic medications can be helpful for pregnancy-related and postoperative nausea. Preferred agents include metoclopramide and prochlorperazine. For stress ulcer prophylaxis, sucralfate and histamine blockers are considered safe. Proton pump inhibitors (PPIs) lack evidence, but newer generation PPIs are likely safe in pregnancy.

Infection and sepsis

Sepsis is approached with the same key principles in pregnant and nonpregnant patients, with early resuscitation and antibiotic initiation. Penicillins, cephalosporins, erythromycin, and clindamycin are safe in pregnancy. Aminoglycosides, sulfonamides, quinolones, and metronidazole are commonly used with caution because they may result in fetal toxicity. Tetracyclines are contraindicated.

Common pregnancy-related infections include chorioamniotis and pyelonephritis in the antepartum period, as well as endometritis, wound infection, clostridial myometritis, and *Clostridium difficile* in the postpartum period. A common initial antibiotic regimen includes ampicillin plus gentamycin.

Pre-eclampsia and eclampsia

Pre-eclampsia is defined by proteinuria and hypertension after 20 weeks gestation. Eclampsia is defined by pre-eclampsia plus seizures. These syndromes may be severe and complications including neurologic dysfunction, renal or hepatic failure, pulmonary edema, HELLP (hemolysis elevated liver enzymes low platelet count) syndrome, and disseminated intravascular coagulopathy necessitate ICU care with standard supportive therapy. The definitive treatment is delivery of the fetus and should be considered when the fetus is viable.

Refractory or severe hypertension (> 160 SBP or > 110 DBP) is treated with intravenous beta blockers, hydralazine, nifedipine, or nicardipine. Nitroprusside should be avoided due to toxicity and reduced uterine blood flow.

Patients may also develop elevated intracranial pressure (ICP) and intracranial hemorrhage. Management is similar to nonpregnant patients and may require measures to reduce ICP. For patients with hemorrhage, treatment is reversal of coagulopathy and cessation of anticoagulants.

Patients with seizures should receive a magnesium sulfate bolus of 4–6 grams and remain on a continuous magnesium drip of 2 g/hr. Patients with severe pre-eclampsia (severe hypertension, HELLP, pulmonary edema) should also be given magnesium supplementation for prophylaxis.

Approach to the pregnant trauma patient

Trauma affects 5% of pregnant women with a 1% maternal and 6% fetal mortality. The principles of Advanced Trauma Life Support hold true in the pregnant patient.

Mechanisms

Motor vehicle crashes are the most common cause of nonobstetric maternal and fetal mortality. Placental abruption occurs with blunt trauma and is the leading cause of fetal death with maternal survival. Ejection from a vehicle is associated with uterine rupture and a high rate of fetal demise.

Penetrating injury is usually associated with domestic violence. Direct fetal injury increases with gestational age as the uterus occupies more of the abdomen.

Monitoring

Beyond 20 weeks, CFHR monitoring should be instituted. Bradycardia is a sign of severe fetal distress (normal 120–160 bpm). Clinicians experienced with CFHR monitoring should be available to address fetal distress, particularly late decelerations. Similarly, regular ultrasound evaluation of the fetus can provide gestational age, heart activity, position, and potential injuries such as abruption.

Imaging

Concern for radiation to the fetus must be weighed against the harm of undiagnosed injuries in the mother. Diagnostic tests should be performed as indicated. A lead apron may be placed over the lower abdomen when appropriate to shield the fetus. Limiting radiation is most important during organogenesis (< 8 weeks). Exposure < 0.1 Gy is safe (CT abdomen/pelvis = 0.09 Gy). If diagnostic peritoneal lavage is indicated, an open supraumbilical approach is used.

Abruption

Placental abruption may occur with minimal trauma to the mother. Abruption > 50% usually results in fetal death. Minor abruption is managed with fluid resuscitation and serial ultrasonographic monitoring. As noted above, CFHR monitoring is mandatory and cesarean delivery is indicated for fetal distress.

Fetomaternal transfusion

Fetal hemorrhage into maternal circulation occurs in 25% of trauma. In addition to fetal hypoperfusion, fetomaternal hemorrhage can result in isoimmunization in an Rh- mother. Although the Kleihauer-Betke test can detect fetomaternal hemorrhage, it is not sensitive enough to detect the amount that can result in isoimmunization, thus all at-risk pregnant women sustaining abdominal trauma should undergo Rh immune globulin administration (50 µg < 16 weeks; 300 µg ≥ 16 weeks).

Premature labor

Contractions resulting in cervical dilation and effacement prior to 36 weeks define premature labor. Early involvement of obstetric specialists is required to determine the need for tocolysis, which is contraindicated in the setting of fetal distress. Vaginal delivery is preferred if possible, as cesarean delivery may increase blood loss by 1–1.5 liters.

Intrauterine fetal demise

Labor usually ensues within 48 hours after fetal demise. If labor does not spontaneously occur within 48 hours or coagulation studies demonstrate worsening coagulopathy, immediate delivery is indicated, as maternal disseminated intravascular coagulation (DIC) may rapidly develop.

Cesarean delivery

Emergent cesarean delivery can be life-saving for both mother and fetus, with a 45% fetal survival and 72% maternal survival. Fetal survival increases to 75% when gestational age is ≥ 26 weeks and fetal heart tones are present. A specialized neonatal resuscitation team is essential. Indications for immediate cesarean delivery include

- Refractory maternal shock or exsanguination
- Risk of fetal distress exceeds risk of prematurity
- Significant placental abruption
- Uterine rupture
- Inadequate exposure for maternal injuries
- Unstable thoracolumbar spine fractures

Perimortem delivery can be considered when the fetus is ≥ 26 weeks and occurs within 15 minutes of maternal demise.

Cardiac arrest

Standard Advanced Cardiac Life Support (ACLS) principles apply; however, some adaptations are necessary. Immediate involvement of obstetricians is mandatory when the fetus is considered viable, with rapid delivery the goal. If not already instituted, CFHR monitoring is not recommended as it is of little value under arrest circumstances.

Airway

Failed intubation of pregnant patients occurs in 1 in 500 compared to 1 in 2000 in the general surgical population. It is essential that advanced airway equipment is available, and a 0.5–1cm smaller endotracheal tube is placed. Cricothyrotomy equipment must be immediately available. Continuous cricoid pressure during laryngoscopy is recommended due to increased aspiration risk.

Advanced Cardiac Life Support

Defibrillation should be utilized as in the nonpregnant patient. It does not harm the fetus; however, fetal monitoring equipment should be removed prior to defibrillation. ACLS resuscitation drugs reduce fetal blood supply; however, there are no alternatives and standard adult doses should be given per protocol. Venous access above the diaphragm should be used to deliver resuscitation drugs as they may not reach the mother's heart otherwise due to inferior vena cava compression by the uterus.

Compressions

A roll or "bump" should be placed under the right side of the patient to displace the uterus to the left and allow venous return. Compressions are performed at the midsternal position and should be deeper than usual due to elevated diaphragms and decreased chest-wall compliance.

Early delivery

When the fetus is > 23 weeks and > 1000 grams, cesarean should be initiated within 4 minutes and delivery within 5 minutes of arrest. Not only have these targets shown improvement in fetal survival and neurologic outcome, but they improve venous return and effectiveness of compressions in the mother. Frequently the mother's condition improves rapidly after delivery; however, prognosis is closely related to the underlying cause of arrest.

Key references

American College of Obstetricians and Gynecologists. Clinical management guidelines: Critical care in pregnancy. *Obstet Gynecol.* 2009;113(2):443–450.

American College of Obstetricians and Gynecologists. Critical care obstetrics: preventing maternal morbidity and mortality. Safe Motherhood Initiative. http://mail.ny.acog.org/website/CriticalCare.pdf. Accessed June 7, 2011.

American Heart Association. Cardiac arrest associated with pregnancy. *Circulation.* 2005;112:IV150–IV153.

Clardy PF, Reardon CC. Critical illness during pregnancy and the peripartum period. In: Basow DS, ed. *UpToDate.* Waltham, MA: UpToDate; 2011.

Hemmila MH. Trauma in pregnancy. In: Flint L, Meredith JW, Schwab CW, Trunkey DD, Rue LW, Taheri PA, eds. *Trauma: Contemporary Principles and Therapy.* Philadelphia, PA: Lippincott Williams and Wilkins; 2008:595–603.

Tinkoff G. Care of the pregnant trauma patient. In: Peitzman AB, Rhodes M, Schwab CW, Yealy DM, Fabian TC, eds. *The Trauma Manual: Trauma and Acute Care Surgery.* 3rd ed. Philadelphia, PA: Lippincott Williams and Wilkins; 2008:515–523.

Chapter 25

Geriatric trauma critical care

Gary T. Marshall

Introduction

Incidence

Over the last century there has been an 11-fold increase in the elderly population. This trend continues, and by the year 2040, 20% of the population will be over age 65 years. Our population is enjoying a longer life expectancy and a more active lifestyle. Unfortunately, the declines in motor and cognitive function associated with aging have combined to create an ever enlarging group of geriatric patients experiencing trauma. As such, the ICU population is made up of an enlarging proportion of injured, elderly patients requiring specially tailored care.

Evaluation

Evaluation of the injured geriatric trauma patient presents several challenges. Falls, even from the same level, are the source of significant morbidity and mortality. The injury severity is often disproportionate to an apparently benign mechanism of injury. Head, chest, pelvic, and extremity injuries are all more common in the elderly fall victim compared with a younger cohort. Injury Severity Scores (ISS) have been shown to be twice as high in older patients as compared with younger ones, and the fall-associated mortality is significantly higher. In addition, significant injuries, including cervical spine fractures, may be asymptomatic. Initial evaluation may also be complicated by the frequent occurrence of occult hypoperfusion in the setting of normal vital signs. One study found elevated lactate and base deficit in 42% of injured elderly trauma patients despite vital signs considered normal. These patients had increased length of stay, and outcomes similar to patients with overt shock. Keeping these facts in mind, it is important to have a high index of suspicion for injury, even with normal vital signs and minor mechanism. The evaluation of these patients should be thorough, and imaging should be used liberally.

Impact of complications and comorbidities

Mortality is increased at all phases of the death curve in geriatric trauma patients: prehospital, early, and late. Early mortality can be reduced by early, aggressive resuscitation, thorough radiographic evaluation, monitoring, and operation. Late death in the elderly is reduced by meticulous attention to detail and subtle changes in patient status. Complication rates of 33% are reported in the elderly, compared with 19% in younger patients. Cardiovascular events (23%) and pneumonia (22%) are the most common and significant complications. These should be identified and treated early and aggressively. The role of comorbidities is also significant; these should be managed with fine attention to detail as well.

Age-related changes in physiology and intensive care management

Proper resuscitation and intensive-care management of the elderly requires an understanding of the changes in physiology associated with normal aging. In general, there is age-related decline in the function of all major organ systems.

Cardiovascular system

The cardiac system undergoes changes related to both aging and to the effects of cardiovascular disease. Silent myocardial ischemia is present in up to 40% of the elderly population. The arterial structures undergo progressive thickening and loss of elasticity. Changes in the arterial pressure transmission combine with the effect of sclerotic vessels to decrease coronary blood flow. When combined with preexisting ischemic heart disease and the stress of major injury, coronary flow may be seriously impaired in the setting of high physiologic need.

Maximal heart rate, ejection fraction, and cardiac output are all decreased with age. In addition, left ventricular hypertrophy occurs and ventricular relaxation is impaired. Diastolic dysfunction is compounded in critical illness by hypoxemia. The elderly heart is less responsive to sympathetic stimulation. Consequently, cardiac output can only be augmented by increasing preload and stroke volume. Minor hypovolemia may result in significant hemodynamic compromise; however, overzealous fluid resuscitation more frequently results in pulmonary edema in older patients compared with younger patients. Therefore, fluid administration must be meticulously managed. When providing volume resuscitation, especially in the unstable elderly, blood transfusion should be considered early, as hemorrhagic shock results in significant mortality. Restrictive transfusion strategies may not be appropriate in the elderly. Large trials of lower transfusion triggers excluded patients with chronic anemia, a frequent finding in the elderly. Other studies have found that hematocrit < 30% leads to increased mortality in patients with myocardial infarction, and is more frequently associated with delirium in postoperative patients. Low hematocrit also predicts functional decline. Left-atrial augmentation of ventricular filling significantly helps cardiac output in the elderly. As a result, atrial fibrillation is poorly tolerated. Thus, maintenance of sinus rhythm or, at a minimum, adequate rate control is critical in managing the elderly.

Pulmonary

Age-related decline in pulmonary function is secondary to changes in both the chest wall and the lung. Chest wall compliance decreases from structural changes in the spine and chest wall. Maximum inspiratory and expiratory force declines by as much as 50%. The lungs have decreased elasticity, with collapse of small airways. This leads to ventilation-perfusion mismatch and subsequent hypoxia. Dead space is also increased. Finally, central control in response to hypoxia and hypercarbia is altered and the ventilatory responses to these stimuli reduced significantly. In general, the ventilator strategies in geriatric patients should make use of positive end-expiratory pressure (PEEP) while limiting FiO_2, avoid over-distention of better aerated alveoli, and allow sufficient expiration time to avoid auto-PEEP and breath stacking.

Renal

Over the course of normal aging, approximately 40% of nephrons become sclerotic by age 85. Renal blood flow is decreased nearly 50% by progressive arterial changes. The serum creatinine remains unchanged due to concomitant losses of lean body mass. As the renal tubular function declines, the capacity to conserve sodium and eliminate acid is diminished. This places the elderly at high risk for dehydration. In the intensive care unit (ICU), careful attention to volume loss and replacement is needed. In addition, the glomerular filtration rate (GFR) should be determined so that drug dosage can be altered appropriately.

Of special concern for the injured patient is the prevention of contrast-induced nephropathy during the initial diagnostic evaluation and during the subsequent hospital stay. Numerous strategies exist, including using low-volume nonionic agents; avoiding repeated, closely-spaced studies; and ensuring adequate hydration. The use of sodium bicarbonate or N-acetylcysteine seems to be of limited value.

With the occurrence of oliguric acute renal failure, up to 85% of the elderly may require renal replacement therapy. The usual indications for renal replacement therapy apply in the elderly. Decisions should be made in conjunction with the appropriate specialists regarding dialysis timing and modality. Although outcomes after initiation of renal replacement therapy are poor, age alone does not determine the outcome, which is similar to younger patients, and should not be used a contraindication. The need for dialysis does, however, frequently represent a branch point in the decision process regarding goals of care. A frank discussion with the patient and surrogates should take place before initiating dialysis.

Neurocognitive function

Delirium is an acute state of confusion that develops over a short period of time and fluctuates in course. This must be distinguished from dementia, which has a more chronic, stable course. Delirium occurs in over 70% of elderly patients during admission, and is even higher in patients with preexisting dementia.

Table 25.1 Predisposing factors for delirium in the ICU

Host Factors	Critical Illness Related Factors	Iatrogenic Factors
Age	Acidosis	Immobilization
Alcoholism	Anemia, Fever/infection/sepsis	Catheters
Apolipoprotein E4 polymorphism	Hypotension	Medications
Cognitive Impairment	Metabolic disturbances	Sleep disturbance
Depression	Fever/hypothermia	
Hypertension	End organ dysfunction	
Smoking	Respiratory disease/hypoxia	
Vision or Hearing Loss	High severity of illness	

Delirium has been found to increase ICU and hospital costs. In addition, it is associated with cognitive decline after discharge from the hospital. Assessing for delirium in the ICU can be challenging due to the severity of disease and lack of verbal communication. One tool for detecting is the Confusion Assessment Method (CAM)-ICU. First, a standardized assessment of sedation is employed. For patients not determined to be comatose, the diagnosis of delirium is based on the following features: (1) acute onset of mental status changes or a fluctuating course and (2) inattention; and either (3) disorganized thinking or (4) altered level of consciousness.

There are numerous predisposing factors for delirium (Table 25.1), which may be present on admission or occur during the course of illness. The factors that may be important after admission allow for therapeutic or prophylactic intervention.

Sedative and analgesic medications are usually required in the ICU setting, but may have detrimental effects, including prolonging the need for mechanical ventilation, especially with continuous rather than intermittent administration of these medications. Daily interruption of sedative agents can decrease these complications. Benzodiazepines and anticholinergics are consistently linked with delirium. The linkage with opioids is less clear; more liberal use of these agents to ensure adequate analgesia may be protective against the development of delirium. Meperidine is the exception, as it is consistently linked to delirium, especially in the elderly.

Once identified, the first step in management of delirium is identification of any underlying organic source for the change in mental status. Careful history and physical examination are required because the altered state of consciousness may herald underlying infection or metabolic derangements. Multi-component regimens of nonpharmacologic measures have been shown to reduce delirium and should be initiated in the ICU. These interventions include repeated reorientation, cognitive stimulation, nonpharmacologic sleep protocol, early mobilization, prompt removal of restraints and catheters, use of eyeglasses and hearing aids, and early correction of dehydration. Pharmacologic intervention should also be considered. Current Society of Critical Care Medicine guidelines recommend haloperidol, beginning with 2 mg dose and repeating every 15–20 minutes with escalating (usually doubled) doses until agitation resolves. Scheduled doses are then initiated every 6 hours and tapered over several days. Newer atypical antipsychotic agents such as risperidone, ziprasidone, quetiapine, and olanzapine may have a role in the management of delirium. Although no placebo-controlled trials have been conducted, data suggests these agents are at least as effective as haloperidol, with fewer side effects. Once initiated, these agents are continued until the patient has shown no delirium for 48–72 hours. They can then be tapered.

Metabolic and endocrine changes

Body composition changes with aging. Up to 40% of lean body mass is lost, with corresponding loss of strength and decrease in resting energy expenditure by up to 15%. As a result of this loss of muscle mass, an elderly patient may rapidly develop protein-energy malnutrition during acute illness and trauma. Ideally, nutritional support should be initiated within 24 hours of admission. Enteral delivery is the preferred method. Early feeding decreases infection and results in lower mortality. Feeding should be adjusted to meet caloric needs, avoiding overfeeding, which may result in longer mechanical ventilation and fat synthesis. Micronutrients are frequently deficient and should be supplemented as well.

The incidence of impaired glucose tolerance increases with age, with nearly 40% of the U.S. population over age 60 having impaired glucose tolerance or type II diabetes mellitus. This occurs due to a decline in insulin secretion with age. Strict glycemic control, as indicated for younger patients, should be employed in the elderly as well.

Management of traumatic injuries

Traumatic brain injury

Traumatic brain injury (TBI) is common, affecting approximately 1.4 million Americans annually, and leads to over 13,000 U.S. deaths in patients aged 65 years and older. Age predicts both higher mortality and disability. The frequent use of anticoagulant and antiplatelet medications presents a challenge in these patients. As many as 9% of elderly TBI patients are anticoagulated with warfarin on presentation. Intracranial hemorrhage in these patients is not reliably predicted by either the presenting symptoms or International Normalized Ratio. Expedited computed tomography (CT) of the head should be obtained in all of these patients to rule out TBI. Once identified, patients should undergo rapid reversal of anticoagulation with fresh frozen plasma. The use of antiplatelet agents, including clopidogrel and aspirin, is widespread in the elderly. Unfortunately, less is known about the impact of these agents on outcome in TBI patients. Reversal of these agents is also unproven. Potential strategies include administration of platelets, desmopressin, and factor VII. The benefit of these strategies is under investigation. All elderly TBI patients should be admitted to the hospital and observed carefully, as clinical deterioration is frequent and subsequent mortality is high.

Thoracic trauma

Thoracic trauma, especially rib fractures, is common in the elderly. Unlike in younger patients, these are a source of significant morbidity and mortality for older patients. Even with lower injury-severity scores, the mortality associated with rib fractures in patients over 65 years is twice that seen in younger patients. The incidence of pneumonia also increases. Both of these are directly related to the number of ribs fractured. Any elderly patient with $\geq$ 3 fractured ribs should be admitted for observation. Pain control is paramount in these patients. Regional techniques such as epidural analgesia and paravertebral blocks should be employed, as they have been documented to significantly decrease mortality, pneumonia rate, and number of ventilator days. Nonsteroidal anti-inflammatory drugs are also beneficial, but attention must be paid to renal function when used. Pain control should be combined with aggressive pulmonary hygiene measures such as incentive spirometry and intermittent positive-pressure breathing.

Solid organ injury

Solid organ injury in the elderly may be managed in the same fashion as in younger patients. Advanced age (> 55 years) is a risk factor for the failure of nonoperative management, and outcomes may be worse after failure. Most failures occur in the first 48–72 hours. Patients should be observed closely for any change in hematocrit, increase in pain, persistent unexplained tachycardia, and hemodynamic decompensation or instability that may indicate the need for operation. Angiography is a reasonable option when a contrast blush or extravasation is seen on imaging, but other sources of blood loss must be ruled out prior to transport to angiography.

Pelvic fractures

Pelvic fractures are a frequent source of morbidity and mortality in the elderly. The lateral compression type fracture is more common among the aging population and is associated with an increase in hemorrhagic complications. This type of fracture is unfortunately not amenable to external fixation. Patients admitted with pelvic fracture should have blood sent for type and crossmatch. Serial hematocrit levels should be obtained. Retroperitoneal hemorrhage is common, and well-suited for angiographic intervention. Indications for angiography include hemodynamic compromise, large pelvic hematoma on CT, and transfusion of more than 4 units of blood. Mortality is decreased by the employment of angiographic embolization. The timing of operative fixation is difficult. One must assess and optimize comorbid conditions quickly, as early operative complications arise from comorbid disease. However, early fixation in < 48 hours has been documented to reduce mortality and morbidity in hip fractures.

Key references

Bulger EM, Edwards T, Klotz P, Jurkovich GJ. Epidural analgesia improves outcome after multiple rib fractures. *Surgery*. 2004;136(2):426–430.

Cheung CM, Ponnusamy A, Anderton JG. Management of acute renal failure in the elderly patient: a clinician's guide. *Drugs Aging.* 2008;25(6):455–476.

Girard TD, Pandharipande PP, Ely EW. Delirium in the intensive care unit. *Crit Care.* 2008;12(suppl 3):S3.

Ivascu FA, Howells GA, Junn FS, Bair HA, Bendick PJ, Janczyk RJ. Rapid warfarin reversal in anticoagulated patients with traumatic intracranial hemorrhage reduces hemorrhage progression and mortality. *J Trauma.* 2005;59(5):1131–1137; discussion 1137–1139.

Martin JT, Alkhoury F, O'Connor JA, Kyriakides TC, Bonadies JA. 'Normal' vital signs belie occult hypoperfusion in geriatric trauma patients. *Am Surg.* 2010;76(1):65–69.

McMillian WD, Rogers FB. Management of prehospital antiplatelet and anticoagulant therapy in traumatic head injury: a review. *J Trauma.* 2009;66(3):942–950.

Peters CW, Beyth RJ, Bautista MK. The geriatric patient. In: Gabrilli A, Layon AJ, Yu M, eds. *Civetta, Taylor, & Kirby's Critical Care.* 4th ed. Philadelphia, PA: Lippincott Williams & Wilkins; 2009:1505–1533.

Sterling DA, O'Connor JA, Bonadies J. Geriatric falls: injury severity is high and disproportionate to mechanism. *J Trauma.* 2001;50(1):116–119.

Chapter 26

Toxicology

Kenneth D. Katz

General approach

Poisonings, intoxications, and withdrawal states are frequently encountered in the trauma patient; consequently, the clinician must be familiar with the general approach to diagnosis and treatment of common toxicological entities. Furthermore, the initial traumatic injury, treatment, or diagnostic studies may mask or delay recognition of an underlying overdose, which can easily impact outcome.

The initial approach to the poisoned patient focuses primarily on history, physical examination, and targeted diagnostics. Because the patient may not be able to give a history due to trauma or altered mental status, it is paramount to gather information from paramedics, family, friends, or even text messages or similar means. Often key historical facts can be obtained regarding the following: the last time the patient was seen in usual state of health, the physical environment in which the patient was found, history of substance abuse or recent cessation, mental illness, or the existence of a suicide note. Particular attention should be paid to the patient presenting with clinical findings incongruous with the history, physical examination, or diagnostic studies. This may signal the presence of an underlying poisoning or withdrawal state blanketed by an apparent injury.

As in all cases, immediate attention to airway, breathing, circulation, and disability is paramount regardless of clinical etiology. Regarding the intoxicated or poisoned patient, physical examination focuses primarily on vital signs, as well as neurologic and dermatologic abnormalities. Furthermore, grouping of abnormalities can collectively illustrate the presence of a particular toxidrome.

Routine diagnostic studies for the toxicology patient are often intertwined with those for the trauma patient, including serum chemistries, in which particular attention is paid to the presence of anion gap metabolic acidosis, as well as glucose, ethanol, and lactate levels; electrocardiogram; and urine studies. However, more specific laboratory testing should be guided by clinical presentation and suspicion.

Diagnostic considerations

The presence, and especially persistence, of an unexplained anion gap metabolic acidosis should always be noted and, at minimum, rechecked after initial resuscitative efforts. This may indicate an initially overlooked toxin such as a toxic alcohol. Serum acetaminophen and salicylate levels should be measured if there is suspicion of ingestion since these medicines are easily obtained and frequently implicated in overdose. Complete blood counts can indicate indices of chronic alcoholism. Routine urine drug screen testing is generally unhelpful for either diagnosis or management of the patient given that the test has many false positives and negatives. Specific drug or poison levels, such as lithium or carbon monoxide, should be guided by patient history, medical record, or high clinical suspicion. Various causes of delirium should be considered in these patients (Table 26.1).

Table 26.1 Common causes of delirium

Cause	Rapidity of Onset	Key Clinical Features	Examples
GABA-agonist withdrawal	Hours to days depending on agent (e.g., onset shorter with shorter-acting drugs, such as alprazolam)	Tachycardia, hypertension, fever, tremulousness, diaphoresis, **visual/tactile hallucinations**, seizure	Ethanol, benzodiazepines, carisoprodol
Anticholinergic	Hours	Tachycardia, hypertension, fever, **dry mucous membranes/ axilla, mumbling/ picking behavior**, mydriasis, seizures	Tricyclic antidepressants, diphenhydramine, cyclobenzaprine, clozapine.
Sympathomimetics	Hours	Tachycardia, hypertension, fever, mydriasis, **diaphoresis**, seizure	Cocaine, amphetamines
Serotonin Syndrome	Hours	Autonomic instability, **lower extremity clonus/ hyper-reflexia**	Serotonin reuptake inhibitors, monoamine oxidase inhibitors, dextromethorphan, cocaine, lithium
Neuroleptic Malignant Syndrome (NMS)	Days	Autonomic instability, **"lead-pipe rigidity,"** catatonia	Atypical/typical neuroleptics, abrupt cessation dopaminergic agents
Malignant Hyperthermia	Minutes/Hours	Autonomic instability, fever (can be late), elevated CO_2, **masseter spasm**	Inhaled anesthetics, succinylcholine

Common toxidromes and clinical syndromes

Sympathomimetics

Excessive sympathetic nervous system stimulation leads to: tachycardia, hypertension, agitation, delirium, mydriasis, and diaphoresis. Examples include illicit drugs, such as cocaine and amphetamines, and medications used to treat attention deficit disorder, appetite suppressants, and decongestants. Furthermore, the clinical entity of "excited delirium" is often found in the young trauma patient in the presence of cocaine. Failure to aggressively sedate and resuscitate these patients can result in fatality.

The sign most closely linked to mortality after sympathomimetic poisoning is hyperthermia. Treatment should focus on reducing muscular rigidity and hyperactivity with benzodiazepines, rehydration, and active cooling for severe cases. In general, large doses of a benzodiazepine may be necessary to achieve an appropriate level of sedation (e.g., lorazepam 2 mg IV every 5 minutes). Though benzodiazepines are the drugs of choice for these patients, an antipsychotic, such as haloperidol (5 mg IV), can often augment sedation due to its ability to block the dopamine surge seen after sympathomimetic poisoning. Physical restraints should only be used as a temporary measure until the patient has been adequately sedated chemically. Severe cases of sympathomimetic poisoning may also present with multi-system organ dysfunction (i.e., cardiomyopathy, renal dysfunction, rhabdomyolysis, etc.).

Anticholinergics

Antimuscarinics are extremely commonly prescribed medications that include tricyclic antidepressants, antihistamines, muscle relaxants, antipsychotics, antiepileptics and antispasmodics. Clinical findings include: tachycardia, low-grade fever, delirium, seizures, mydriasis, dry mucous membranes, flushed skin, picking behavior, and in some instances, ventricular arrhythmias.

In severe cases of anticholinergic toxicity, the patient is often extremely agitated. Benzodiazepines are the drug of choice for agitation. Physostigmine (1–2 mg IV once) can also be used to abruptly improve anticholinergic delirium, but its effects are short-lived and can have detrimental consequences (i.e., bronchorrhea and bradycardia).

Many anticholinergic drugs (particularly tricyclic antidepressants) can cause cardiac dysrhythmias from sodium channel blockade. An electrocardiogram (ECG) should be monitored on all patients. Sodium bicarbonate should be administered if the QRS exceeds 120 ms. The goal with sodium bicarbonate is to raise serum pH to 7.5, reduce the QRS to below 120 ms, and achieve hemodynamic stability. Other dysrhythmics, preferably Class Ib agents (such as lidocaine), which do not worsen the QRS widening, may be necessary in cases refractory to bicarbonate therapy. In addition, a Foley catheter should be placed due to urinary retention, and a total creatine kinase (CK) should be measured to monitor for rhabdomyolysis.

Opiates/Opioids

The findings of coma, respiratory depression, and miosis define the opiate/opioid toxidrome. Meperidine can cause mydriasis and anticholinergic effects. Tramadol, propoxyphene, and meperidine can all cause seizures. Methadone is associated with dose-dependent QTc prolongation and increased risk of Torsades de Pointes.

Naloxone is the antidote for opiate/opioid toxicity. The goal of naloxone reversal is adequate breathing, not wakefulness. Large doses of naloxone often result in rapid induction of opiate withdrawal, which frequently leads to a belligerent patient. Commonly, 0.4 mg of naloxone is drawn up with 10 cc of saline. Then 1 cc of the diluted naloxone is administered every few minutes until the desired effect is achieved. This technique will often prevent the precipitation of acute withdrawal. If a continuous infusion of naloxone is needed for treatment of long-acting opioids, two-thirds of the effective naloxone dose is administered continuously per hour. Naloxone can precipitate seizures in some opioid overdoses, such as meperidine and tramadol. Intubation may be necessary for treatment of these opioid overdoses rather than reversal with naloxone.

Sedative/Hypnotics

These medications are often γ-aminobutyric acid (GABA) agonists, causing lethargy and obtundation, often with relatively preserved vital signs. Many agents, such as eszopiclone, zaleplon, and zolpidem, rarely require any intervention when ingested alone. Ethanol poisoning can cause hypoglycemia, hypotension, and hypothermia in severe cases. Barbiturates, on the other hand, may require intubation and vasopressor support in severe cases.

In general, flumazenil should be avoided as a reversal in sedative/hypnotic overdose. As opposed to opiate/opioid withdrawal, inducing acute GABA-agonist withdrawal may be life-threatening and difficult to treat. In general, airway monitoring/support is the best approach when treating sedative/hypnotics overdose.

Serotonin syndrome

This clinical syndrome should be suspected in patients prescribed serotonergic agents who exhibit the following signs and symptoms: relatively abrupt onset and termination of autonomic instability, delirium, and lower extremity hyper-reflexia/clonus. Most commonly the syndrome occurs in the presence of two serotonergic agents, including some of the following: serotonergic reuptake and monoamine oxidase inhibitors, dextromethorphan, lithium, cocaine and amphetamines.

Although some recommend cyproheptadine as the antidote for serotonin syndrome, there is no evidence to support its use and the medication must be administered by mouth. Because serotonin syndrome most commonly resolves within 24 hours of cessation of the offending agent, treating delirium with a short-acting benzodiazepine works well. These patients also often require hydration and monitoring for rhabdomyolysis due to their level of agitation. Because serotonin syndrome is a diagnosis of exclusion, the physician should maintain a low suspicion to treat and evaluate for other illnesses.

Neuroleptic malignant syndrome

Patients suffering from neuroleptic malignant syndrome (NMS) are exposed to neuroleptics and exhibit gradual onset of autonomic instability, hyperthermia, and "lead-pipe" rigidity. Differentiation from other clinical syndromes can be made by the medication(s) involved prior to onset and also rapidity of onset.

NMS is a rare illness with no gold standard for diagnosis or treatment. This syndrome is best treated with good supportive care and by discontinuing the suspected agent. Unlike serotonin syndrome, NMS symptoms may continue for as long as 10 days despite good supportive care. Benzodiazepines are considered first-line treatment for this syndrome. Although there is no good evidence to support the use of bromocriptine for NMS, it might act as an acceptable adjunctive treatment. Bromocriptine can only be given by mouth and is dosed at 2.5–10 mg 4 times per day.

Malignant hyperthermia

Patients exposed to inhaled anesthetics or succinylcholine can develop malignant hyperthermia. They exhibit elevated pCO_2, autonomic instability, fever, muscle rigidity (especially masseter spasm). Malignant hyperthermia must be treated immediately to reduce the risk of rhabdomyolysis, cardiovascular collapse, and mortality. As soon as the syndrome is recognized, the patient should receive dantrolene, intravenous fluids, active cooling, and correction of electrolytes. Dantrolene is given 2–3 mg/kg IV bolus every 15 minutes until clinical improvement or a total dose of 10 mg/kg has been administered.

Common specific poisonings

Nonopioid analgesics (acetaminophen, salicylates, and nonsteroidal anti-inflammatory drugs)

Some of the most common agents involved in poisonings are analgesics such as acetaminophen and salicylates, which are found either singularly or in combination with other medications, such as opioids. Acetaminophen causes a non-specific gastrointestinal disturbance followed by hepatic necrosis as the parent compound is metabolized to its toxic metabolite, N-acetyl-p-benzoquinone imine (NAPQI). Unexplained, worsening transaminitis in the trauma patient should warrant investigation of acetaminophen exposure.

Treatment of acetaminophen toxicity is largely based on the measurement of the aspartate aminotransferase (AST) and serum acetaminophen level. When the ingestion time is unknown or has been staggered over several hours, an acetaminophen level > 10 μg/mL or an elevated AST warrants treatment with n-acetylcysteine (NAC). When the time of ingestion is known and the entire dose was ingested at the same time, the acetaminophen level should be plotted on the Matthew-Rumack nomogram. Any acetaminophen level exceeding the line starting at 150 µg/mL at 4 hours merits NAC treatment. Currently, intravenous NAC (Acetadote) is the preferred dosing method due to the poor palatability of oral NAC. In addition, intravenous NAC is the only method that has been studied in patients with fulminant hepatic failure. NAC is administered at 150 mg/kg over 1 hour followed by 50 mg/kg over 4 hours then finally 100 mg/kg over 16 hours. If the patient's AST, alanine aminotransferase (ALT), prothrombin time (PT), renal function, and acid-base status remain normal at the conclusion of this dosing regimen, then no further NAC doses are typically necessary. If the patient's labs are worsening or the patient remains clinically ill, 100 mg/kg over 16 hours of additional NAC is continued until the patient shows signs of clear clinical and laboratory improvement.

Depending on acuity of ingestion, salicylism is generally associated with the following: tachycardia, hyperthermia (uncoupling of oxidative phosphorylation), tinnitus, gastrointestinal disturbance, coma, seizure, and both primary respiratory alkalosis and anion gap metabolic acidosis. Salicylate toxicity treatment begins with careful monitoring of serum salicylate levels, electrolytes, and serum pH every 2–3 hours. Patients cannot be safely discharged until two or more salicylate levels have been measured, the last level is < 25 mg/dL, and the level is decreasing. Many salicylate-poisoned patients are 4 to 6 liters volume-depleted at the time of presentation. The first treatment goal should be aggressive IV fluid resuscitation to maintain a brisk urine output. Alkalinization of the blood, using IV doses of sodium bicarbonate to produce a blood pH of 7.5–7.55, will encourage distribution of salicylate out of the brain (the location of salicylate's most significant toxicity) and into the blood. Blood alkalinization should lead to urinary alkalinization, which will increase urinary elimination of salicylate as well. In severe cases (e.g., acute and chronic serum salicylate levels > 100 mg/dL and > 60mg/dL, respectively, noncardiogenic pulmonary edema, renal failure, altered sensorium, or seizures), hemodialysis may be indicated as well.

Massive overdoses of nonsteroidal anti-inflammatories, such as ibuprofen or naproxen, are associated with coma, metabolic acidosis, and renal insufficiency.

Antidepressants

Tricyclic antidepressants and serotonergic agents were previously discussed. Many antidepressants are fairly innocuous in overdose. Certain serotonin reuptake inhibitors, however, such as citalopram, bupropion, and venlafaxine are also associated with seizures and cardiac conduction disturbances, as well as increasing morbidity and mortality. Patients should be monitored for delirium and seizures and treated with benzodiazepines as needed. Administration of Intravenous Lipid Emulsion therapy (ILE) for severe, refractory tricyclic antidepressant and bupropion toxicity has also been reported.

Neuroleptics

Both typical and atypical neuroleptic toxicity can cause tachycardia, lethargy, coma, and QTc prolongation. Clozapine is associated with excessive drooling, anticholinergic delirium, and agranulocytosis. Olanzapine causes anticholinergic delirium and miosis. Treatment for this class is largely supportive, including the use of benzodiazepines for delirium and monitoring of the QT for dysrhythmias.

Cardiovascular agents

Beta antagonists cause bradycardia, hypotension, coma, hypoglycemia, and hyperkalemia. Calcium channel blockers can cause a very similar clinical picture, except for hyperglycemia due to blockade of insulin release, and in the case of the dihydropyridine class, reflex tachycardia due to peripheral vasculature vasodilatation. However, massive dihydropyridine toxicity can also cause bradycardia. The 1A and 1C antidysrhythmics, such as quinidine and propafenone, respectively, can cause both cardiac sodium influx and potassium efflux blockade. The class III agent sotalol is associated with bradycardia, QTc prolongation, and Torsades de Pointes. Cardiac glycosides, such as digoxin, are associated with hyperkalemia (serum K^+ > 5.5 mEq/L directly correlates with mortality in acute poisoning) and a myriad of cardiac conduction disturbances due to its Na^+/K^+ ATPase blockade, enhanced automaticity, and, paradoxically, delayed conduction. Although premature ventricular contractions are often the earliest and most common electrocardiographic abnormality, suspicion for glycoside poisoning should be heightened in patients with atrial fibrillation with slow ventricular response or bidirectional ventricular tachycardia. Antihypertensives, such as angiotensin converting enzyme inhibitors, can cause hypotension and relative bradycardia. Clonidine is associated with transient hypertension followed by hypotension, bradycardia, and miosis.

Despite the differences in classes of agents, therapy for cardiovascular drug toxicity is fairly uniform. Glucagon, classically considered the "antidote" for β-blocker toxicity, has also been shown to have some benefit in studies of calcium channel blocker toxicity. The initial dose of glucagon for cardiovascular effect is 5–10 mg IV followed by an infusion of 5–10 mg/hr if the initial dose generates an effect. Glucagon therapy is limited by vomiting, modest benefits, cost, and availability. Intravenous calcium administration, as either calcium chloride or calcium gluconate, may result in minimal improvement, but is rarely sufficient in treating significant toxicity. The choice of vasopressor best suited to treat toxicity has not been proven, though norepinephrine, epinephrine, and phenylephrine are commonly utilized. Dopamine, specifically, is generally a poor choice for a vasopressor due to its primarily indirect activity, which may be impaired by presynaptic reuptake inhibition common to many psychiatric medications. Direct-acting vasopressors are typically required to overcome the competitive inhibition of the agent. Once a vasopressor is chosen, the dose may require rapid escalation, potentially beyond the usual "maximum" dose. Adequate tissue perfusion, as evidenced by normalization of mental status and urine output, as well as improvement in acid-base status, is the goal. Additional benefit may be gained by the addition of hyperinsulinemia-euglycemia (HIE) therapy. Initially recommended for calcium channel blocker toxicity, animal studies have also shown benefit in β-blocker toxicity. High-dose insulin, 0.5–1 unit/kg/hr, is infused with dextrose containing fluids meant to maintain euglycemia. Use of ILE for severe toxicity due to verapamil and propranolol poisoning has also been reported.

Treatment of antidysrhythmic toxicity is primarily guided by the patient's ECG in addition to the clinical presentation. Prolongation of the QRS duration beyond 120 ms resulting from sodium channel blockade should prompt initiation of serum alkalinization with sodium bicarbonate to serum pH of 7.5. Ventricular dysrhythmias refractory to appropriate serum alkalinization may be safely treated with lidocaine. Potassium channel blockade manifests in prolongation of the QTc interval and risk of torsades de pointes. Magnesium sulfate, 2–4 g IV, may be given in an attempt to avert potentially fatal arrhythmias.

Finally, digoxin is inactivated by digoxin-specific antibody fragments. The most specific indication for treatment is an elevated serum potassium level (K^+ > or =− 5.5 mEq/L) following acute ingestion. Otherwise, administration is based on the patient's clinical status and the presence of life-threatening arrhythmias or hypoperfusion following suspected acute digoxin ingestion or chronic toxicity. The specific serum level of digoxin does not indicate the need for treatment in the absence of hyperkalemia, clinically significant arrhythmia, or cardiovascular compromise. Empiric dosing in acute toxicity is 10 vials and 3–6 vials for chronic exposures. In patients with a known digoxin level, a formula to calculate the dose is: # of vials = [weight (kg) × level (ng/mL)]/100. Rapid reversal of the effects of chronic digoxin use may precipitate acute exacerbations of congestive heart failure or atrial fibrillation with rapid ventricular response.

Toxic alcohols

Ingestion of toxic alcohols, such as ethylene glycol, propylene glycol, and methanol, cause coma, profound anion gap metabolic acidosis, acute tubular necrosis (ethylene glycol) and retinal toxicity (methanol) due to parent compound degradation via alcohol dehydrogenase to oxalic, lactic, and formic acid, respectively. Patients can exhibit life-threatening poisoning even without detectable parent compound or the presence of an osmolal gap due to complete metabolism prior to seeking medical care. Bedside urine illumination using a Wood's lamp may reveal fluorescein in ethylene glycol poisoning; however, its absence does not absolutely rule out exposure. Isopropyl alcohol ingestion causes inebriation, coma, hemorrhagic gastritis, ketosis *without* metabolic acidosis (due to metabolism to acetone directly) and falsely elevated serum creatinine.

Suspicion of toxic alcohol ingestion should prompt administration of fomepizole, 15 mg/kg IV, in order to inhibit any further alcohol dehydrogenase metabolism of the alcohol to toxic metabolites. Osmotic diuresis prompted by the presence of the parent compound results in volume depletion, which typically requires several liters of crystalloid resuscitation. Sodium bicarbonate infusion is indicated for significant metabolic acidosis. Hemodialysis is indicated for evidence of end-organ damage, significant acidemia upon presentation demonstrating production of toxic acidic metabolites, renal failure, or significant osmotic burden. Hemodialysis may also be considered in patients with extremely elevated toxic alcohol levels with elongated half-lives despite fomepizole administration.

Additionally, vitamin therapy may provide incremental benefit by aiding in the metabolism of toxic acids to nontoxic metabolites. For methanol toxicity folic or folinic acid, 50 mg IV every 4 hours, is recommended. Following ethylene glycol administration, thiamine and pyridoxine, 100 mg IV every 8 hours and 50 mg IV every 6 hours, respectively, are given.

Diabetic agents

Both insulin and sulfonylurea toxicity will manifest as hypoglycemia—the duration of which is dependent on the specific agent involved. Treatment with dextrose and somatostatin should *only* be administered with documented hypoglycemia, not empirically.

Frequent measurements of serum glucose concentration are required in the management of exogenous insulin or sulfonylurea toxicity. Typical recommendations suggest hourly glucose measurements while the patient is sleeping alternated with 2-hour intervals when awake. A normal diet should be permitted during the observation period. Once hypoglycemia has been documented, intravenous dextrose should be administered, usually as a bolus of 25 g followed by an infusion of 5% dextrose-containing fluids. Recurrent hypoglycemia should prompt increases in the dextrose concentration of IV fluid. Importantly, if a 20% dextrose infusion is necessary, central venous access should be obtained due to the risk of phlebitis. Octreotide, 50 mcg subcutaneously every 8 hours, may reduce dextrose requirements and episodes of hypoglycemia following sulfonylurea ingestion, and, potentially, even following exogenous insulin administration. Prolonged observation is necessary in these patients owing to the long half-life of sulfonylureas and large stores of deposited subcutaneous insulin.

Biguanide toxicity (e.g., metformin) is hallmarked by profound metabolic acidosis, especially in the presence of renal or liver insufficiency; because these drugs are not insulin secretagogues like the sulfonylureas, hypoglycemia is generally not observed. Treatment is with sodium bicarbonate infusion titrated to normalizing pH; however, large doses of bicarbonate are often necessary. Some severely intoxicated patients benefit from hemodialysis clearance of metformin. Following metformin ingestion, patients should be observed with serial serum chemistry and lactic acid measurements.

Antiepileptics

Antiepileptic medications include a diverse range of drugs and toxicities. Antiepileptic toxicity generally manifests with lethargy and coma due to the mechanism of drug action, which is neuronal inhibition. A few medications—tiagabine, lamotrigine, and carbamazepine—can paradoxically cause agitation or delirium, as well as seizures. Carbamazepine is also associated with anticholinergic delirium, cardiac sodium channel blockade, and erratic gastrointestinal absorption and hyponatremia. Phenobarbital toxicity can cause coma, hypotension, bradycardia, hypothermia, and respiratory depression. Valproic acid may cause a hyperammonemic encephalopathy, which may respond to therapy with L-carnitine given as a 100 mg/kg IV loading dose (max 6 g) followed by 15 mg/kg every 4 hours. Topiramate ingestion has been associated with angle-closure glaucoma and, more frequently, a nonanion gap metabolic acidosis of unclear significance. Bicarbonate therapy is generally unnecessary due to the mild nature of the acidosis.

Anticonvulsant Hypersensitivity Syndrome (AHS) affects people with a specific enzyme deficiency resulting in a global inflammatory response leading to fever, dermatitis, nephritis, and hepatitis, which resolves with cessation of the anticonvulsant and administration of steroids, though the specific dose of steroids is debated. The agents most associated with this syndrome are phenobarbital, phenytoin, lamotrigine, felbamate and carbamazepine.

Beyond the treatment of specific syndromes, anticonvulsant toxicity primarily requires supportive care.

Methylxanthines

Both caffeine and theophylline can cause profound gastrointestinal disturbance, supraventricular dysrhythmias, seizures, metabolic acidosis, and hypokalemia due to excessive β-adrenergic receptor stimulation.

Methylxanthine toxicity results in tachycardia, hypotension, vomiting, tremor, confusion, and potentially in seizures. Short-acting β-blocker administration, such as esmolol, will often actually improve hypotension, because of the underlying mechanism of β-receptor agonism. Prior to β-blocker administration a pulmonary history and examination should be performed because patients prescribed theophylline frequently have underlying bronchospastic pulmonary disease. Phenylephrine represents a reasonable alternative, particularly when the precise etiology of hypotension is unclear. Benzodiazepine administration is recommended for the treatment of seizure activity. Methylxanthines can be removed by dialysis, if necessary, in patients suffering severe toxicity.

Organophosphate pesticides

Both carbamate and organophosphate poisoning inhibit acetyl cholinesterase activity and demonstrate a "DUMBELS" clinical syndrome, including defecation, urination, miosis, bronchorrhea, bradycardia, excessive lacrimation, and salivation. Seizures may also be seen, and a garlic odor may accompany the exposed patient.

Patients exposed to organophosphates should first be decontaminated to prevent any further inhalational or transdermal exposure. Symptoms related to excess muscarinic receptor stimulus are treated with repeat doses of atropine or glycopyrrolate to improve airway pressure and bronchorrhea. Beneficial effects at the remaining peripheral muscarinic receptors are secondary. Large doses of atropine are frequently required in patients suffering organophosphate toxicity. In order to prevent aging of the bond created between organophosphates and cholinesterase enzymes, pralidoxime, 1–2 g IV followed by 500 mg/hr, is recommended. Failure to administer pralidoxime in a timely fashion, within 24 hours of exposure, results in prolonged toxicity. Pralidoxime is likely not necessary in the treatment of carbamate toxicity, but if the source of muscarinic symptoms is unknown, pralidoxime should be given empirically.

Toxic gas exposure

A high clinical index of suspicion is required to consider the diagnosis of toxic gas exposure. The primary treatment is removal from the source while rescue personnel take precautions to prevent additional exposures.

Cyanide, hydrogen sulfide, and carbon monoxide inhibit cellular respiration by disrupting the electron transport chain. Poisoning should be suspected in the critically ill smoke inhalation patient, especially with soot around the nares and airway, with severe metabolic acidosis and cardiovascular collapse. A plasma lactate > 10 mmol/L in this population has relatively highly sensitive and specificity for a blood cyanide level of > 39 μmol/L. Cherry-red skin is generally a postmortem finding for carbon monoxide poisoning and, therefore, unreliable.

Patients in whom cyanide toxicity is suspected due to a history of exposure combined with severe metabolic acidosis and cardiovascular toxicity can be treated empirically. Historically, the cyanide antidote kit comprised amyl nitrite, sodium nitrite, and sodium thiosulfate. However, nitrite administration is relatively contraindicated in patients with smoke inhalation injury and hypoxemia because the intended production of methemogloginemia, while beneficial in removing cyanide from cytochrome oxidase, may further worsen tissue oxygen delivery. Recently approved for use in the United States, hydroxocobalamin, a vitamin B_{12} precursor, offers a simple alternative therapy when given as a single 5 g IV injection. Adverse effects include deep-red discoloration of secretions and urine as well as interference with colorimetric laboratory tests such as creatinine. The dose may be repeated if necessary.

Hydrogen sulfide poisoning, clinically similar to that of cyanide, should be suspected in sewer workers, especially with multiple victims at the scene. Generally foul, rotten-egg smelling in lower concentrations, hydrogen sulfide paradoxically exhibits olfactory fatigue at high and potentially fatal concentrations. Interestingly, suicide with hydrogen sulfide has gained popularity in some countries. Treatment is primarily supportive.

Optimal therapy for carbon monoxide poisoning is unclear. Following removal from the source and administration of high-flow oxygen, most patients will experience resolution of symptoms without further sequelae. In a select group, toxicity may be more severe leading some to recommend hyperbaric oxygen therapy (HBO). Theoretical benefits of HBO include rapid removal of any remaining CO as well as prevention of long-term neurologic complications; however, data are equivocal that there is any significant benefit. HBO is generally reserved for patients with severe end-organ toxicity.

Miscellaneous drugs of abuse

Gamma hydroxybutyrate (GHB) is commonly used at rave parties, causing sedation and even respiratory failure requiring intubation and mechanical ventilation; classically, patients exhibiting respiratory failure awaken fairly quickly allowing rapid extubation even in the emergency department. Ketamine and dextromethorphan are dissociative agents that can cause similar clinical syndromes of tachycardia, mydriasis, catatonia, or agitation via inhibition of N-Methyl-D-aspartate (NMDA) glutamate receptors. Ecstasy (MDMA, or 3,4 Methylenedioxymethamphetamine), is an amphetamine derivative known for its hallucinogenic effects. Interestingly, severe, life-threatening hyponatremia has been associated with its use.

Acute intoxication can manifest in a variety of presentations. Patients may be agitated, delirious, somnolent, or comatose. Agitated intoxicated patients are most appropriately treated with titrated doses of benzodiazepines in order to prevent seizures, psychomotor agitation, and cardiovascular toxicity, as well as self-injurious behavior. Physical restraint should only temporarily be employed while chemical sedation is optimized due to the associated risk of injury and rhabdomyolysis. Somnolent patients must be closely monitored for respiratory depression as well as aspiration. Naloxone may be considered in patients with an unknown, or polypharmacy, ingestion exhibiting signs of respiratory insufficiency. Otherwise, the goal of therapy is supportive care.

Common withdrawal states

Opiate/Opioid

Withdrawal from opiates or opioids is associated with a flu-like illness: gastrointestinal disturbances, piloerection, excessive yawning, and myalgias. Although uncomfortable, it is not life-threatening. Of critical importance is to realize that the sensorium is *preserved*.

Management of opioid withdrawal focuses on the management of symptoms that might otherwise complicate underlying medical or trauma pathology. Opioid replacement with a long-acting μ receptor agonist, such as methadone, adequately controls physiologic withdrawal at a dose of 10–30 mg daily titrated to amelioration of symptoms. Intravenous methadone, at 50% of the oral dose, is also available for critically ill or intubated patients. When opioid therapy is not a viable option for medical or psychosocial reasons, symptomatic care can be provided for the most predominant symptoms.

Sedative/Hypnotic

Unlike narcotics, sedative/hypnotic withdrawal can manifest with *clouded sensorium*, delirium, and autonomic instability. Careful attention should be given to those patients who are chronically prescribed short-acting benzodiazepines, such as alprazolam, because withdrawal can be fairly abrupt and clinically stormy if not recognized. Clearly, ethanol withdrawal in the trauma patient is quite common. However, it is important to recognize the different stages depending on time from last ethanol ingestion. Early manifestations within the first 24–48 hours include alcoholic tremulousness (diaphoresis, tremulousness, tachycardia), hallucinosis (preserved sensorium, tactile/visual hallucinations) and withdrawal seizures (generalized, tonic-clonic, rarely status). The most feared and also latest manifestation of ethanol withdrawal (72–96 hours) is delirium tremens, which includes clouded sensorium and inattention along with severe autonomic instability.

Predicting which patients will experience complicated sedative/hypnotic or alcohol withdrawal can be difficult. No reliable prediction rule exists. However, a detailed history of previous episodes of withdrawal may provide an indication of the patient's current withdrawal risk. Once a risk of withdrawal has been identified, careful observation and frequent examinations focusing on vital-sign abnormalities and neurologic changes including tremor, hyper-reflexia, clonus, hallucinations, and confusion should be performed. Several validated scoring systems, for example the Withdrawal Assessment Score (WAS), have been developed to assign a standardized score that can be used to trend the severity of withdrawal as well as to trigger interventions. These scales are limited, however, due to a heavy reliance on subjective symptoms and lack of specificity for withdrawal in patients suffering from acute traumatic injuries.

Benzodiazepines remain the mainstay in the treatment of sedative/hypnotic and alcohol withdrawal. In particular, diazepam has a favorable pharmacologic profile because it is long-acting and has active metabolites allowing for a prolonged self-tapering effect. Additionally, the peak effect is rapidly achieved allowing rapid titration of dosing. Patients with mild withdrawal or who have not yet shown signs of withdrawal are most appropriately treated by a symptom-triggered approach in order to avoid unnecessary benzodiazepine administration and sedation. Therapy may be triggered based on a withdrawal scale or based on changes in examination. Dosing can vary, but 10–20 mg of IV diazepam can be safely given with further increases in dose based upon response. Once a patient has demonstrated a need for repeated benzodiazepine doses, a standing dose can be given based on individual requirements followed by a taper over several days. In patients suffering from moderate-to-severe withdrawal at the time of presentation, aggressive titration of IV diazepam with rapidly increasing doses, or "front loading," until symptoms are controlled is recommended. Again, 10–20 mg of IV diazepam is a reasonable starting dose, which can then be doubled every 5–10 minutes as needed. Some patients may require several hundred milligrams or more. The endpoint of therapy is light sedation, cessation of tremors, and improvement in hemodynamic abnormalities.

Alternative agents should be considered in patients who are resistant to benzodiazepines. Phenobarbital may prove more effective in these patients, but has a narrow therapeutic index and should be given in a critical care setting with hemodynamic and respiratory monitoring. Intubated patients can also be effectively treated with propofol. However, due to the short duration of action of propofol, the addition of a long-acting agent prior to discontinuation of propofol is advisable. Alternative classes of agents such as antihypertensives, antipsychotics, and anticonvulsants are not recommended as primary agents in the treatment of sedative/hypnotic/ethanol withdrawal due to the potential obfuscation of signs of worsening withdrawal, lowering of the seizure threshold, and inability to treat the underlying pathophysiology. Interestingly, ketamine infusion has recently been reported as a successful adjunct to benzodiazepine therapy for severe alcohol withdrawal.

Key references

Alarie Y. Toxicity of fire smoke. *Crit Rev Toxicol*. 2002;32(4):259–289.

Boyer EW, Shannon M. The serotonin syndrome. *N Engl J Med*. 2005;352(11):1112–1120.

Brooks DE, Levine M, O'Connor AD, French, RNE, Curry, SC: Toxicology in the ICU: Part 2: specific toxins. *Chest*. 2011;140(4):1072–1085.

Buckley NA, Eddleston M. The revised position papers on gastric decontamination. *Clin Toxicol*. 2005;43(2):129–130.

Ghatol A, Kazory A. Ecstasy-associated acute severe hyponatremia and cerebral edema: A role for osmotic diuresis? *J Emerg Med*. 2012;42(6):e137–e140.

Kraut JA, Kurtz I. Toxic alcohol ingestions: clinical features, diagnosis, and management. *Clin J Am Soc Nephrol*. 2008;3(1):208–225.

Marzuk PM, Tardiff K, Leon AC, et al. Ambient temperature and mortality from unintentional cocaine overdose. *JAMA*. 1998;279(22):1795–1800.

O'Connor PG, Fiellin DA. Pharmacologic treatment of heroin-dependent patients. *Ann Intern Med*. 2000;133(1):40–54.

Pentel PR, Benowitz NL. Tricyclic antidepressant poisoning—management of arrhythmias. *Med Toxicol*. 1986;1:101–121.

Reulbach U, Dutsch C, Biermann T, et al. Managing an effective treatment for neuroleptic malignant syndrome. *Crit Care*. 2007;11:R4.

Romanelli F, Smith KM. Dextromethorphan abuse: clinical effects and management. *J Am Pharm Assoc*. 2009;49(2):e20–e25.

Sarff M, Gold JA. Alcohol withdrawal syndromes in the intensive care unit. *Crit Care Med*. 2010;38(suppl 9):S494–S501.

Stotts AL, Dodrill CL, Kosten TR. Opioid dependence treatment: options in pharmacotherapy. *Expert Opin Pharmacother*. 2009;10(11):1727–1740.

Wade JF, Dang CV, Nelson L, Wasserberger J. Emergent complications of the newer anticonvulsants. *J Emerg Med*. 2010;38(2):231–237.

Wilson E, Waring WS. Severe hypotension and hypothermia caused by acute ethanol toxicity. *Emerg Med J*. 2007;24(2):e7.

Winecoff AP, Hariman RJ, Grawe JJ, et al. Reversal of the electrocardiographic effects of cocaine by idocaine. Part 1. Comparison with sodium bicarbonate and quinidine. *Pharmacotherapy*. 1994;14:698–703.

Zed PJ, Krenzelok EP. Treatment of acetaminophen overdose. *Am J Health Syst Pharm*. 1999;56(11):1081–1091.

Chapter 27

Rehabilitation considerations of trauma patients

Kerry Deluca and Amy Wagner

Assessment of the rehabilitation needs of the trauma patient begins in the Trauma Intensive Care Unit (ICU). Physiatrists, specialists in the field of Physical Medicine and Rehabilitation (PM&R), focus on a patient's current and potential functional impairment(s) with the goal of maximizing functional ability despite physical and cognitive limitations.

In addition to the physiatrist, the rehabilitation team caring for the patient in the Trauma ICU often consists of physical therapists, occupational therapists, speech language pathologists, and discharge planning specialists. Physical therapists evaluate many aspects of the patient's function, including strength, joint range-of-motion (ROM), mobility, some activities of daily living (ADLs), gait, and balance. Occupational therapists evaluate multiple aspects of the patient's function, including upper limb strength and ROM, performance and capacity for ADLs, cognitive function, splinting, and positioning needs. Speech and language pathologists evaluate swallow, language, and cognition. Functional evaluation from each therapist includes a description of baseline level of function.

To best determine the appropriate level of postacute therapies, the physiatrist considers prior level of function, living situation, and level of social support as well as the patient's current medical needs, functional level, and therapy needs. Care managers, social workers, and rehabilitation liaisons evaluate the patient's social supports and prior function. They facilitate the transition of patients from acute care in the hospital to the postacute rehabilitation program. Common venues for postacute rehabilitation care include acute inpatient rehabilitation programs, subacute rehabilitation programs (often at skilled nursing facilities), and long-term acute care facilities. If the patient is safe to return home, home therapies or outpatient therapies may be options for continued rehabilitation. Studies in some populations suggest that early rehabilitation involvement in patient care leads to better acute outcomes and decreased length of stay in acute care.

General rehabilitation issues

Rehabilitation evaluation and management in the Trauma ICU focuses broadly on issues common to all ICU patients and on issues that are specific to those with spinal cord injury (SCI) or traumatic brain injury (TBI). Bed rest, often necessary in the trauma ICU setting due to medical and surgical issues following trauma, causes a number of adverse conditions that have significant functional consequences. These include skeletal muscle atrophy, decreased endurance, joint contracture, pressure ulcer formation, and nerve compression injuries. Attention to proper positioning and splinting of the patient in bed can help decrease these complications and maximize the patient's functional outcome.

Skin protection

Patients in the Trauma ICU are at increased risk for skin breakdown *and* pressure ulcer formation because of poor bed mobility, impaired sensation, and poor nutritional status, as well as tissue-shearing stresses associated with positioning. Emergency ICU admission and an ICU stay of more than 7 days in elderly patients increase risk for pressure ulcer formation. One strategy for skin protection is to turn the patient every 2 hours while in bed, if medical condition allows. Turning techniques should limit friction and shear. Adequate pressure-relieving mattresses can be used, as well as proper pillow placement with positioning.

Skin should be assessed frequently. Common sites of skin breakdown for patients in bed include occiput, scapula, sacrum, coccyx, trochanters, ankles, and heels. Once the patient begins sitting, skin over the ischial tuberosities is also at risk for breakdown. Patients with spinal cord injury who are able to sit up in a chair should be instructed (as able) to perform pressure reliefs every thirty minutes. Those patients unable to perform their own pressure relief independently should be assisted in this task and placed on pressure-relieving cushions when out of bed.

Prevention of joint contractures

Joint contractures can have significant functional implications. Prevention of contractures is accomplished by gentle range-of-motion through all major joints on a daily basis. In addition, proper splinting and positioning prevent contracture formation. Pressure-relieving ankle foot orthoses (PRAFOs) provide the heels with pressure relief while preventing Achilles contracture. Physiatrists may consider serial casting to increase range of motion and prevent contracture in patients with more severe ROM deficits and spasticity.

Spasticity

Spasticity, a velocity-dependent increase in muscle tone that is a sign of upper motor neuron injury, often develops in patients with spinal cord injury and acquired brain injury. Spasticity may result in decreased joint motion, pain, or decreased function. At times, spasticity may be functionally useful, as in performing stand-pivot transfers, therefore treatment decisions must be individualized to the patient. Daily range-of-motion of each joint (passive or active, depending on the patient's situation and within the parameters of allowable ROM due to orthopedic injuries) is the cornerstone of treatment in controlling spasticity and preventing joint contracture. Medications to decrease spasticity can be considered but most act centrally and can cause sedation. The choice of medication to manage spasticity should be based on the patient's cognitive status as well as neurologic and medical considerations.

Deconditioning

Hospital-associated deconditioning is a multifactorial phenomenon with significant functional implications. The rehabilitation team initially works to minimize the effects of immobility by assisting the patient with exercise at the bedside. Once the patient is cleared for out-of-bed activity, physical and occupational therapists assess functional activity including bed mobility, ability to sit at the edge of bed, transfers, gait, and balance. A growing body of literature documents the beneficial effects of mobility and exercise early in ICU admissions. Much of this investigation has been done in medical ICU settings, but strategies can be adapted to the needs of the Trauma ICU patient.

Heterotopic ossification

Patients with traumatic brain injury, spinal cord injury, and burns are at increased risk for developing heterotopic ossification (HO). Characterized by abnormal periarticular growth of bone, HO often results in decreased ROM and pain. Clinically, the area is often swollen and warm, and the first clinical signs of HO are often noted by physical and occupational therapists during treatment. Decreased ROM may have functional implications. Elevated alkaline phosphatase is not specific in the early stages of this condition because it may be elevated by other orthopedic conditions. Plain radiograph findings may significantly lag behind the development of symptoms. Thus, triple-phase bone scan is the preferred method of confirming the diagnosis.

Rehabilitation issues in specific populations

Patients with spinal cord injury

Spinal cord injuries are classified according to the American Spinal Injury Association (ASIA) Impairment Scale (AIS) In this scale, the neurologic level of injury is considered to be the lowest level with normal function (provided that all rostral levels are normal), and the completeness of injury (graded A [most severe] through E [no injury]) is based on sensory/motor function at the sacral segments, as well as strength in muscle groups below the neurologic level of injury. Ideally, AIS measurement should be done at 72 hours postinjury, after respiratory and cardiovascular stabilization and after resolution of spinal shock. Clinical factors including intubation, sedation, and medical instability may delay full assessment (Figure 27.1).

Accurate AIS classification early after injury enables correct evaluation of changes in neurologic function over time and allows clinicians to predict eventual

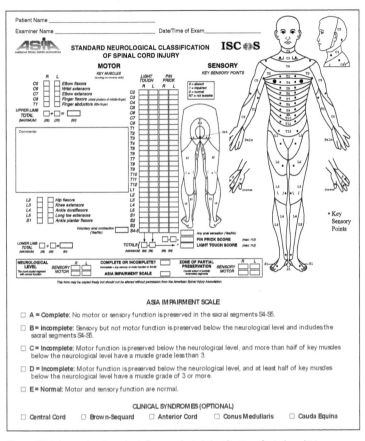

Figure 27.1 International standards for neurological classification of spinal cord injury

---

ASIA IMPAIRMENT SCALE

☐ **A = Complete:** No motor or sensory function is preserved in the sacral segments S4-S5.

☐ **B = Incomplete:** Sensory but not motor function is preserved below the neurological level and includes the sacral segments S4-S5.

☐ **C = Incomplete:** Motor function is preserved below the neurological level, and more than half of key muscles below the neurological level have a muscle grade less than 3.

☐ **D = Incomplete:** Motor function is preserved below the neurological level, and at least half of key muscles below the neurological level have a muscle grade of 3 or more.

☐ **E = Normal:** Motor and sensory function are normal.

CLINICAL SYNDROMES (OPTIONAL)

☐ Central Cord   ☐ Brown-Sequard   ☐ Anterior Cord   ☐ Conus Medullaris   ☐ Cauda Equina

---

function. Patients with AIS Grade A complete SCI may have small improvements over time, but generally there is not dramatic change in neurological function. However, patients with incomplete SCI (AIS Grades B through D) can have significant neurological improvement over time. When considering future function in a patient with cervical SCI, key levels to consider are: elbow flexion with intact C5 (allowing patient to bring hand to mouth for feeding and orofacial hygiene), wrist extension with intact C6 (allowing patient to use tenodesis grip to accomplish feeding and orofacial hygiene), and elbow extension with intact C7 (enabling independent transfers in most patients). Clinicians use the patient's AIS and related motor score at 1 month to predict long-term function and orthotic needs.

Spinal shock

Immediately following a traumatic SCI, patients may be in what is termed "spinal shock," with temporary loss or depression of spinal reflexes below the level of injury. The pathology associated with this phase is not entirely understood, may last from days to weeks, and ends with the return of elicitable muscle spindle reflex arcs. Throughout the period of spinal shock, distal reflexes such as the bulbocavernosus may never be absent, even in cases of verified cord transection. The development of spasticity, referred to in an earlier section, is also seen as the patient emerges from spinal shock. Spasticity can be a major functional issue in patients with SCI, and must be managed on an individual basis, given that it may have both positive and negative effects on function.

Neurogenic shock and cardiovascular instability

Neurogenic shock, which is a separate entity from spinal shock, describes the severe hypotension and bradycardia that are seen immediately following a SCI. After cervical and high-thoracic SCI, the vagus nerve produces unopposed parasympathetic stimulation as sympathetic input to the vessels below the level of the injury is lost. The resultant loss of sympathetic tone leads to neurogenic shock, which manifests as decreased cardiovascular contractility and bradycardia, sometimes necessitating pressor support for hypotension and temporary pacing for cardiac arrhythmia. Orthostatic hypotension can be a problem in the ICU when patients are transferred out of bed. Often compression stockings, abdominal binders, and medications such as midodrine must be utilized to maintain blood pressure. Autonomic dysreflexia (AD) is a secondary complication seen in patients with SCI at T6 level and above. AD generally develops after the period of spinal shock has resolved and presents as an acute elevation in blood pressure due to noxious stimuli below the level of the injury. Because AD can be life-threatening, it requires immediate intervention.

Rehabilitation recommendations for respiratory management

The most frequent pulmonary complications in SCI are atelectasis and pneumonia. Respiratory complications occur most frequently in patients with high-cervical (C1–C4) SCI due to both inspiratory and expiratory muscle weakness. However, respiratory complications are also common in patients with lower cervical (C5–C8) and thoracic (T1–T12) injuries because paralysis of abdominal muscles results in ineffective cough to clear secretions. Those with significant chest trauma and thoracic vertebral fractures may also have concomitant damage to lung parenchyma.

Mucus hypersecretion occurs as a result of unopposed vagal stimulation of the submucosal glands in the lungs. Management of secretions in patients with both cervical and thoracic SCI is critical, as tracheal suctioning alone may be insufficient for secretion mobilization. Expiratory aids to mobilize bilateral bronchial secretions include mechanical insufflation/exsufflation, manual-assisted cough, and pulmonary hygiene with nebulizer treatments.

In order to prevent pneumonia in patients with SCI, current clinical practice guidelines suggest the use of large tidal volumes (15 mL/kg of ideal body weight, based on height) to keep the lungs inflated. Higher tidal volumes have been shown to reduce atelectasis and facilitate weaning from the ventilator. The risk of barotrauma can be reduced if the peak airway pressure is kept under 40 cm of water. Caution should be used when increasing tidal volumes in patients with acute respiratory distress syndrome (ARDS) or pneumothorax. If the SCI involves cervical levels C3, C4, or C5, phrenic nerve loss results in weakness or paralysis of the diaphragm. Despite this, a certain percentage of patients with C3 level injuries and a majority of patients with C4 level injuries should eventually be weaned from the ventilator. Patients with injuries at C5 level and below are routinely weaned from the ventilator. Ventilator weaning after SCI is more successful when using periods of progressive ventilator-free breathing instead of synchronized intermittent mandatory ventilation.

When a tetraplegic patient begins to sit upright, an abdominal binder should be applied. The binder forces abdominal contents upward and increases vital capacity by placing the diaphragm in a better position for inspiration.

Dysphagia

Patients with traumatic tetraplegia are at increased risk for dysphagia. Risk factors for dysphagia after SCI include increased age, tracheostomy, mechanical ventilation, and spinal surgery via anterior approach. Early evaluation for dysphagia helps to minimize aspiration risk.

Management of neurogenic bladder

Initial management of neurogenic bladder after SCI is typically with a Foley catheter. Transition to an intermittent catheterization program can be considered if the patient is unable to void spontaneously, and when total daily fluid intake is approximately 2000 cc. Catheterizing the bladder every 4–6 hours with a goal of obtaining volumes less than or equal to 500 cc per catheterization prevents overdistension of the bladder and the development of upper-tract complications. In persons who void after Foley catheter removal, postvoid residuals should be checked to ensure that urine output is not a result of overflow voiding.

Management of neurogenic bowel

Ileus is the most common gastrointestinal complication occurring during the acute stage of SCI. Once intestinal peristalsis has resumed, a bowel management program can be initiated. Neurogenic bowel following SCI can be classified as "upper motor neuron" (for lesions above the conus medullaris) or "lower motor neuron" (for lesions at the cauda equina). Upper-motor-neuron bowel programs typically consist of stool softeners and a laxative. Reflex emptying of the colon is elicited by digital stimulation of the external anal sphincter following suppository insertion. Lower motor neuron neurogenic bowel is managed with bulking agents and intermittent manual disimpaction. Patients with incomplete SCI often recover bowel and bladder function over time.

Pain in patients with spinal cord injury

Patients with SCI may experience pain from a number of sources. Nociceptive pain above the level of injury, due to fracture or other sources of tissue injury, may be treated with local blocks or opioid medications. Patients may experience neuropathic pain, characterized as burning or tingling, in dermatomes at or below the level of injury. They may experience allodynia at the level of injury. These patients often respond well to medications that specifically target neuropathic pain, such as gabapentin, an anticonvulsant.

Dual diagnosis—head injury and spinal cord injury

Up to 40%–50% of patients who have sustained traumatic SCI have also sustained a concomitant TBI. Cognitive delays in these patients can affect their ability to learn new information while undergoing rehabilitation and may limit their functional gains.

Patients with traumatic brain injury

Traumatic brain injury diagnosis and disorders of consciousness

Traumatic brain injury diagnosis in the critically injured patient is not always clear. Careful serial examinations while off sedation, drug screening, and repeat imaging may be needed to verify the diagnosis.

Some patients with severe TBI have prolonged periods of depressed consciousness. The ICU-based physiatric evaluation of patients with depressed consciousness involves brainstem reflexes such as corneal responses, gag reflex, and oculocephalic reflexes, referred to as *doll's eyes*. The presence of these reflexes reflects intact brainstem pathways. Direct and consensual papillary responses and response to visual threat should be examined. Spontaneous activity and responses to environmental stimuli are important. During the exam, it is important to optimize environmental conditions and patient positioning and avoid sedating medications. In addition to clinical examination and scales, somatosensory-evoked potentials (SSEPs) may be requested for some patients with severe TBI to help to further evaluate posttraumatic coma and persistent vegetative states.

The Trauma ICU team, including the physiatric consultant, is often asked to provide input on outcome prognostication, particularly for severely injured patients. An accurate understanding of clinical classification is vital for appropriate prognostication. *Coma* is a state of pathologic unconsciousness in which the eyes remain closed, and there is no purposeful motor activity. A *vegetative state* may follow coma. With the vegetative state is some evidence of wakefulness but no consistent response to the environment. Vegetative states should be described in relation to the length of time since injury. Patients in a *minimally conscious state* (MCS) have severely depressed consciousness but demonstrate definite, reproducible evidence of self-awareness and/or interaction with the environment. Typical interactions might include verbalizations, purposeful nonverbal and/or motor responses, or emotional responses. As patients emerge from the MCS, they interact more with their environment and start participating in functional activities. Physiatrists can then begin to set goals and discharge planning for a trial of acute inpatient rehabilitation.

Cognition and neuropharmacology

Intervention with neurostimulants can help improve arousal, facilitate transition from a vegetative state or MCS, facilitate weaning from ventilator support, and increase participation with therapies performed in the ICU, which may impact discharge planning and qualification for inpatient rehabilitation services.

Multiple neurotransmitter systems, particularly monoamines such as dopamine, affect arousal. These may be altered in humans after TBI. Consequently, dopamine agonists can be beneficial in attenuating cognitive deficits. A recent evidence-based guideline recommended methylphenidate as a neurostimulant to improve cognition, particularly attention. There is also support for the use of amantadine to enhance general cognition and attention.

Despite evidence of effective treatment with neurostimulants, the optimal timing to initiate treatment is unclear. Experimental work suggests that dopamine agonists such as amantadine, methylphenidate, and bromocriptine can be initiated during the acute stages of injury without negative effects. However, most physiatric consultants will defer the use of neurostimulants until after the acute resuscitation and postoperative period has passed. Careful attention should be paid to drug-drug interactions, potential risk for post-traumatic seizures (PTS), and other adverse effects when beginning neurostimulant medications in this population.

Medical rehabilitation and management

Agitation

Agitation is a common symptom in the acute phase of recovery for many patients with TBI. Management of agitation can be a significant challenge in the ICU. Post-traumatic agitation is defined as excessive and/or aggressive physical and verbal behaviors, associated with restlessness and disinhibition, often with an altered state of consciousness, including post-traumatic amnesia. Pain and other noxious stimuli can increase agitation in these patients. Because environmental factors can worsen agitation, bright lights and loud noises should be reduced when possible. When a patient must be physically restrained, physiatric recommendations often include abdominal binders to protect feeding tubes, protective coverings for intraluminal access ports, and hand mitts, prior to moving into more restrictive interventions.

Pharmacologic treatment for agitation can be helpful for symptom management. Heavily sedating medications can prolong agitation duration and slow cognitive recovery; however, they may be required to decrease agitated behaviors. Medications should be chosen carefully and used in conjunction with other environmental and behavior management techniques for maximum effect. In elderly patients, agitation may be due to TBI or may represent an exacerbation of pre-existing behaviors related to dementia or other cognitive impairment. Older individuals are also likely to experience delirium related to medical issues, such as urinary tract infection, anesthesia, medications, or pain.

Classic antipsychotics, such as haloperidol, which carry strong dopamine 2 receptor antagonism, can have adverse effects on neurologic recovery. Atypical antipsychotic (AAP) drugs are better choices for TBI-related agitation because of their more favorable side-effect profile. Some AAP medications may also negatively impact recovery; however, quetiapine is frequently selected as first-line AAP treatment for its favorable side-effect profile and ability to reduce agitation while improving cognition. Propranolol and other β-blockers can help manage TBI-related agitation and restlessness, with minimal side effects, by decreasing agitation intensity and need for physical restraints. Agitated patients frequently have disordered sleep-wake cycles and insomnia in the ICU. Thus, improving sleep duration and quality may also improve agitation. Antidepressants, such as trazodone, are sometimes recommended in the ICU for their low side-effect profile, limited interactions with other neurostimulants or antidepressants, and positive effects on sleep-wake cycles and sleep architecture.

Neuroendocrine dysfunction

Neuroendocrine disorders affect a significant portion of the population with TBI. Up to 100% of patients surviving acute severe TBI develop hypogonadism, and a significant portion of long-term survivors have pituitary dysfunction. Injury to the hypothalamus and pituitary gland is one mechanism for acute neuroendocrine dysfunction. Acute hypogonadism occurs in the setting of an acute stress response associated with the trauma. Acute peripheral synthesis of gonadal hormones is implicated as a part of this stress response and is indicative of poor outcomes in those with severe TBI. Early intervention is not required for acute hypogonadism; however, acute and postacute monitoring may be informative in identifying patients who may have persistent hormone deficits that require ongoing hormone replacement. Additional neuroendocrine disorders, including hypothyroidism and growth hormone deficiency may also be monitored as patients progress through the recovery phase.

Although less common than anterior pituitary dysfunction, posterior pituitary-mediated neuroendocrine dysfunction may occur in the ICU after TBI or during subsequent rehabilitation. Vasopressin, also called *antidiuretic hormone* (ADH), regulates water retention. Neurogenic diabetes insipidus (DI) is caused by ADH deficiency and is associated with elevated plasma sodium and excretion of large amounts of dilute urine that is refractory to fluid restriction. Vasopressin replacement is effective therapy. In contrast, the syndrome of inappropriate antidiuretic hormone is characterized by excessive ADH secretion accompanied by excess natiuresis and low plasma sodium. Fluid restriction and ADH inhibitors are a part of the therapeutic approach to this disorder. Management for each of these disorders may begin in the ICU.

Dysautonomia

Dysautonomia can occur in up to a third of patients with severe TBI. The pathology underlying TBI-induced dysautonomia is not well-understood, and theories suggest a disconnection between brainstem and higher cortical centers. Dysautonomia is caused by excessive sympathetic outflow, and symptoms often become clinically apparent as sedation is weaned. Common symptoms include tachycardia, tachypnea, pyrexia, hypertension, and excessive perspiration. These autonomic symptoms are often accompanied by motor findings such as decerebrate or decorticate posturing, dystonia, rigidity, and spasticity. Dysautonomia is a diagnosis of exclusion, and other medical sources for the presenting symptoms should be evaluated. Left unaddressed, symptoms associated with dysautonomia can potentially increase the morbidity associated with severe TBI. Given the increased sympathetic output, beta-blockers, (particularly propranolol), are a mainstay of treatment. Bromocriptine treatment is linked to anecdotal evidence of symptomatic improvements. Gabapentin has recently been identified as a useful agent in reducing dysautonomia, and refractory patients have had some relief with intrathecal baclofen.

Traumatic brain injury considerations for spasticity management

Patients with severe TBI are often at risk for developing spasticity, and spasticity can contribute to other comorbidities such as heterotopic ossification. In the ICU, active range of motion (AROM), positioning, and splinting are the mainstay for nonpharmacological treatments of spasticity in patients with TBI. When systemic pharmacological management is required early after injury, physiatric recommendations typically include nonsedating medications such as dantrolene, which act at the muscular level by targeting calcium efflux in the endoplasmic reticulum.

Patients with multiple orthopedic trauma

Patients who have sustained fractures as part of their injury complex are also assessed for rehabilitation needs. Location of fracture determines whether or not the patient will be able to use an assistive device with the affected limb. Patients with proximal upper limb fractures cannot bear weight through the affected arm, but if the fracture is in the hand or wrist, the patient can often use a platform walker, bearing weight through the elbow. Weight-bearing status, including number of limbs affected and whether the patient is cleared to ambulate, determines the patient's rehabilitation goals. In general, if the patient is non-weight-bearing on 3 or 4 limbs, he/she will not be a candidate for inpatient rehabilitation. Therapy needs are met with 1–2 hours of therapies per day in a skilled nursing facility setting until weight-bearing restrictions are lifted. Once the patient is cleared to bear weight on at least 2 limbs, intensive inpatient rehabilitation can be considered.

Patients with peripheral nerve injury

If motor weakness is noted in a patient who has sustained trauma, evaluation should be done to determine presence and location of nerve injury. Fractures may result in nerve laceration, and traction injuries may result in neuropraxic nerve injuries. In situations where it is important to define a nerve injury early, initial electrodiagnostic studies done 7–10 days postinjury can help localize the lesion and distinguish conduction block from axonal injury. If clinically appropriate, studies done 3–4 weeks from the time of injury will provide more diagnostic and prognostic information. Early rehabilitation of patients with peripheral nerve injury includes proper splinting, positioning, and exercise to maintain joint ROM and prevent contracture.

Patients with traumatic amputation

Initial management of patients with traumatic amputation focuses on wound healing, edema control, and pain management. Phantom limb sensation and pain are normal and common sequelae. Phantom limb pain can be managed with desensitization and with use of agents to address neuropathic pain including anticonvulsants and antidepressants.

Maintaining good joint range-of-motion of the unaffected joints on the amputated limb is of critical importance for eventual prosthetic fit and function. Pillow placement under the knee should be avoided to prevent knee flexion contractures for transtibial amputation. Knee immobilizers prevent knee flexion contracture in these patients. Similarly, placement of pillows between the legs should be avoided to prevent hip abductor contracture after transfemoral amputation. Once the lower extremity amputee is cleared to lie prone, these patients should spend time daily in this position to avoid hip flexor contracture.

Key references

Baguley IJ, Heriseanu RE, Cameron ID, et al. A critical review of the pathophysiology of dysautonomia following traumatic brain injury. *Neurocrit Care.* 2008;8(2):293–300.

Campagnolo DI, Merli GJ. Autonomic and cardiovascular complications of spinal cord injury. In: Kirshblum S, et al, eds., *Spinal Cord Medicine.* Philadelphia, PA:Lipincott Williams & Wilkins; 2002: 123–134.

Consortium for Spinal Cord Medicine. *Neurogenic Bowel Management in Adults with Spinal Cord Injury: A Clinical Practice Guideline for Health-Care Professionals.* Washington, DC: Paralyzed Veterans of America; 1998.

Consortium for Spinal Cord Medicine. *Respiratory Management Following Spinal Cord Injury: A Clinical Practice Guideline for Health-Care Professionals.* Washington, DC: Paralyzed Veterans of America; 2005.

Consortium for Spinal Cord Medicine. *Bladder Management for Adults with Spinal Cord Injury: A Clinical Practice Guideline for Health-Care Professionals.* Washington, DC: Paralyzed Veterans of America; 2006.

Needham DM. Mobilizing patients in the intensive care unit. *JAMA*. 2008;300(14): 1685–1690.

Neurobehavioral Guidelines Working Group: Warden D L, Gordon B, McAllister TW, et al. Guidelines for the pharmacologic treatment of neurobehavioral sequelae of traumatic brain injury. *J Neurotrauma*. 2006;23:1468–1501.

Wagner AK, Fabio A, Zafonte RD, Goldberg G, Marion DW, Peitzman A. Physical medicine and rehabilitation consultation: relationships with acute functional outcome, length of stay and discharge planning after traumatic brain injury. *Am J Phys Med and Rehabil*. 2003;82(7):526–536.

Wagner J, Dusick JR, McArthur DL, et al. Acute gonadotroph and somatotroph hormonal suppression after traumatic brain injury. *J Neurotrauma*. 2010;27(6):1007–1019.

Section 3

Other Issues

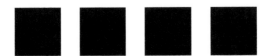

Chapter 28

Legal issues in trauma intensive care

Richard P. Kidwell

Critically ill trauma patients are at high risk for complications and death. The fact that there may be legal proceedings related to the original injury further adds to the fear of litigation for physicians caring for trauma patients. Most of this fear is ungrounded, however. There is a paucity of reported appellate court opinions regarding trauma cases. Thus, there is little guidance from courts to delineate with any degree of clarity the expected standard of care with respect to trauma patients in the Intensive Care Unit (ICU).

A successful malpractice case for the critically ill trauma patient, as with any medical malpractice case, must allege and prove: (1) a duty owed by the physician to the patient; (2) a breach of that duty; (3) which caused; (4) injury to the patient. (*Stimmler v. Chestnut Hill Hosp.*, 981 A.2d 145, 154–55 [Pa. 2009] citing [*Quinby v. Plumsteadville Fam. Prac.*, 907 A.2d 1061, 1070–71 (Pa. 2006)]). The first element is easily proven and is evidenced by the care rendered to the patient by the intensivist. Proof of the second element requires expert testimony to establish the standard of care and how the intensivist failed to meet that standard. The expert must also opine that the patient sustained an injury separate and apart from the harm that placed the patient in the ICU in the first place and that this distinct injury was due to substandard care. Most states have established restrictions on who may serve as an expert witness and under what conditions such testimony is admissible. For example, in Pennsylvania, the testifying expert must meet the qualifications of Pennsylvania's Medical Care Availability and Reduction of Error (MCARE) Act, namely: be in active practice or teaching within the five (5) years prior to testifying; be in the same specialty as the defendant physician; and be board certified if the defendant physician is. (40 Pa.C.S. § 1303.512; see *Hyrcza v. W. Penn Allegheny Health Sys., Inc.*, 978 A.2d 961, 972–73 [Pa. Super. 2009].)

Although most potential medical malpractice matters regarding trauma patients would focus on the emergency department physicians and trauma surgeons, some may also spill over to intensivists. For example, trauma patients are more likely than any others to have retained objects from surgery (usually sponges), but an intensivist's failure to consider such a cause for an ongoing infection in an ICU patient may ultimately drag him or her into litigation once the retained object is discovered.

Other issues regarding infections are whether an infection was hospital-acquired versus an infection from the trauma event itself. Whether hospital or event associated, an ongoing infection may form the basis for a lawsuit if the intensivist either fails to diagnose that infection or fails to timely diagnose it. Trauma intensivists are also subject to medical malpractice claims alleging a failure to recognize a complication, or failure to timely recognize a patient's deterioration. Even if a physician does timely discern a new problem for a trauma ICU patient, the physician may also be accused of either failing to treat the condition or failing to treat it timely and appropriately. Thus, even a timely diagnosis can be the basis for a medical negligence case if the intensivist is alleged to have failed to treat the infection appropriately; for example, by choosing a less effective antibiotic. This fallback approach to malpractice litigation is one used repeatedly by patients' attorneys and experts. They argue that a diagnosis was missed or even if not missed, the diagnosis was not made timely, or even if timely, the treatment ordered was not carried out, not timely carried out, or the treatment plan was suboptimal.

Even if a plaintiff attorney gets it right, meaning that the care a patient received was substandard, the ICU physician, his counsel, and his expert can respond that the patient suffered no harm because of the negligent care. A badly injured trauma patient may very well be no worse off no matter what happens in the ICU. Some states, such as Pennsylvania, however, do have an anomaly in medical malpractice law known as the increased risk of harm. (Vicari v. Spiegel, 936 A.2d 503, 510 [Pa. Super. 2007]). A cagey plaintiff counsel, therefore, can assert that the inappropriate care, even though it may have, in and of itself, caused no additional harm, did increase the risk faced by the patient, such as potentially delaying his or her recovery.

Much of what an expert (plaintiff or defendant) has to say seems highly speculative and indeed it is. Judges, nonetheless, permit experts to extrapolate what could have been based on the course of care and the expert's training, experience, and knowledge.

Many other decisions by intensivists are subject to scrutiny by patients' attorneys. Postoperative monitoring is a frequent focus of litigation where patients survive their accidents and surgery but then decompensate in the ICU. Intensivists contribute to their own downfall in this area by the lack of documentation. Despite rounding on an ICU patient every day, if an intensivist does not chart his or her activities, plaintiff counsel can allege that the physician was not there, or even if there, did not appreciate the patient's deteriorating condition until it was too late to prevent further injury or death. This scenario underscores the old maxim that if it is not written down, then it did not occur. It is imperative that intensivists, indeed all providers, document their patient interactions even when there is no change in the patient's current status. The note in these circumstances need only be a sentence or two reflecting the status quo. That note, though, will serve to establish the ongoing presence and care that an intensivist, many years later at a deposition or trial, will have to substantiate his or her ongoing oversight of the trauma patient who takes a turn for the worse in the ICU.

Other issues likely to lead to litigation are anticoagulation, pain control, or early discharges. Anticoagulation care in a trauma patient carries the concerns of balancing the need to prevent pulmonary emboli while also avoiding further bleeding in a critically ill postsurgical patient. Timely testing and reaction to test results to maintain therapeutic levels must be done when appropriate. An attorney and an expert will presume negligence in a patient who develops clots or bleeding and then the burden shifts to the physician to justify his or her anticoagulation care.

Likewise, if a patient receives too much pain medication and suffers a setback or dies, litigation will likely ensue. Although patient-controlled analgesia is more of an issue outside the ICU, whether the pain medications are patient-controlled or solely administered by personnel in the ICU, dosages and frequency must be constantly monitored.

Pressure to turn over ICU beds can never justify premature patient discharge. The plaintiff expert will always, with the benefit of hindsight, be able to demonstrate that the patient who suffers a setback when he or she goes to a step-down unit or regular floor was moved too swiftly from the ICU.

Many other likely legal issues can be categorized as communication concerns. Nursing care may be subject to attack for not notifying intensivists about changes in a patient's status or for failing to call a code when warranted, but these same scenarios can also lead to physician liability. Residents who allegedly fail to alert fellows or attendings about a patient's problems, whether because the residents missed something or because the residents thought they could handle, or should be able to handle, a situation on their own, lead to ominous outcomes for patients and physicians. Attendings need to be available and accessible at all times. They must also create a culture where it is not a sign of weakness for residents to ask questions or to seek assistance. Advocating ongoing communication among all levels of providers will enable the care team to deal with concerns in real time instead of sorting out what led to an adverse event and disclosing shortcomings in care to a grieving family. (See below)

Part of that culture of communication is encouraging providers to call codes or conditions to bring a rapid response team when needed. Chastising a resident or nurse who sought the assistance of a rapid response team will only discourage codes from being called even when they are necessary, resulting in missed opportunities to intervene to prevent poor results.

Communication after a bad outcome is also extremely important. Physicians who cared for the patient should discuss the course of the care with each other but must do so in the appropriate peer review context. Conversations and documents are privileged when undertaken under the peer review protection and are not discoverable in litigation. Nor can a physician be compelled to testify about such matters. Thus, what is discussed at morbidity and mortality conferences stays in that meeting room. Conversations outside of that context, however, are not protected and are fair game for questioning during depositions or trial or both. Physicians must refrain from comparing notes or engaging colleagues in a discourse about a situation other than in peer-review-protected venues.

Promptly reporting an event to the risk management or legal department is prudent. Risk management or legal personnel can offer advice (again protected by peer review or attorney-client privilege) on how to deal with distraught families. These people can also help those families with simple things like writing off bills, arranging complimentary meals or parking, or assisting with the finances of follow-up care. Simple gestures can diffuse the anger of families and keep the focus on the patient's ongoing care and recovery.

In the unfortunate circumstance of a physician error leading to a patient's death or disability, after consulting with risk management or legal personnel, a physician should disclose what happened to the patient or family or both. Indeed, under these circumstances the patient or family arguably is most in need of open and continuing dialogue with a physician. People, for the most part, understand that physicians are human and can make mistakes in the complex care of an ICU patient. Those same people, however, are not accepting of physicians who ignore or, worse yet, cover up medical mistakes. The deliberate decision to cover up an initial unintentional error is the second mistake families will not forgive.

When a patient has been harmed by erroneous care, the patient or family expects to receive and should receive three (3) responses from a physician. First, the physician should apologize and take responsibility for what happened. Most states, unlike Pennsylvania, have apology laws, which protect such disclosures from being used as evidence in a subsequent medical malpractice case, if any is filed. Whether or not a state has such an apology law, however, should not be the deciding factor on whether or not to deliver an apology. An apology should be offered regardless, because it is the right thing to do. An apology serves to stabilize an otherwise volatile situation. It also starts the healing process for patients, families, and physicians themselves. Institutions should have programs to assist physicians through these anxious situations. There is even some evidence that prompt, complete, and sincere disclosure reduces the likelihood of litigation, but that, too, should not be the motivating factor in apologizing. (Jennifer K. Robbennolt, Attorneys, Apologies, and Settlement Negotiations, 13 Harv. Negot. L. Rev. 349, 359 [2008]).

Second, the patient or family expects an explanation of what happened. Physicians should let them know what occurred and why to the extent it is known. Physicians should refrain from speculating, however. If there is uncertainty about what happened or why, then the patient or family should be told so, but they should also be told they will be kept in the loop and informed of the results of the root cause analysis to be undertaken. There must be restraint from finger pointing or blaming a particular person for what happened. Most likely, a system flaw, and not an individual, led to the error.

Third, the patient or family should be assured that corrective actions will be undertaken to prevent a recurrence or to minimize the chance that another patient or family will suffer in the same way. Physicians should explain any changes to practice, procedure, or policy to be made. This can be done without worry that such conversations will be repeated to a jury. Such assurances are termed subsequent remedial measures and are not admissible in a later lawsuit. (Pa. R. Evid. 407.) Regardless, physicians should be candid and forthright and remain accessible to patients and families during these emotionally charged circumstances.

Even if the patient's adverse outcome is a progression of his or her traumatic injuries and not the result of a medical mistake, the intensivist should still be sympathetic. The intensivist can revisit any early discourse with the family about the patient's likely struggle to recover, yet still provide an empathetic explanation of the course of the patient's ICU care.

Another recent and frequent subject of litigation involves bed sores or pressure ulcers developed by patients, including ICU trauma patients. This has been fueled by Medicare labeling such sores as Never Events. (Centers for Medicare and Medicaid Services, Bed Sores and Other "Never Events" Medicare Will Not Pay For, http://www.24–7pressrelease.com/press-release/bed-sores-and-other-never-events-medicare-will-not-pay-for-187274.php [Dec. 18, 2010]). Despite best efforts and optimal care, patients who are immobile and suffering from various comorbidities are prone to develop this condition. Although most of these claims are directed against nursing care and the hospitals, ICU physicians can also be named as defendants. Documentation is even more important in these cases than any other. Demonstrating skin assessment and attempts to prevent such sores, or once developed, to aggressively treat them, is essential to defending these claims.

Intensivists may also be sued to put their insurance coverage into play. Intensivists and all physicians must have separate insurance coverage from the hospitals in which they work. Naming both the hospital and any physician as defendants gives multiple targets for the plaintiff to attack. This may also cause in-fighting among the defendants, especially if the hospital and doctors are insured by different insurance companies. When nurses and doctors try to blame each other for any negligence, the defendants undercut their ability to defend the overall care, much to the benefit of the plaintiff. When the intensivist and hospital have the same insurance carrier, a united defense can be mounted.

One other legal matter involves reports to the National Practitioner Data Bank. If a lawsuit is settled and money is paid to the plaintiff on behalf of a defendant physician, then the insurance company making the payment must file a report of the outcome with the National Practitioner Data Bank. There is no *de minimus* amount exception so any sum paid to settle a case or a jury verdict results in a report. When a physician is initially credentialed or is recredentialed, a hospital must query the data bank to determine the existence of any entries against the physician and to take such entries into consideration when deciding whether to grant privileges to the physician. Most, if not all, physicians dread a data bank report, but in actuality a single entry in the data bank will have no impact on a medical career. Given the current climate in medicolegal matters, entanglement in litigation is almost inevitable and credentialing personnel understand and appreciate this sad state of affairs. A physician does have an opportunity to submit his or her own statement regarding this specific case to the data bank. A physician should always take advantage of this opportunity.

Trauma intensivists face a myriad of ethical issues as well as the aforementioned legal ones. They range from determining who may visit a patient to who may make life or death decisions for a patient. The clearest situation arises when a patient with an advance directive is in the ICU post-trauma and the directive is provided to the physician. If the patient cannot make decisions for himself or herself, then the directive will contain either instructions on what care may or may not be rendered in specific circumstances or appointment of a healthcare agent to make such decisions or both. In these instances, the physician's duty is to abide by the patient's previously penned limitations or to deal with the agent and abide by his or her directions, including end-of-life decisions. The most difficult situations arise when a trauma patient without an advance directive is admitted to the ICU and is unable to make his or her own decisions. Most states have laws that prioritize which relatives, and in limited situations nonrelatives, may become surrogate decision makers for the patient. In order of priority, the listing of surrogate decision makers usually is: (1) spouse; (2) adult child; (3) parent; (4) adult sibling; (5) adult grandchild; and (6) close friend (i.e., individual who is knowledgeable of the patient's preferences and values).

When there is more than one person in the highest level of priorities, a physician must follow the decision of the majority. A physician cannot substitute his or her own judgment for that of the surrogate decision maker. Nor may a physician permit a healthcare agent to override the express wishes of a patient's advance directive. A physician does have immunity, however, for abiding by the decisions of the surrogate or for following the dictates of a patient's advance directive if one exists. When an even number of surrogates exist within a class and they are evenly split, then the physician must use his or her powers of persuasion and perhaps an ethics consult to try to help the family reach a consensus regarding the patient's care.

In very unusual circumstances, if a physician thinks the surrogate is not acting in the best interest of the patient (e.g., advocating for care not in the best interest of the patient) then the physician could, after discussion with hospital counsel, initiate guardianship proceedings to have a judge appoint someone else to make decisions on behalf of the patient and to have such decisions made by a court-appointed guardian overseen by the Court.

Some states recognize a definite distinction between a healthcare agent appointed by a patient and a healthcare representative who becomes the decision maker when no advance directive exists. An agent can make any and all end-of-life decisions, but a representative may direct the withholding or withdraw of care necessary to preserve life only when the patient is permanently unconscious or has an end-stage medical condition. (20 Pa.C.S.A. § 5462(c); see 20 Pa.C.S.A. § 5422 [definition of healthcare agent and healthcare representative]).

There is one other approach to be considered when the care team concludes that further care is futile and the family insists that everything be done for the patient. The attending intensivist can tell the family that such future care is indeed futile and that he or she will assist the family in transferring the patient to a facility that will abide by their requests, but if after a brief period of time to they are unable to find such a facility, a "do not resuscitate" order will be written and care will be withdrawn. This places the burden on the family to confront the patient's dire circumstances and to find an accommodating facility or to seek a court hearing if they desire to continue all avenues of care against medical advice.

Recent regulations from the federal government require hospitals to allow certain visitors to see patients. This directive was aimed at permitting same sex partners of patients to spend time with each other in the hospital. An ethical conflict will exist, however, when a patient unable to make decisions has no advance directive and a family member becomes his or her surrogate, who then insists that the hospital forbid the patient's partner to visit [42 CFR, parts 482 and 485]. The new regulation is designed to have gay or lesbian partners treated like heterosexual, unmarried partners. Following that reasoning the hospital should honor the surrogate's request to bar visitation by the partner. That is the result under existing law, no matter the sexual orientation of the partner.

Caring for trauma patients in an ICU setting is a tough task made even tougher by the legal and ethical issues intensivists confront each day. A touchstone for each decision facing an intensivist is, of course, to do what is best for the patient. Guided by this and with some education and advice from counsel, intensivists can maintain their focus on helping the trauma patient recover.

Definitions

End-stage medical condition:
An incurable and irreversible medical condition in an advanced state caused by injury, disease, or physical illness that will, to a reasonable degree of medical certainty, result in death, despite the introduction or continuation of medical treatment.

Permanently unconscious:
A medical condition in which the patient has total and irreversible loss of consciousness and capacity for interaction with the environment, such as an irreversible vegetative state or an irreversible coma. A diagnosis that the patient is permanently unconscious must be made in accordance with currently accepted medical standards and to a reasonable degree of medical certainty.

Key references

Boothman RC, Blackwell AC, Campbell DA Jr, Commiskey E, Anderson S. A better approach to medical malpractice claims? The University of Michigan Experience *J Health Life Sci Law*. 2009. www.healthlawyers.org/bookstore.

Wu AW. Medical error: the second victim. The doctor who makes the mistake needs help, too. *BMJ*. 2000; 320:726–727.

Index

Page numbers followed by *f* or *t* indicate figures or tables, respectively.